Current Research in Medicinal Plants

Current Research in Medicinal Plants

Edited by **Holly Philips**

SYRAWOOD
PUBLISHING HOUSE

New York

Published by Syrawood Publishing House,
750 Third Avenue, 9ᵗʰ Floor,
New York, NY 10017, USA
www.syrawoodpublishinghouse.com

Current Research in Medicinal Plants
Edited by Holly Philips

© 2016 Syrawood Publishing House

International Standard Book Number: 978-1-68286-172-1 (Hardback)

Printed in the United States of America.

Contents

Preface

This book aims to highlight the current researches and provides a platform to further the scope of innovations in this area. This book is a product of the combined efforts of many researchers and scientists from different parts of the world. The objective of this book is to provide the readers with the latest information in the field.

Medicinal plants are used traditionally for preparing herbal medicines and remedies. They are also used in manufacturing and developing contemporary medicines. This book attempts to compile the current researches and experiments in the field of medicinal plants that focus on identifying new species of herbal plants, analyzing their characteristics and properties, and examine their emerging applications. Some of the important topics elucidated herein are plant nutrition and physiology, phytochemical properties, pharmacognosy, etc. Researchers and students engaged in this field will find this book helpful.

I would like to express my sincere thanks to the authors for their dedicated efforts in the completion of this book. I acknowledge the efforts of the publisher for providing constant support. Lastly, I would like to thank my family for their support in all academic endeavors.

Editor

Application of RSM and Multivariate Statistics in Predicting Antioxidant Property of Ethanolic Extracts of Tea-Ginger Blend

Solomon Akinremi Makanjuola[1*], Victor Ndigwe Enujiugha[1], Olufunmilayo Sade Omoba[1] and David Morakinyo Sanni[2]

[1]Department of Food Science and Technology, Federal University of Technology, Akure, Nigeria.
[2]Department of Biochemistry, Federal University of Technology, Akure, Nigeria.

Authors' contributions

This work was carried out in collaboration between all authors. Author SAM carried out the research, statistical analysis and wrote the first draft of the manuscript. Author VNE reviewed the first draft of the manuscript. All authors read and approved the final manuscript.

Editor(s):
(1) Marcello Iriti, Department of Agricultural and Environmental Sciences, Milan State University, Italy.
Reviewers:
(1) Atef Mahmoud Mahmoud Attia, Biochemistry Department, Biophysical laboratory, National Research Centre, Egypt.
(2) N. Srividya, Sri Sathya Sai Institute of Higher Learning, India.

ABSTRACT

The optimum conditions for ethanolic extraction of antioxidants from tea-ginger blend were determined using response surface modelling. The relationship between the colour, hue index and antioxidant properties of the extracts were also expressed as multivariate models using ordinary least square, principal component and partial least square regressions (OLSR, PCR, and PLSR). Results from the multi-response optimisation revealed the optimum conditions for the extraction as temperature of 50.16°C, concentration of 2.1 g $(100\ ml)^{-1}$ and time of 5 minutes with a desirability of 0.68. The PLSR gave the most preferable model among the three multivariate regression techniques investigated. Hue index, A510 and a* were able to predict total flavonoid content (R^2 = 0.933, Q^2 = 0.905) and diphenyl-picrylhydrazyl (DPPH) radical activity (R^2 = 0.945, Q^2 = 0.919). The a*, A510, hue Index and hue were able to predict iron chelating activity (R^2 = 0.854, Q^2 = 0.794). The study revealed that colour and hue index property could give an indication of some antioxidant properties of ethanolic extracts of tea-ginger blend.

Corresponding author: E-mail: makakins2001@yahoo.com

Keywords: Antioxidants; tea-ginger blend; ethanolic extraction; optimisation; multivariate statistics.

1. INTRODUCTION

Ginger has gained popularity worldwide for its culinary and nutraceutical usage. Ginger root is one of the most heavily consumed dietary substances in the world [1,2]. The health benefits of ginger are derived mainly from its antioxidant property. Rats fed with ginger extract and methotrexate have been reported to have enhanced antioxidant levels compared with rats fed with methothrexate only which experienced a decline in antioxidant levels [3]. This indicates that ginger could play a role in reducing the effect of oxidative stress. Ginger contains many bioactive phenolic compounds, including non-volatile pungent compounds such as gingerols, paradols, shogaols and gingerones [4]. Tea (*Camellia sinensis*) is the most widely consumed beverage in the world after water [5]. Flavonoids are one of the major antioxidant components of tea. Tea flavonoid consumption has been linked to lower incidences of chronic diseases such as cardiovascular disease and cancer [6].

Antioxidants came to public attention in the 1990s, when scientists began to understand that free radical damage was involved in the early stages of artery clogging atherosclerosis and may contribute to cancer, vision loss, and a host of other chronic conditions [7]. Antioxidants have been known to prevent degenerative oxidative reactions. The antioxidant property confers on ginger and tea their ability to prevent oxidation of cells thus hindering malignant reactions. With the increase in oxidative stress in humans as a result of globalization and industrialization, the need to increase the consumption of antioxidants is quite germane. A combination of different antioxidants can help increase protection against free radical reaction. According to Halvorsen et al. [8], a combination of different redox-active compounds (ie, antioxidants) may be needed for proper protection against oxidative stresses.

Various novel techniques have been employed to recover phenolics from plant matrices but from an industrial production point of view, solvent extraction is commonly chosen due to simplicity, efficiency of the procedure, and low investment costs required in terms of equipment [9]. Parameters having a great impact on the amount and composition of antioxidants in extracts, and thus on the measured antioxidant capacity, notably include the extraction solvent composition, temperature, extraction time (duration), solvent-to-solid ratio, and storage conditions [10].

Quality control is an essential part of the food manufacturing chain. An important quality check for ginger and tea is their antioxidant property. The measurement of quality parameters (i.e. antioxidants) is generally, carried out using traditional analytical techniques whose application in the food industry poses several problems: they require very long duration, are expensive and destructive [11]. Colour can be an important indication of the antioxidant properties of foods. An understanding of this relationship can help present a rapid analytical technique for the evaluation of the antioxidant content of tea-ginger extracts. This is possible because many food components – such as xanthophylls, lycopenes, tannins, anthocyanins and β-carotenes – are responsible for the colour of the food. The colour of foods will usually change when these food pigments undergo degradation. Degradation of these pigments can occur due to storage method used and processing method applied. It was reported that canned whole tomatoes packed in $CaCl_2$ juice were lighter than tomatoes packed in ordinary juice [12]. The advantage of relating colour property of food to their antioxidant property centres on the opportunity of doing rapid online in-process check in the factory to have an indication of the antioxidant property of the extract being produced. This means that the time for reagent preparation, sample preparation and incubation time are eliminated. The other advantage that would be presented by this new approach will be the reduced frequency in the use of analytical reagents. This means a reduced cost of evaluation. Another positive this approach offers is environmental friendliness – as the volume of reagent that will be used for antioxidant analysis will be reduced. It has been demonstrated that the antioxidant activity and total phenol content of carrots can be predicted from their colour [11]. Also colour measurements of intact tomatoes have been used as a non-destructive method to assess total antioxidant capacity of tomatoes [13].

In this study, we seek to: i) determine the optimum condition for ethanolic extraction of antioxidants from tea-ginger blend using response surface methodology (RSM), ii) investigate the relationship between colour, hue index and antioxidant properties of the ethanolic

Application of RSM and Multivariate Statistics in Predicting Antioxidant Property...

3

tea-ginger extracts using multivariate statistics (ordinary least square regression – OLSR, principal component regression, PCR and partial least square regression – PLSR).

To our knowledge, this is the first study looking at extraction of antioxidants from tea-ginger blend. Futhermore we are not aware of studies that have tried to predict antioxidant properties of tea, ginger and tea-ginger extracts from their colour property.

2. MATERIALS AND METHODS

2.1 Plant Material and Processing

Tea leaves were obtained from Obudu Mountain in Cross River state in Nigeria. The tea leaves were sun-dried, ground and passed through a 1.4 mm sieve. Ginger rhizomes were obtained from Kaduna state. Kaduna state is the leading ginger producing state in Nigeria. The ginger rhizomes were peeled, sun-dried and ground. The powder samples were passed through a 1.4 mm sieve. The obtained powders were packed in aluminium foil and stored under refrigerated condition until analysis.

2.2 Extraction

The extraction was done in a conical flask placed on temperature controlled magnetic stirrer (UC 152, Bibby Scientific, UK). The stirrer speed was set at scale 3. Ethanol was then introduced into the conical flask. The flask was covered with aluminium foil to minimize light penetration. To ensure the accuracy of the extraction temperature, a temperature controller (SCT 1, Bibby Scientific, UK) was placed inside the conical flask and connected to the temperature controlled magnetic stirrer. Once the required extraction temperature was reached, the required weight of blended powder sample of tea-ginger (2:1) was introduced into the conical flask. Tea-ginger (2:1) powder was selected after some preliminary investigation which revealed that the tea-ginger (2:1) powder had a higher total flavonoid content compared to the tea-ginger (1:1) and tea-ginger (1:2) extracts. The extraction was continued until the required extraction time was achieved. The extract was then filtered to remove the residues.

2.3 Response Surface Methodology

A face centered central composite design with three independent variables was used. The design consisted of 20 experiments: 8 factorial

points, 6 axial points and 6 central points. The range of the independent variables investigated were: extraction temperature (TEM: 30-70 $^\circ$C), powder to solvent ratio (CON: 0.12-2.10 g/100 ml), extraction time (TIM: 5-90 min). The response variables consisted of selected antioxidant properties of the extracts. The antioxidant properties were: total flavonoid content (TFC), total phenol content (TPC), 2,2′-azinobis (3-ethylbenzothiazoline sulfonate (ABTS) radical activity, diphenyl-picrylhydrazyl (DPPH) radical activity, peroxide scavenging activity (PSA) and iron chelating activity (ICA). Data were fitted to different models. Models considered were linear, 2 factor Interaction and quadratic. Analysis of variance (ANOVA) was carried out to select the best model. The best model selected was further subjected to backward regression to remove redundant variables. Both single response and multi-response optimisation were done using the desirability concept. The optimisation was set to maximise all the antioxidant properties and the process conditions were set to be within the experimental range. The antioxidant properties were all given an equal weighting of 1 for the optimisation. The quality of the model was determined by evaluating the lack-of-fit, the coefficient of determination (R^2), Adjusted R^2, Predicted R^2, and adequate precision.

2.4 Prediction of Antioxidant Properties from Colour and Hue Index Properties of the Extract

Colour (CIE L*, a*, b*), sample absorbance at 510 nm (A510) and 610 nm (A610) of the extracts were determined. L* is a measure of lightness with value ranging from 0 to 100. The a* and b* are chromaticity coordinates. From the a* and b* values, the hue and chroma of the extract were estimated. The hue index value was also estimated from A510 and A610. The hue index has been used in the caramel industry as an indicator of its colour [14]. The suitability of hue index in evaluating colour of tea has also been reported [15]. A multivariate regression was conducted on the obtained data. The dependent variables were the antioxidant properties. The independent variables were: L*, a*, b*, hue, chroma, A510, A610, A510/A610 and hue index. The multivariate statistics used were: ordinary least square regression (OLSR), principal component regression (PCR) and partial least square regression (PLSR). The data were scaled and centered before running the regression analysis. In the PCR analysis, the regression was run for components that explain between 90 to 99% of the variation in the independent variables. The dependent variables were also subjected to some transformation ($\log_{10}$, square root and inverse square root) to check if it improves the quality of the model.

2.5 Antioxidant Analysis

ABTS was assayed using the improved technique of Miliauskas et al. [16], as described by Spradling [17]. A phosphate buffer solution (PBS) was prepared by mixing 95 ml of sodium phosphate monobasic (2.98 g 100 ml^{-1}) and 405 ml of sodium phosphate dibasic (15.6 g 500 ml^{-1}), followed by 8.04 g of sodium chloride and filled to volume (1 l), lastly the pH was adjusted to 7.4 with 2M NaOH. The ABTS mother solution was prepared by mixing 44.8 mg of ABTS, 8.12 mg potassium persulfate, and 20 ml of distilled water. The solution was allowed to react in the dark for 12 h. The ABTS working solution was prepared by mixing 145 ml of PBS with 5 ml of the ABTS mother solution. Trolox was used as standard. To 2900 μl of the ABTS working solution, 100 μL of each extract or standard was added and allowed to react for 15 min before reading spectrophotometrically (Spectrumlab 23A, England) at 734 nm against a blank solution.

DPPH was measured as described by Sompong et al. [18]. The reaction mixture contained 1.5 ml DPPH working solution (4.73 mg of DPPH in 100 ml ethanol HPLC-grade) and 300 μl extract. The mixture was shaken and left to stand for 40 min in the dark at room temperature. The absorbance was read at 515 nm relative to the control (as 100%) using a spectrophotometer. The percentage of radical-scavenging ability was calculated by using the formula:

DPPH scavengingability (%)=

$$[(A_{control} - A_{sample}) / A_{control}] \times 100 \qquad (1)$$

where A $_{control}$ = Absorbance at 515 nm of control, A$_{sample}$ = Absorbance at 515 nm of sample.

Iron chelating activity was measured by the method of Dinis et al. [19] as described by Ozena et al. [20]. The samples were added to a solution of 2 mM $FeCl_2$ (0.05 ml). The reaction was initiated by the addition of 5 mM ferrozine (0.2 ml) and the mixture was shaken vigorously and incubated at room temperature for 10 min. The absorbance of the resulting solution was then measured at 562 nm. The iron chelating activity was calculated by the given formula:

Iron chelating activity (%)=

$$[(A_{control} - A_{sample}) / A_{control}] \times 100 \qquad (2)$$

where A $_{control}$ = Absorbance at 562 nm of control, A$_{sample}$ = Absorbance at 562 nm of sample.

Peroxide scavenging activity was measured by the method of Smirnoff and Cumbes [21] as described by Ozena et al. [20]. Peroxide radicals were generated by mixing of $FeSO_4$ and H_2O_2. The reaction mixture contained 1 ml $FeSO_4$ (1.5 mM), 0.7 ml H_2O_2 (6 mM), 0.3 ml sodium salicylate (20 mM) and appropriate volume of extracts. This was followed by incubation for 1 h at room temperature. The absorbance of the hydroxylated salicylate complex was measured at 562 nm. The percentage scavenging activity was calculated as:

The peroxide scavenging activity (%) =

$$[1 - (A_1 - A_2) / A_0] \times 100 \qquad (3)$$

Where A_0 is the absorbance of the control (without extract or standards), A_1 is the absorbance including the extract or standard and A_2 is the absorbance without sodium salicylate.

Total flavonoid content was measured as described by Prommuaka et al. [22]. A 0.5 ml of the extracted samples or catechin solutions was mixed with 1.5 ml of 95% ethanol (v/v), 0.1 ml of 10% aluminum chloride - $AlCl_3.6H_2O$ (m/v), 0.1 ml of 1 M of potassium acetate, and 2.8 ml of distilled water, and the mixture was incubated at room temperature for 30 min. The absorbance of the mixture was then measured against a blank using a spectrophotometer at 415 nm. The blank contained all the reagents except the extract. Catechin was used as standard.

Total phenol was measured as described by Waterhouse [23], using the method of Slinkard and Singleton [24]. From the calibration solution, extract, or blank, 50 μl volume was taken and added to 1.58 mL water, and 100 μl of Folin-Ciocalteu reagent, and mixed well. After 8 min, 300 μl of the sodium carbonate solution was added. The solutions were left at room temperature for 1 h and absorbance of each solution was determined at 765 nm against the blank. The sodium carbonate solution was prepared by dissolving 200 g of anhydrous sodium carbonate in 800 ml of water and brought to boil. After cooling, a few crystals of sodium carbonate powder were added. After 24 h, the solution was filtered and made up to 1 l. Gallic acid was used as standard.

2.6 Colour and Hue Index Analysis

Colour was measured with a spectrophotometer CM-700d (Konica Minolta Sensing). The spectrophotometer was calibrated against a white plate. The extracts were placed in a cuvette for the measurement. The CIE L*, a* and b* values were read from the spectrophotometer. Readings were taken in triplicate. Hue was calculated as θ using eq. 4.

$$\Theta = \tan^{-1}(b^*/a^*) \tag{4}$$

The following transformation were applied to the calculated θ [25]

$$\text{If } a^* > 0 \text{ and } b^* > 0 \text{ then hue} = \theta \tag{5}$$

$$\text{If } a^* < 0 \text{ and } b^* > 0 \text{ then hue} = 180 + \theta \tag{6}$$

$$\text{If } a^* < 0 \text{ and } b^* < 0 \text{ then hue} = 180 + \theta \tag{7}$$

$$\text{If } a^* > 0 \text{ and } b^* < 0 \text{ then hue} = 360 + \theta \tag{8}$$

Chroma was calculated with eq. 9.

$$\text{Chroma} = \sqrt{(a^{*2} + b^{*2})} \tag{9}$$

The hue index was calculated from eq. 10.

$$\text{Hue index} = (10 * \log (A510/A610)) \tag{10}$$

The A610 and A510 values were determined by measuring the absorbance of the extracts against a distilled water blank in a spectrophotometer.

2.8 Software

The response surface analysis was carried out using Design Expert v 7.0.0 (Stat-Ease). The multivariate statistics was done with XLSTAT Pro, 2013 (Addinsoft)

3. RESULTS AND DISCUSSION

3.1 Single Response Optimisation

Table 1 shows the regression parameters for the extraction of antioxidants. The very low P-values ($P < 0.05$) demonstrate that all the antioxidant extraction models were significant. An insignificant lack-of-fit ($P > 0.05$) indicates that the entire extraction model fits the data well. The

R^2 is a measure of the ratio of the mean sum of squares to total sum of squares (MSS/TSS). This gives a measure of the amount of variation in the data explained by the model. A value closer to one indicates that the model has a very good fit. However, the R^2 tends to increase with an increase in the number of variables in the model. With this situation a case may arise such that a model may have a very high R^2 but a low predictive quality. To compensate for the weakness in R^2, another parameter used to assess a model is the adjusted R^2. The adjusted R^2 does not necessarily increase with an increase in the number of variables in the models. The adjusted R^2 only increases if the new variable added to the model has a significant contribution to the model. The R^2 for the extraction models in this investigation range from 0.5410 to 0.9212 and the adjusted R^2 range from 0.4550 to 0.8848. This means that the extraction model with the least adjusted R^2 was able to explain 45.5% of the extraction process. The adjusted R^2 from this study indicates that the parameters included in the different extraction models could explain the various extraction process but this does not in any way tell us about the predictive ability or quality of the model. The predicted R^2 is a measure of the predictive quality of model. It measures the ability of a model to predict from new data. From Table 1, it is observed that the predictive quality of TPC and ABTS are very low with predicted R^2 of 0.1271 and 0.1779, respectively. The extraction models for TFC, PSA. ICA and DPPH have good predictive quality, with predicted R^2 of 0.8325, 0.5379, 0.6333 and 0.7396, respectively. The adequate precision is a measure of signal to noise ratio of the model. It is a measure that indicates if the model generated can be used to navigate the design space. The Design Expert software suggested that a value greater than 4.0 can be used to navigate the design space.

A square root transformation was used for the extraction model for TFC, as it gave a better model ($R^2 = 0.8982$, adjusted $R^2 = 0.8791$, predicted $R^2 = 0.8325$) compared to the untransformed model ($R^2 = 0.8326$, adjusted $R^2 = 0.8129$, predicted $R^2 = 0.7545$). Similar pattern was also observed in the TPC models and a square root transformation was found to give the best model. Temperature, concentration and quadratic effect of concentration had significant influence ($P < 0.05$) on the extraction of flavonoids. Temperature, concentration and interaction of temperature and concentration had significant influence on extraction of phenolics.

The ABTS of the extract was influenced by temperature, concentration, time and quadratic effect of temperature. Temperature, concentration, time, temperature-concentration interaction, temperature-time interaction and quadratic effect of temperature had significant influence on peroxide scavenging activity of the extracts. The iron chelating activity of the extracts was significantly influenced by temperature, concentration, temperature-concentration interaction and quadratic effect of temperature. Temperature, concentration, time, temperature-concentration interaction, concentration-time interaction and quadratic effect of concentration had significant influence on the DPPH activity of the extracts. A look at the regression coefficients for all the extraction models indicated that concentration had the most significant impact on the antioxidant property of the extracts.

The response surface graphs for the models are shown in Fig. 1. From Figs. 1a and c, the optimum temperature to maximise TFC and ABTS are around 60°C and 50°C, respectively. A numerical optimisation approach using the desirability factor approach was used to obtain the optimum conditions for the antioxidant extractions (Table 2). Using a central composite design model [26], the optimal conditions for extraction of total flavonoid from green tea using the desirability function was achieved at the extraction time of 32.5 min, ethanol concentration of 100% (v/v) and solid-to-liquid ratio of 1:32.5 (m/v). This extraction was performed at the boiling point of ethanol. In our study, the optimum condition for extraction of total flavonoids from tea-ginger was 58.14°C, 2.10 and a time of 9.99 min. The desirability for the single response optimisation extraction was defined to maximise each of the antioxidant properties in this study.

Table 1. Response surface model for ethanolic tea-ginger (2:1) extraction

Source	TFC	TPC (mg)	ABTS	PSA	ICA	DPPH
Transformation	Square root	Square root				
INTERCEPT	-70.3393[a]	36.8798	0.9615	30.3143	57.8835	111.6115
TEM	3.1403	-0.08268	2.1437E-3	1.7701	0.3980	-0.9668
CON	30.5182	-7.7515	-0.01279	12.4191	-0.04034	-0.9648
TIM			-2.031E-4	0.1749		-4.353E-3
TEM*CON		0.2211		-0.2913	0.06233	-0.1244
TEM*TIM				-4.907E-3		
CON*TIM						-0.05581
TEM²	-0.02700		-2.482E-5	-0.01724	-3.7205E-3	9.192E-3
CON²						
TIM²						
P-value Model	<0.0001	0.0051	0.0033	0.0008	<0.0001	<0.0001
Lack of fit	0.1577	0.3123	0.4551	0.6915	0.6082	0.1958
R²	0.8982	0.5410	0.6298	0.7898	0.7815	0.9212
Adjusted R²	0.8791	0.4550	0.5311	0.6928	0.7232	0.8848
Predicted R²	0.8325	0.1271	0.1779	0.5397	0.6333	0.7396
Adequate precision	20.759	7.762	9.872	11.160	11.750	18.615

[a] Regression coefficients are in actual factors.

Table 2. Optimised conditions for ethanolic tea-ginger (2:1) extraction

Source	TFC	TPC	ABTS	PSA	ICA	DPPH
TEM (°C)	58.14	nd	nd	30.00	67.14	30.00
CON (g 100 ml⁻¹)	2.10	nd	nd	2.10	2.10	0.12
TIM (min)	9.99	nd	nd	90.00	5.20	5.35

nd = optimised conditions not determined due to the low predictive R^2

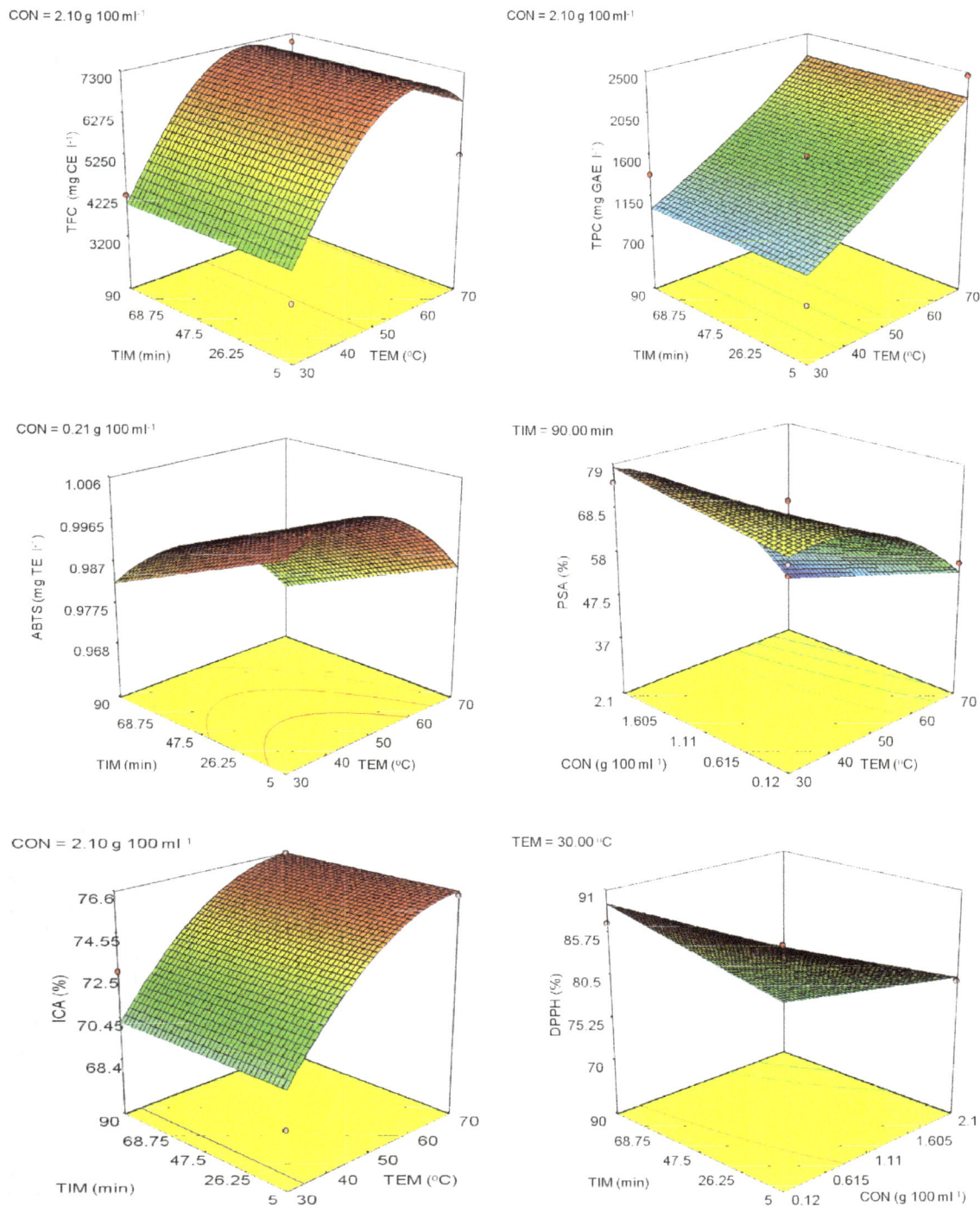

Fig. 1. Response surface graphs showing effect of extraction variables on antioxidant properties (a), total flavonoid content (b), total phenol content (c), ABTS (d), peroxide scavenging activity (e), iron chelating activity (f), DPPH

3.2 Multi-Response Optimisation

The different antioxidant properties have varied optimum regions (Table 2). This has an implication such that a particular antioxidant property might have reached its maximum and begins to degrade, whereby another antioxidant property may just start approaching its maximum. To resolve this kind of issue, the multi-response optimisation using the desirability approach was used. The desirability for the multi-response optimisation was defined to maximise all the antioxidant properties. The process variables were set to be within the range used in the investigation. The response surface graph for the multi-response optimisation is shown in Fig. 2. The required process condition for the multi-response optimisation is a temperature of 50.16°C, concentration of 2.1 g 100 ml^{-1} and time of 5 min. This process condition resulted in a desirability of 0.68.

The confirmation run was done at 50.00°C, concentration of 2.1 g 100 ml^{-1} and time of 5 min. The temperature was approximated to the nearest whole number by taking into account the operating convenience of the temperature controller. The values obtained from the confirmation runs were similar to the predicted values (Table 3).

3.3 Prediction of Antioxidant Properties from Colour and Hue Index Properties of the Extract

The OLSR, PCR and PLSR were run for all the antioxidant properties and a comparative analysis was done between the regression models. Multivariate model obtained by multiple linear regressions has been used for the prediction of antioxidant properties [11]. The PCR model having the highest adjusted R^2 was selected as the most preferred model among the PCR models. A sample of a PCR analysis is shown in Table 3. In most cases it was observed that the PCR with the highest adjusted R^2 had the lowest root mean square error (RMSE) and PRESS root mean square error (PRESS RMSE). The three components PCR for DPPH had higher adjusted R^2, lower RMSE and PRESS RMSE compared to the five components PCR (Table 4).

A comparative analysis of the different data mining technique is shown in Table 5. The extraction models for TFC, DPPH and ICA, gave good predictive quality with a R^2 that range from

0.591 to 0.960 and Q^2 that range from 0.461 to 0.919 (Table 5). The OLSR models had the highest R^2 values and the PLSR models had the highest Q^2 values for all the models. The PCR models recorded the lowest R^2 and Q^2 values among the regression techniques. These results indicated that the PLSR model has the highest predictive quality among the regression techniques due to its higher Q^2 values when compared to OLSR and PCR. The lower R^2 and Q^2 values of the PCR models can be attributed to the way the independent variable are selected. The PCR is an unsupervised regression technique [27], as it focuses on explaining the variability in the independent variables. The PLSR is a supervised regression technique [27], because the independent variables are selected in such a way that these selected variables are also able to explain the dependent variables [28]. The OLSR could be regarded as an all inclusive supervised technique because all the measured independent and dependent variables are involved in building the regression model. The OLSR extraction models of TPC and PSA had a good R^2 of 0.755 and 0.789, respectively, but a low Q^2 of 0.068 and -0.530, respectively. This infers that we have an OLSR model that is able to predict the current data well but has poor predictive quality with new data. This is a demerit of the OLSR technique. Hence, there is need to use other quality parameters (other than R^2) to assess the quality of regression models. The PLSR models had the lowest RMSE for the TFC and DPPH prediction and the OLSR model had the lowest RMSE for the prediction of ICA (Table 5). In terms of model simplicity, the PCR and the PLSR gave the most parsimonious models. One of the considerations in model building is simplicity. In most cases, the rule of Occam's Razor, which states that the simpler explanation is the preferable one, is very useful, and is now applied to data analysis or data mining techniques in building models [27]. The PCR was able to predict TFC with a combination of: a*, hue index, hue, though with a very high RMSE of 1404.897 mg CE l^{-1}. The PLSR was able to predict TFC with a combination of: a*, A510, hue index with a low RMSE of 552.706 mg CE l^{-1}. Pace et al. [11], were able to predict the antioxidant activity and total phenol content of pigmented carrots using a regression equation built from L*, a* and b* properties of the carrots. Also Wold [13] reported that colour measurements of intact tomatoes can be used as a non-destructive method to assess total antioxidant capacity of tomatoes. They reported that a high negative correlation existed between high values of L*, b* and ferric reducing ability of plasma (FRAP), and a high positive correlation between a*, hue, a*/b and FRAP values. A comparative analysis of the 3 regression techniques revealed the PLSR models as the most preferred model due to its higher R^2, higher Q^2, and low RMSE and less number of independent variables in the model. We have chosen the word preferred and not the best models because all the models have their merits and demerits. For example a look at the ICA extract models showed that the PLSR gave the highest R^2 and Q^2, the OLSR gave the lowest RMSE.

Table 3. Confirmation runs under multi-response optimisation conditions

Response	Prediction	95% PI low	95% PI high	Validation (n = 3)
DPPH (%)	70.51	62.90	78.13	78.08±1.74
TPC (mg GAE / L)	1579.44	883.49	2476.12	1266.61±44.19
TFC (mg CE / L)	6943.83	4008.13	10681.13	4725.00±530.33
ABTS (mg TE / L)	0.98	0.95	1.01	0.97±0.03
PSA (%)	70.78	55.75	85.81	76.62±1.21
ICA (%)	74.96	71.03	78.90	81.82±0.17

PI = Prediction interval

Table 4. Model quality parameters for principal component regression of DPPH

Number of components	% Variation explained	P-value for model	R^2	Adjusted R^2	MSE	RMSE	PRESS RMSE
3	91.128	0.000583	0.653	0.588	31.204	5.586	7.646
5	99.463	0.00156	0.667	0.579	31.916	5.649	9.454

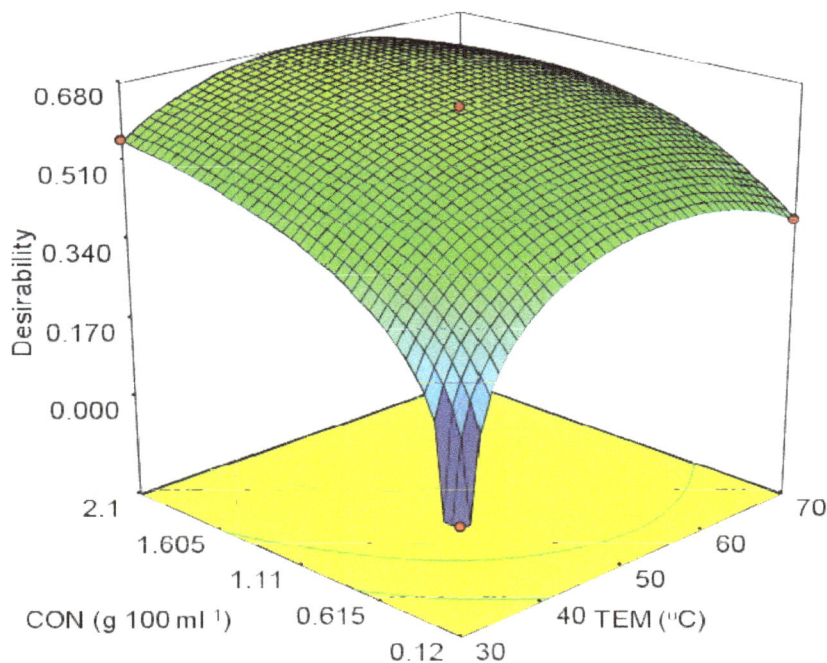

Fig. 2. Response surface graph for multi-response optimisation of antioxidant extraction

Table 5. Comparative analysis of regression techniques for antioxidant prediction

	Components	R^2	Q^2	RMSE
TFC				
OLSR	L*, a*, b*, hue, chroma, A510, A610, A510/610, hue index	0.939	0.749	745.061
PCR	a*, hue index, hue	0.655	0.561	1404.897
PLSR	a*, A510, hue index	0.933	0.905	552.706
1 /TPC^2				
OLSR	L*, a*, b*, hue, chroma, A510, A610, A510/610, hue index	0.755	0.068	4.015E-07
PCR	a*, hue index, hue, L*	0.397	-0.030	5.141E-07
PLSR	-^{c}	-	-	-
DPPH				
OLSR	L*, a*, b*, hue, chroma, A510, A610, A510/610, hue index	0.960	0.814	8.937
PCR	a*, hue index, hue,	0.653	0.543	5.586
PLSR	hue index, A510, a*	0.945	0.919	1.984
1 / ABT S^2				
OLSR	L*, a*, b*, hue, chroma, A510, A610, A510/610, hue index	0.434	-1.031	0.106
PCR	a*, hue index, hue	0.186	-0.260	0.101
PLSR	-	-	-	-
1 / PSA^2				
OLSR	L*, a*, b*, hue, chroma, A510, A610, A510/610, hue index	0.789	-0.530	0.0000790
PCR	a*, hue index, hue	0.109	-0.157	0.000128
PLSR	-	-	-	-
ICA				
OLSR	L*, a*, b*, hue, chroma, A510, A610, A510/610, hue index	0.944	0.743	1.047
PCR	a*, hue index, hue	0.591	0.461	2.232
PLSR	a*, A510, hue index, hue	0.854	0.794	1.190

^{c} no suitable model was found because the antioxidant property had no positive Q^2 with any of the PLSR components

4. CONCLUSION

This work has identified optimum conditions for extraction of antioxidants from tea-ginger (2:1) blend using ethanol. Rapid procedures that could be useful for predicting the TFC, DPPH and ICA of ethanolic tea-ginger (2:1) extract have also been identified. A comparative analysis of the regression techniques indicated that the PLSR gave the most preferred models.

CONSENT

Not applicable.

ETHICAL APPROVAL

Not applicable.

COMPETING INTERESTS

Authors have declared that no competing interests exist.

REFERENCES

1. Surh YJ, Lee E, Lee JM. Chemoprotective properties of some pungent ingredients present in red pepper and ginger. Mutation Research. 1998;402:259–267.
2. Surh YJ. Cancer chemoprevention with dietary phytochemicals. Nature Reviews. Cancer. 2003;3:768–780.
3. El Kutry MS. Ginger and honeybee modulates MTX-induced oxidative stress in kidney of rats. European Journal of Medicinal Plants. 2015;5(1):53-65.

4. Shukla Y, Singh M. Cancer preventive properties of ginger: a brief review. Food and Chemical Toxicology. 2007;45(5):683-690.

5. Harbowy ME, Balentine DA. Tea chemistry. Critical Review in Plant Science. 1997;16:415–480.

6. Rusak G, Komes D, Likic' S, Horz˘ic' D, Kovac M. Phenolic content and antioxidative capacity of green and white tea extracts depending on extraction conditions and the solvent used. Food Chemistry. 2008;110(4):852–858.

7. Harvard School of Public Health. The Nutrition Source Antioxidants: Beyond the Type. Available:http://www.hsph.harvard.edu/nutritionsource/what-should-you-eat/antioxidants/ (Accessed on 24 October 2011)

8. Halvorsen BL, Carlsen MH, Phillips KM, Bohn SK, Holte K, Jacobs Jr DR, Blomhoff R. Content of redox-active compounds (ie, antioxidants) in foods consumed in the United States. American Journal of Clinical Nutrition. 2006;84:95–135.

9. Xu P, Bao J, Ghao J, Zhou T, Wang, Y. Optimization of phenolic antioxidant extraction from tea (Camellia Sinensis L.) fruit peel biomass using response surface methodology. BioResources. 2012;7(2): 2431–2443.

10. Michiels JA, Kevers C, Pincemail J, Defraigne JO, Dommes J. Extraction conditions can greatly influence antioxidant capacity assays in plant food matrices. Food Chemistry. 2012;130(4):986-993.

11. Pace B, Cefola M, Renna F, Renna M, Serio F, Attolico G. Multiple regression models and computer vision systems to predict antioxidant activity and total phenols in pigmented carrots. Journal of Food Engineering. 2013;117:74–81.

12. Makanjuola SA, Akanbi CT, Enujiugha, V.N.Sensory characteristics and sterilization value of unpeeled whole tomato in juice. Agricultural Engineering International: CIGR Journal. 2010;12(2):117-123.

13. Wold A, Rosenfeld HJ, Holte K, Baugerød H, Blomhoff R, Haffner K. Colour of post-harvest ripened and vine ripened tomatoes (Lycopersicon esculentum Mill.) as related to total antioxidant capacity and chemical composition. International Journal of Food Science and Technology. 2004;39:295–302.

14. Kamuf W, Nixon A, Parker O, Barnum GC. Overview of caramel colors. Cereal Foods World. 2003;48(2):64-69.

15. Goodner KL, Wampler B. Measuring tea colour using a simple spectrometric assay. Sensus Technical Note (SEN-TN-0002); 2008. Available:http://www.synergytaste.com/sites/synergytaste.com/files/SEN-TN-0002-Measuring_Tea_Color_Using_A_Simple_Spectrometric_Assay.pdf

16. Miliauskas G, Venskutonis P, Van Beek T. Screening of radical scavenging activity of some medicinal and aromatic plant extracts. Food Chemsitry. 2004;85:231-237.

17. Spradling VB. Phenolics in Red Wine Pomace and their Potential Application In Animal and Human Health. M.Sc Thesis, Department of Food Science, University of Missouri; 2008.

18. Sompong R, Siebenhandl-Ehn S, Linsberger-Martina G, Berghofer E. Physicochemical and antioxidative properties of red and black rice varieties from Thailand, China and Sri Lanka. Food Chemistry. 2011;124:132–140.

19. Dinis TCP, Madeira VMC, Almeida LM. Action of phenolic derivatives (acetaminophen, salicylate and 5-aminosalicylate) as inhibitors of membrane lipid peroxidation as peroxyl radical scavenging effects. Chemical &Pharmaceutical Bulletin. 1994;36:2090–2097.

20. Ozena T, Demirtas I, Aksit H. Determination of antioxidant activities of various extracts and essential oil compositions of Thymus praecox subsp. skorpilii var. Skorpilii. Food Chemistry. 2011;124:58–64.

21. Smirnoff N, Cumbes QJ. Hydroxyl radical scavenging activity of compatible solutes. Phytochemistry. 1989;28(4):1057–1060.

22. Prommuaka C, De-Eknamkulb W, Shotipruka A. Extraction of flavonoids andcarotenoids from Thai silk waste and antioxidant activity of extracts. Separation and Purification Technology. 2002;62: 444–448.

23. Waterhouse, A.L. Determination of Total Phenolics. Current Protocols in Food Analytical Chemistry. 2001;111-118.

24. Slinkard K, Singleton VL. Total Phenol Analysis: Automation and comparison with manual methods. American Journal of Enology and Viticulture. 1977;28:49-55.

25.   McGuire, R.G. Reporting of objective color measurements. Horticultural Science. 1992;27(12):1254-1255.

26.   Savić IM, Nikolić VD, Savić IM, Nikolić LB, Stanković MZ, Moder K. Optimization of total flavonoid compound extraction from *Camellia sinensis* using the artificial neural network and response surface methodology. Hemijska. Industrija. 2013; 67(2):249–259.

27.   Nsofor GC. A Comparative Analysis of Predictive Data-Mining Techniques. M.Sc Thesis, Department of Industrial and Information Engineering, University of Tennessee, Knoxville; 2006.

28.   Wold S, Sjostrom M, Eriksson L. PLS-regression: a basic tool of chemometrics. Chemometrics and Intelligent Laboratory Systems. 2001;58:109-130.

2

Preliminary Investigation of the Antibacterial Activity of *Psidium guajava* Extracts

Iroha Ifeanyichukwu[1], Ejikeugwu Chika[2*], Nwakaeze Emmanuel[1], Oji Anthonia[1], Afiukwa Ngozi[1] and Nwuzo Agabus[1]

[1]*Department of Pharmaceutical Microbiology and Biotechnology, Nnamdi Azikiwe University, P.M.B 5025, Awka, Nigeria.*
[2]*Department of Applied Microbiology, Ebonyi State University, P.M.B 053, Abakaliki, Nigeria.*

Authors' contributions

This work was carried out in collaboration between all authors. Authors II and NE designed the study and wrote the protocol. Author EC wrote the first draft of the manuscript and took care of all correspondence. Authors OA, AN and NA managed the analyses of the study and the literature searches. All authors read and approved the final manuscript for publication.

Editor(s):
(1) Shanfa Lu, Institute of Medicinal Plant Development, Chinese Academy of Medical Sciences & Peking Union Medical College, China.
(2) Ghalem Bachir Raho, Biology department, Sidi Bel Abbes University, Algeria.
(3) Marcello Iriti, Department of Agricultural and Environmental Sciences, Milan State University, Italy.
Reviewers:
(1) Anonymous, Austria.
(2) Mohamed E. Hamid, Microbiology, King Khalid University, Saudi Arabia.
(3) Muhammad Tahir Haidry, Institute of Molecular Biology and Biochemistry University of Lahore, Punjab, Pakistan.
(4) Anonymous, South Africa.

ABSTRACT

Psidium guajava (guava tree plant) is widely used in Nigerian communities as food and for medicinal purposes to treat some bacterial and non-bacterial related diseases. Increase in the rate at which pathogenic bacteria develop resistance to some available synthetic drugs calls for urgent action to turn the search lights on natural products such as plants for bioactive compounds needed to develop novel antimicrobials. This study evaluated the antibacterial activity of ethanolic and methanolic crude leaf and bark extracts of *P. guajava* against pathogenic strains of *Escherichia coli, Staphylococcus aureus, Klebsiella pneumoniae, Pseudomonas aeruginosa* and *Streptococcus pneumoniae* by the agar well diffusion technique. Ethanolic and methanolic leaf extracts of *P. guajava* produced inhibitory zones of 15-22 mm and 13-20 mm against the test bacteria respectively. Inhibitory zones of 16-19 mm and 13-23 mm was recorded against the test bacteria for methanolic and ethanolic bark extracts respectively. The observed antibacterial activities of *P. guajava* further explain the use of guava tree plant for medicinal purposes in this part of the world. And further research is necessary to characterize the bioactive compounds of *P. guajava*.

Keywords: Extracts of Psidium guajava; antibacterial activity; microorganisms.

1. INTRODUCTION

Psidium guajava plant possesses diverse medicinal values, and it has been used since time immemorial to manage several human ailments including stomach problems, diarrhea and other bacterial related diseases [1]. In many rural parts of Africa and even in some metropolitan towns in Nigeria, natural products especially those of plant origin (including *P. guajava*) are often resorted to for medicinal purposes. *P. guajava* belongs to the plant genus *Psidium* and family *Myrtaceae*; and its leaves contain numerous essential oils rich in phytochemicals such as tannins, mineral salts, fats and flavonoids amongst others [1]. Though considered to have originated from Central and Southern America, *P. guajava* is now grown in virtually all parts of the world (Nigeria inclusive). *Psidium guajava* commonly known as the guava tree plant is a widespread plant (native to Tropical America); and it is used for culinary and medicinal purposes, and its fruits are eaten for nutritional purposes. Guava peels are chewed in most parts of the world to freshen-up breath and treat some oral-related ailments; and the phytochemicals present in guava plant gives scientific credibility to its usage in traditional medicine or folk practices across the globe. The biological and antimicrobial activities of *P. guajava* include antioxidant properties, anti-diarrheal effect, antibacterial and anti-cough activity [2]. It is one of the plants used in folk medicine for the management of various disease conditions and is believed to be active against various infections such as malaria, gastroenteritis, coughs, and sore throat [1,3,4,5]. Guavas are rich in dietary fiber, vitamin, potassium, copper and manganese; and these compounds are vital for the body's metabolic activities [6,7,8,9,10,11]. Antibiotics and other antimicrobial agents have always played significant roles in the treatment and management of many infectious diseases but the emergence and spread of some resistant microbial strains have compromised the antimicrobial activity of some antimicrobial drugs. This preliminary study was undertaken to evaluate the antibacterial activity of ethanolic and methanolic crude extracts of *P. guajava* leaves and bark against some selected pathogenic bacteria.

2. MATERIALS AND METHODS

2.1 Collection of Plant and Preparation

The *Psidium guajava* leaves and bark were collected from a garden at Amike-Aba community in Ebonyi Local Government Area of Ebonyi State, Nigeria between January and March, 2014; and identified by the Applied Biology Department of Ebonyi State University Abakaliki, Nigeria. The leaves and bark of *P. guajava* collected were cleaned, washed and dried in shade at room temperature for 2 weeks. Upon drying, the plant material was pounded using mortar and pestle into smaller particles and then blended to powder with an electric blender. Powered samples of the plant were stored in an air tight container until use.

2.2 Extraction

Twenty grams (20 g) each of the dried *Psidium guajava* sample was used for solvent extraction, and these were percolated in 200 ml methanol and ethanol and allowed for two days. The resulting extract was filtered through Whattman filter paper No 2 and evaporated to give crude extract. The extracted compound of *P. guajava* was used for the antimicrobial assay.

2.3 Test Organisms

The selected bacterial pathogens used in this study include *Staphylococcus aureus*, *Escherichia coli*, *Klebsiella pneumoniae*, *Pseudomonas aeruginosa* and *Streptococcus pneumoniae*; and they were collected from the culture preservation unit of the Microbiology laboratory of Ebonyi State University Abakaliki, Nigeria.

2.4 Determination of Antibacterial Activity

The methanol extracts of *Psidium guajava* were screened for antibacterial activity by agar well diffusion method as was previously described

[6,7]. Briefly, 100 mg/ml crude extracts of the plant were each tested on 6 mm punctured wells or holes on Mueller Hinton agar plates (Oxoid, UK) that were previously swabbed with the test bacteria. Zones of inhibition were recorded to the nearest millimeter (mm) after 24 hrs of overnight incubation at 37°C. Chloramphenicol was used as the positive control drug.

3. RESULTS

Table 1 shows the results of the methanol and ethanol leave extracts against the test bacteria. Dimethyl sulphoxide (DMSO) was used as the solvent for the plant extracts, and as negative control. DMSO did not inhibit the test bacteria. It could be deduced from our result that the methanol and ethanol extracts showed considerable levels of antibacterial activities against the test pathogens. The diameter of inhibition zone of the methanolic leaf extracts against the test bacteria ranged between 13 mm-20 mm. The largest zone of inhibition (20 mm) was recorded against *Escherichia coli* while the least inhibition zone diameter (13 mm) was recorded for *Pseudomonas aeruginosa*. On the other hand, ethanolic leaf extracts inhibited the test bacteria at 18 mm (*E. coli*), 23 mm (*S. aureus*), 19 mm (*S. pneumoniae*), 15 mm (*K. pneumoniae*) and 22 mm (*P. aeruginosa*). The ethanolic leave extracts inhibited the growth of the test bacteria more than the methanolic leave extracts (Table 1).

The ethanolic and methanolic bark extracts of *P. guajava* had appreciable antibacterial effect against the test bacterial pathogens. Ethanolic bark extract inhibited the test bacteria at 19 mm (*E. coli*), 23 mm (*S. aureus*), 13 mm (*S. pneumoniae*), 14 mm (*K. pneumoniae*) and 20 mm (*P. aeruginosa*). For the methanolic bark extracts, the zones of inhibition recorded against the pathogenic bacteria were 19 mm (*E. coli*), 18 mm (*S. aureus*), 16 mm (*S. pneumoniae*), 18 mm (*K. pneumoniae*) and 19 mm (*P. aeruginosa*). Both Gram positive and Gram negative bacterial pathogens as used in our study were considerably inhibited by the methanolic and ethanolic leave and bark extracts of *P. guajava* (Tables 1 and 2).

4. DISCUSSIONS

Some plants contain many biologically active compounds which are widely used to meet certain primary healthcare needs especially in most rural communities. They could serve as sources of lead compounds for the development of putative antimicrobial agents especially now that some synthetic drugs are barely efficacious against some pathogenic bacteria. In this study, the ethanolic and methanolic leaf and bark extracts of *Psidium guajava* (commonly known as the guava tree plant) was investigated against

Table 1. Antibacterial activity of methanolic and ethanolic leaf extracts of *P. guajava* against pathogenic bacteria

Test organisms	Zones of inhibition (mm)		
	Methanolic leaf extract	Ethanolic leaf extract	Chloramphenicol (10 mg)
Escherichia coli	20	18	20
Staphylococcus aureus	19	23	28
Streptococcus pneumoniae	18	19	25
Klebsiella pneumoniae	16	15	26
Pseudomonas aeruginosa	13	22	24

Table 2. Effect of ethanolic and methanolic bark extracts of *P. guajava* against pathogenic bacteria

Test organisms	Zones of inhibition (mm)		
	Ethanolic bark extract	Methanolic bark extract	Chloramphenicol (10 mg)
Escherichia coli	19	19	16
Staphylococcus aureus	23	18	26
Streptococcus pneumoniae	13	16	23
Klebsiella pneumoniae	14	18	21
Pseudomonas aeruginosa	20	19	18

some selected pathogenic bacteria. The notable antibacterial activities of guava tree plant (as obtainable in this present study) have been previously reported [4,8,9,10,11,12,13]. Generally, the observed results in this study showed that both the methanolic and ethanolic leaf and bark extracts of *P. guajava* had considerable antibacterial activities against the test bacterial pathogens. The ethanolic leaf extracts of *P. guajava* had an inhibitory zone of 15-22 mm against the Gram positive and Gram negative bacteria when compare to the control drug (chloramphenicol) which produced similar antibacterial activity. Methanolic leaf extracts also showed inhibition zones against the test pathogens at 13-20 mm (Table 1). It has been previously reported that the ethanolic and methanolic crude extracts of *P. guajava* possess antimicrobial activity and inhibited both Gram positive and Gram negative bacteria [1,6]. This broad spectrum activity of *P. guajava* extracts against pathogenic microorganisms (as obtainable in our study) have been linked to the presence of bioactive compounds that they possess [6,8,10,12]. In a related development, the broad spectrum activities of *P. guajava* extracts have also been reported, and these studies opined that guava tree plant possess bioactive compounds that warrants their use for therapeutic measures [1,2,3,4]. The results of the methanolic and ethanolic bark extracts of *P. guajava* produced broad spectrum of antibacterial activities against *E. coli, S. aureus, S. pneumoniae, K. pneumoniae* and *P. aeruginosa*. The inhibitory zones recorded against the test pathogens for the methanolic bark extracts were in the range of 16-19 mm while the ethanolic bark extracts showed inhibition zones that were in the range of 13-23 mm. Ethanolic bark extracts showed better inhibitory effects against the Gram positive and Gram negative bacteria used in this study than the methanolic bark extracts (Table 2). The broad spectrum activity of the methanolic and ethanolic bark extracts of *P. guajava* reported in this study are similar to earlier reports that showed similar antibacterial activities of guava tree plant against pathogenic bacteria [6,8,10,13]. Our study provides a preliminary investigation of the antibacterial activities of *P. guajava* plants, and this gives credence to further determine and characterize by molecular studies the other pharmacological properties of the guava tree plant. Based on our findings, *P. guajava* (guava tree plant) possess antibacterial activities, and this justifies their use in most rural communities to meet certain healthcare needs.

5. CONCLUSION

Conclusively, the notable inhibitory activity showed by the ethanolic and methanolic leaf extracts of *P. guajava* against some Gram-positive and Gram-negative bacteria gives impetus to their use for solving some primary health care needs in some rural Nigerian communities.

CONSENT

It is not applicable.

ETHICAL APPROVAL

It is not applicable.

COMPETING INTERESTS

Authors have declared that no competing interests exist.

REFERENCES

1. Biswas B, Rogers K, McLaughlin F, Daniels D, Yadav A. Antimicrobial activities of leaf extracts of guava (*Psidium guajava* L.) on two gram-negative and gram-positive bacteria. International Journal of Microbiology. 2013;1-7.
2. Belemtougri RG, Constantin B, Cognard C, Raymond G, Sawadogo L. Effects of two medicinal plants *Psidium guajava* L. (Myrtaceae) and *Diospyros mespiliformis* L. (*Ebenaceae*) leaf extracts on rat skeletal muscle cells in primary culture. J Zhejiang Univ Sci B. 2006;7(1):56-63.
3. Jairaj, et al. Anticough and antimicrobial activities of *Psidium guajava* Linn Leaf Extract. Journal of Ethnopharmacology. 1999;67:203.
4. Abdelrahim SI, et al. Antimicrobial activity of *Psidium guajava* L. Fitoterapia. 2002;73(7-8):713-715.
5. Lutterodt GD. Inhibition of gastrointestinal release of acetylcholine by quercetin as a possible mode of action of *Psidium guajava* leaf extract in the treatment of acute local disease. Journal of Ethnopharmacology. 1989;25:235-247.
6. Okwute S, et al. Broad spectrum antimicrobial activity of *Psidium guajava* Linn-leaf. Nature and Science. 2010;8(12): 43-50.

7. Sarayo S, et al. Development of guava extract chewabletablet for anticariogenic activity against *Streptococcus mutans*. Journal of Pharmaceutical Sciences. 2010; 35(1-4):18-23.

8. Mukhtar HM, et al. Antidiabetic activity of ethanol extract obtained from the stem bark of *Psidium guajava* (*Myrtaceae*). Pharmaize. 2006;61(8):725-727.

9. Jimenez-Escrig A, et al. Guava fruit (*Psidium guajava* L.) as a new source of antioxidant dietary fiber. Journal of Agricultural and Food Chemistry. 2001; 49(11):5489-5493.

10. Jairaj P, et al. Anticough and antimicrobial activities of *Psidium guajava* Linn leaf extract. Journal of Ethnopharmacology. 1999;67:203.

11. Gutierrez RM, et al. *Psidium guajava* a review of its traditional uses, phytochemistry and pharmacology. J. Ethnopharmacol. 2008;117(1):1-27.

12. Ana K, et al. *In vitro* antibacterial activity of *Psidium guajava* Linn. leaf extract on clinical isolates of multidrug resistant *Staphylococcus aureus*. India Journal of Experimental Biology. 2008;16:41-46.

13. Cruzada, et al. Evaluation of *Psidium guajava* (Guava) Leaf extract against gram-bacteria in planktonic and biofilm lifestyles. Ann Res Rev Biol. 2014;4(24): 4370-4380.

Efficient *In vitro* Micro Propagation of *Andrographis paniculata* and Evaluation of Antibacterial Activity from Its Crude Protein Extract

M. A. Al-Mamun[1], Rafica Akhter[2], A. Rahman[2] and Z. Ferdousi[3*]

[1]Protein Science Lab, Department of Genetic Engineering and Biotechnology, University of Rajshahi, Rajshahi-6205, Bangladesh.
[2]Ali. Mohammad Eunus Laboratory, Department of Genetic Engineering and Biotechnology, University of Rajshahi, Rajshahi 6205, Bangladesh.
[3]Department of Genetic Engineering and Biotechnology, University of Rajshahi, Rajshahi-6205, Bangladesh.

Authors' contributions

This work was carried out in collaboration between all authors. Author MAA and RA contribute equally. Authors MAA and ZF designed the study, performed the statistical analysis, wrote the protocol and wrote the first draft of the manuscript. Author RA and AR managed the analyses of the study and the literature searches. All authors read and approved the final manuscript.

Editor(s):
(1) Marcello Iriti, Department of Agricultural and Environmental Sciences, Milan State University, Italy.
Reviewers:
(1) Anonymous, Malaysia.
(2) Yuan Shiun Chang, Department of Chinese Pharmaceutical Sciences, College of Pharmacy, China Medical University, Taiwan.
(3) Priti Mathur, Amity institute of Biotechnology, Amity University, India.

ABSTRACT

Aims: The current study was designed to establish a cost effective protocol for rapid *in vitro* regeneration of *Andrographis paniculata* (Kalmegh) and also screening the antibacterial activity of its crude protein extracts against five human pathogenic bacteria.
Study Design: The whole investigation of in vitro micro propagation was carried out using three replications. Screening of antibacterial assay was carried out using disc diffusion method and measuring inhibition zone in millimeter.
Place and Duration of Study: The entire study was conducted in Prof. Ali. Mohammad Eunus Laboratory of the Department of Genetic Engineering and Biotechnology, University of Rajshahi,

Corresponding author: E-mail: mamungeb26@gmail.com; ferdousi04@yahoo.com

Efficient In vitro Micro Propagation of Andrographis paniculata and Evaluation...

19

Bangladesh between October 2012 to March 2014.

Methodology: The present research work was undertaken for *in vitro* shoot formation, shoot multiplication, root induction and establishment of whole plantlets from shoot tips and nodal segment of Kalmegh using MS media supplemented with BAP, Kn NAA and IBA, either alone or in combination. The extracted crude protein from the leaf of *Andrographis paniculata* was used for antibacterial screening against three gram negative and two gram positive pathogenic bacteria and measuring the antibacterial activity as zone inhibition in millimeter. Gentamicin was used as standard drug.

Results: BAP alone showed maximum (100%) shoot regeneration from nodal segment at a concentration of 0.5 mg/l. In combination, medium having 0.5 mg/l BAP + 0.1 mg/l NAA was found to be best for auxillary shoot proliferation (90%). Maximum rooting 100% with 12.4 roots per explants were recorded on the medium containing 0.2 mg/l of IBA. The crude extract showed dose dependent strong antimicrobial activity against the entire test organism by showing zone inhibition ranging between 7.91 to 17.5 mm.

Conclusion: The protocol for *in vitro* micro propagation has been described here, is very simple and cost effective, which can be easily utilized for mass regeneration of Kalmegh for the purpose of drug development due to the presence of potential antibacterial polypeptide in its leaf extracts.

Keywords: Andrographis paniculata; disk diffusion; growth regulator; microorganism; micropropagation; zoon inhibition; protein.

ABBREVIATIONS

BAP, *6-Benzylaminopurine;* **Kn,** *kinetin;* **NAA,** *1-naphthaleneacetic acid;* **IBA,** *indole-3-butyric acid.*

1. INTRODUCTION

The growing demands of conventional drugs for maintaining public health from a past century and recent development of microbial resistance to the commercial therapeutic agent have leaded the scientist to explore the antimicrobial activity of herbal products. A range of people in developing countries relies on natural medicine for combating against the invention of micro organism because of their potent medicinal activity, lesser side effect, sufficiency and economic feasibility. A number of medicinal plants have already been evaluated for screening of antimicrobial activity and showing a significant inhibition of microbial growth compared with the conventional drug [1,2]. The medicinal values of plant products are unique to specific plant species or groups because of the disparity in the constituents of their primary and secondary metabolites [3]. Along with these secondary metabolites, recently a considerable attention of professionals is attracted to a specific group of plant polypeptides responsible for the antagonistic action against microbes. Therefore, exploring newer species of medicinal plants and fiund out its cost effective rapid regeneration protocol may play a vital role in the development of potential therapeutic agents for curing infectious disease.

Andrographis paniculata Nees usually known as "King of Bitters" belongs to the family Acanthaceae, an erect annual herb normally 30 to 110 cm in height and widely distributed in southern India and tropical Asia. Traditionally the leaves and aerial parts of this plant have long been used for fighting off colds and infection [4]. Enormous pharmacological implications of kalmegh have already been reported against a range of diseases including hepatitis, bronchitis, colitis, cough, fever, mouth ulcers, tuberculosis, bacillary dysentery, urinary tract infections and acute diarrhoea [5]. The bioactive components of kalmegh showed significant antimicrobial [6], anti-cancer [7], anti-diabetes [8,9], anti-inflammatory [10], antioxidant [11] Anti HIV [12], hepatoprotective [13], cardio-protective [14], anti-protozoan [15] insecticidal [16] and immunostimulatory activity [17]. Antibacterial activity of methanolic, ethanooic, aqueous, acetone and chloroform extracts of *Andrographis paniculata* has been documented by many worker and showing potential inhibition of bacterial growth [18-20]. Among them methanloic extract showed highest antagonist action to pathogenic organism [20]. Hence, the screening of antibacterial activity of crud protein extract of kalmegh may emerge a new prospect to surmount the growing problem of multiple drug resistance and toxicity of commercially available antibiotic. Active crude extracts of *Andrographis paniculata* have already been standardized toward drug development in Nigeria [21]. After finding out the potential natural compound, cost effective mass production of plant material is the subsequent step toward drug development. Clonal regeneration of medicinal plants requires the establishment of successful *in vitro* plant tissue culture methods. A number of potential medicinal plants have already been successfully *in vitro* propagated with greater performance [22,23]. The limitation of plant regeneration through conventional techniques are low germination rate, pathogenic attract, higher life span and insufficiency of germination material [24,25]. Therefore, there is an utmost need to practical understanding of the mass multiplication, conservation, cost effective and sustainable usage of *Androgra phispaniculata* clones within a reasonable time frame [26]. Therefore, the current study was conducted to evaluate comparative response of auxin-cytokinin either alone or in combination on shoot multiplication and root induction from shoot tip and nodal explants of kalmegh and also screening of antibacterial activity of crude protein extract against human pathogenic bacteria.

2. MATERIALS AND METHODS

2.1 *In vitro* Micro Propagation

2.1.1 Collection of plant materials

Entire kalmegh plants were collected from the Botanical garden of Rajshahi University by author. The identity of the plants was verified by a taxonomist professor Mahbubur Rahman at the Department of Botany of Rajshahi University, Bangladesh.

2. 1.2 Maintaining aceptic condition

Sterilization of leaves sample was carried out by washing under running tap water for 30 minutes then taken in a reagent bottle containing distilled water with 1% savlon (v/v) and 4 drops of Tween-80 (wetting agent) with constant shaking for 8 minutes to remove gummy substance. This was followed by second washing with autoclaved distilled water. The explants were kept into 3 sterile conical flasks containing different concentrations of $HgCl_2$ for 1-8 minutes to ensure surface sterilization followed by washing 5-7 times with sterile double distilled water promptly to remove all traces of $HgCl_2$.

2.1.3 Media and culture condition

The culture media containing Murashige and Skoog (MS) salt supplement with different macro and micro element sucrose 3% (w/v) as carbon source and agar 0.8% (w/v) as gelling agent previously described by Murashige and Skoog, [27]. The growth regulators (Auxin and cytokinine) of the culture media were prepared separately as stock solutions for ready use during the preparation of culture media. Sterilization of the media was carried out by adjusting 15-1bs./sq. inch pressure and temperature at 121°C for 20 minutes. The cultures were maintained in the culture room at 25±2°C under a 16h photoperiod (cool-white fluorescent tube supplying). Light intensity varied from 2000-3000 lux.

2.1.4 Shoot initiation and multiplication

For shoot proliferation and multiplication, the explants were cultured on MS medium supplemented with various concentrations of plant growth regulators (cytokines rich) viz.6-Benzylaminopurine (BAP), kinetin (Kn) either alone or in combination with 1-naphthaleneacetic acid (NAA) andindole-3-butyric acid (IBA). Shoots were rescued aseptically from the culture vessels and were cut into several small pieces having auxiliary buds and again cultured to freshly prepared medium containing different combinations of hormonal supplements for multiplication of shoots at regular intervals of every 3 per weeks. Among the regenerated explants which showed adventitious shoots proliferations were recorded after 8 weeks of culture.

2.1.5 Rooting of micro shoot

When *in vitro* raised shoots grew about 4-5 cm in length, they were separated aseptically from the culture vessels and transferred to freshly prepare rooting media containing different combinations of NAA and IBA (0.1, 0.2, 0.5, 1.0, 2.0 µM). Data were also documented on percentage of rooting, number and length of roots after 4 weeks of transferring to rooting media.

2.1.6 Transplantation and acclimatization of plantlets

Plantlets with sufficient rooting system were then transferred carefully from the culture vessels and washed under running tap water followed by transferring to polar pots containing different planting substrates viz. garden soil, sand and compost (2:1:1) under diffuse light (16/8 h photoperiod). All polar pots were covered with a moist polythene bag immediately to prevent desiccation. After 13-14 days the polythene bags were gradually exposed to acclimatization to natural condition. However the plants were successfully adapted to the natural environment and were transferred to the field condition. In this way, the regenerated plants showed 80% success in field condition.

2.2 Antibacterial Assay

2.2.1 Extraction of total protein content

The simplified protocol for extraction of total plant protein described previously Wang et al. [28]. The leaves sample were blended with Tris-hydrochloric acid (Tris-HCl) buffer until making paste with mortar and spatula. Then the paste materials were mixed with Tris-HCl buffer (1 ml/10 mg leaves) as well as β-mercapto ethanol (1 μl) then vortexes for homogenization. The homogenized mixtures were centrifuged at 10000 rpm for 20 minutes. Out of three layers found in the epindroff tube, the middle layer was taken carefully with the help of micropipette and stored in the eppendorf tube at 4°C.

2.2.2 Test microorganism

Antimicrobial activity of *Androgra phispaniculata* protein extracts was investigated against three gram-negative human pathogenic bacteria such as *Escherichia coli*, *Pseudomonas aeruginosa*, *Staphylococcus aureus* and two gram-positive bacteria namely *Bacillus subtilis* and *Mycobacterium smegmatis* collected from the Microbiology laboratory, Department of Genetic engineering and biotechnology, University Rajshahi, Bangladesh.

2.2.3 Agar diffusion assays

The agar diffusion assay was used for screening of antibacterial activities of *A. paniculata*crud protein extract according to the method described by Bagamboula et al. [29]. 6 μm paper disks were punched into the agar media with sterile cork borer containing 0.5, 1, 2 and 4 mg/disccrude protein extracts with micropipette and kept them at laminar air flow hood for dryness (5-10 minutes). The test organisms (100 μL) were inoculated on the surface of the solid agar medium with a sterile spreader. The agar plates inoculated with test organism were incubated for one hour before placing the protein

sample impregnated paper disks on the plates for diffusion. The bacterial plates impregnated with a paper disk containing different concentrations of crude protein were incubated at 37±0.1°C for 24 hours. Gentamicine (30 μg/disc) was used as positive control for comparing the antibacterial assay. Antimicrobial activity was determined by measuring the zone of inhibition in millimeter around each wall (excluding the diameter of the wall).

3. RESULTS AND DISCUSSION

3.1 *In vitro* Micro Propagation of Kalmegh

Different morphogenetic responses with different concentrations and combinations of plant growth regulators were documented from nodal segment and shoot tip of kalmegh.

3.1.1 Standardization of hgcl₂ treatment for field grown explants

We measured the exact time duration of 0.1% $HgCl_2$ treatment with getting the highest number of viable cultures during surface sterilization. Among the different time of treatments with 0.1% $HgCl_2$, the treatment for 5 min produced 100% contamination free cultures and subsequently yielded 95% aseptic plantlets. (Table 1). When treatment duration was more than 5 minutes, the survivability of the culture was also decreased. Neglecting some drawbacks of inhibitory effect, $HgCl_2$ has emerged as a potent surface sterilizing agent in modern plant tissue culture [30].

3.1.2 Shoot multiplication from shoot tips and nodal segments

Nodal segments (1.0-1.5 cm) and shoot tips (1.0 cm) were cultured in MS medium supplemented with BAP and Kn singly or combinely with IBA and NAA for shoot proliferation and multiplication. Among the various cytokinins tested, BAP alone resulted in maximum number of explants initiating the shoots. The highest 100% explants induced multiple shoots from nodal segment in medium containing 0.5 mg/l BAP alone with mean number of shoots per explants was 8.4 and mean length of shoots was 4.7 against 80% from shoot tip for the same concentration of BAP (Table 2). On the other hand, the highest 83% explants induced multiple shoots from nodal segments in medium containing 0.5 mg/l Kn against 70% from shoot tip (Table 2).

Table 1. Effect of 0.1% HgCl$_2$ solution used at varying periods of minutes on surface sterilization of explants and their viability

Duration of treatment in minutes	No. of explants cultured	% of contamination free culture	% of survival cultured explants
3	20	30.03±1.2	15.02±1.0
4	20	60.12±1.5	46.13±0.6
4.3	20	75.10±1.6	60.42±0.8
5*	20	100.00±1.2	95.89±1.2
6	20	100.00±1.8	85.01±1.7
7	20	100.00±2.0	63.12±1.5
8	20	100.00±2.5	50.15±0.9

The airstrike mark in the table mentioned best result in the current study

Table 2. Effects of different concentration of BAP and Kn on shoot multiplication from both the explants. (Data were collected after 6 weeks of culture)

Treatment (mg/l)	Shoot tips			Nodal segments		
	% of culture responde	Mean No. of shoots per explant	Mean length of longest shoot in cm	% of culture responded	Mean No. of shoots per explants	Mean length of longest shoots in cm
BAP						
0.1	50.05±1.6	2.1±0.1	2.0±0.06	72.04±1.2	3.5±0.2	3.5±0.0
0.2	70.12±2.5	4.9±0.3	3.8±0.4	90.09±2.0	6.6±0.2	4.0±0.3
0.5*	80.09±1.9	6.8±0.2	4.0±0.3	100.0±2.3	8.4±0.3	4.7±0.6
1.0	62.02±1.8	4.0±.01	3.0±0.2	83.06±1.9	6.2±0.4	3.8±0.01
2.0	55.01±1.7	3.2±0.2	2.2±0.1	55.11±1.5	4.6±0.2	2.5±0.02
Kn						
0.1	40.12±1.3	1.1±0.3	1.0±0.0	53.15±0.9	2.1±0.2	2.2±0.2
0.2	50.16±1.9	2.0±0.2	2.0±0.1	73.16±1.9	3.1±0.3	3.1±0.1
0.5*	70.10±2.0	2.6±0.4	2.2±0.2	83.11±1.6	4.0±0.1	3.5±0.4
1.0	60.14±1.8	1.2±0.1	1.1±0.1	67.41±1.5	2.3±0.0	1.4±0.3
2.0	30.09±1.6	1.0±0.0	0.9±0.1	30.09±1.8	2.0±0.2	1.2±0.0

The airstrike mark in the table mentioned best result in the current study. Data were presented as Mean±Standard deviation, n=3

The results from the present study were in agreement with the findings reported by Fatima et al. [31] which showed that maximum shoot bud induction and shoot sprouting was obtained on MS medium supplemented with BA (2.5 µM) from both nodal segments and shoot tip explants. Similar results were also obtained during *in vitro* micro-propagation of cotyledon node explants of *Lallemantia iberica* cultured on MS medium containing 0.50 mg/L BAP [32]. The dominance of BAP over Kn as well as other cytokinins has been reported in a number of familier studies using a variety of explants [33]. The stimulatory effect of BAP on multiple shoot induction and proliferation has been reported previously for other medicinal plant [34]. The findings from our current study also indicated that shoot regeneration was partially inhibited by callus regeneration. Highest (100%) shoot multiplication was induced on the medium containing 0.5 mg/L BAP, where there was no callus induction. The possible explanation of more stability of BAP over other cytokinins was mainly attributed due to the presence of naturally occurring ribosides and nucleotides in BAP. Increasing concentration of BAP beyond the optimal level (0.5 mg/L) suppressed the overall shoot proliferation frequency, number of shoot and shoot length probably due to detrimental effect on the cells predetermined to form vegetative buds.

Among different concentrations and combinations of cytokinin (higher) and auxin (lower) were used, BAP and NAA combinations were also proved to be efficient in axillary shoot proliferation from nodal explants and shoot tips. The combined effects of different concentration of Auxin (IBA) and cytokine (BAP) on shoot multiplication of kalmegh were presented Table 3. Among the auxin were used, NAA significantly induced shoot regeneration, number and length of shoots while; IBA did not considerably developed the parameters evaluated. Among all the growth hormone tested, the highest

Table 3. Effects of different concentration and combination of IBA and NAA with BAP on shoot multiplication from both types of explants (Data were collected after 6 weeks of culture)

Treatment (mg/l)	Shoot tips			Nodal segments		
	% of culture responded	Mean No. of shoots per explants	Mean length of longest shoot in cm	% of culture responded	Mean No. of shoots per explants	Mean length of longest shoots in cm
BAP+NAA						
0.2 + 0.1	55.12±1.8	2.8±0.3	2.6±0.3	60.19±2.2	3.0±0.3	2.9±0.4
0.2 + 0.2	30.14±1.1	1.6±0.2	1.0±0.1	40.10±1.1	2.6±0.1	1.4±0.1
0.5 + 0.1*	82.16±2.0	3.4±0.4	3.4±0.6	90.20±1.8	4.2±0.6	3.7±0.3
1.0 + 0.1	70.14±1.2	2.9±0.3	3.0±0.4	80.16±2.5	3.5±0.4	3.2±0.2
1.0 + 0.5	45.1.4±1.7	2.2±0.0	1.8±0.3	51.17±1.3	2.8±0.2	2.0±0.0
2.0 + 0.1	40.0.9±2.1	2.7±0.1	1.5±0.2	45.18±1.6	3.2±0.3	1.8±0.1
BAP+IBA						
0.2 + 0.1	50.21±1.1	2.6±0.3	2.5±0.1	55.15±1.6	3.0±0.3	2.7±0.1
0.5 + 0.1*	70.12±1.8	3.2±0.1	3.0±0.05	80.24±1.9	3.9±0.12	3.3±0.3
0.5 + 0.2	60.22±2.1	2.1±0.0	2.6±0.13	62.22±4.4	3.6±0.08	3.0±0.06
1.0 + 0.1	61.20±1.5	2.3±0.5	2.5±0.2	63.26±1.6	3.3±0.2	2.9±0.04
1.0 + 0.5	45.21±1.9	2.0±0.2	2.3±0.12	50.22±1.6	2.9±0.1	2.7±0.2
2.0 + 0.1	40.14±1.8	2.1±0.1	1.2±0.01	40.24±1.4	2.4±0.04	1.4±0.07

The airstrike mark in the table mentioned best result in the current study. Data were presented as Mean±Standard deviation, n=3

percentage regeneration (90%) and (82%) with the highest (4.2±0.6) and (3.4±0.6) number of shoots were found at 0.5 mg/lBAP+0.1 mg/lNAA from nodal segments and shoot tip explants, respectively. Whereas, 0.5 mg/l BAP + 0.1 mg/l IBA combination showed comperatively lower percentage multiple shoots (80%) then NAA combination from nodal segment. The findings from the observation were in accord with a number of previous literature which indicated that a combination of cytokinin and auxins particularly BAP with low concentration of auxin is essential shoot proliferation and multiplication [35,36]. The efficient combination of BA and NAA for *in vitro* shoot proliferation and multiplication has already been reported by anumber of workers in various medicinal plants such as *Centella asiatica* and *Asteracantha longifolia* [37,38].

3.1.3 Adventitious root induction in microclones

For root induction, successfully grown multiple shoot (4-5 cm in length) were aseptically separated from the primary culture and again cultured on MS media supplemented with IBA and NAA at different concentration 0.1, 0.2, 0.5, 1.0, 2.0 mg/l. The highest recorded rooting (100%) were observed in the media containing 0.2mg/l IBA with mean number of roots per explants was 12.4 and mean length of roots was

3.7 against 90% in the media containing 0.2 mg/l NAA (Table 4). The degree responses of different concentration of IBA and NAA on shoot multiplication and root induction followed by acclimatizing in field condition from nodal segment and shoot tip are shown in Fig. 1. The results from the current study were in agreement with the findings reported by Vijayalaxmi and Hosakatte [39] which demonstrated that maximum rooting was on half strength MS medium supplemented with 2.0 µM IBA. The enhancing effect of NAA over IBA on rooting in microshoots were reported by a range of worker during in vitro micro-propagation of medicinal plant [40], which also contradictory with our present study.

However, stimulatory action of auxin on root induction has widely been documented by a number of worker on various explants. The rooted plantlets were transferred to plastic pots and then acclimatized to field conditions. It was observed that the prevailing atmospheric conditions (humidity and temperature) of the transplanting season greatly influenced the initial survival of potted plantlets. In this regard, the month of October- November and February – March with moderate temperature and low humidity were found to be more suitable than any other months of the year. Similarly plantlets having 2-3 cm roots at their active elongation period survived better than those transferred with much elongated and branched root systems. It was observed that 70.0% and 80% plantlets were established in *ex vitro* conditions when transferred on garden soil and compost potting mix and on garden soil, sand and compost potting mix, respectively.

Table 4. Effect of different concentration of auxins on rooting from regenerated shoots (Data were collected after 30 days of culture)

Treatments (mg/l)	No. of explants inoculation	Days of root initiation	% root induction	Mean No. of root per explants	Mean length of longest root in cm
IBA					
0.1	20	10-15	95.12±1.5	7.5±.8	2.8±0.5
0.2*	20	8-10	100.00±0.9	12.4±0.5	3.7±.0.2
0.5	20	7-12	80.20±1.9	6.5±0.3	2.4±0.05
1.0	20	8-12	70.41±2.5	4.2±0.08	2.2±0.09
2.0	20	-	-	-	-
NAA					
0.1	20	8-12	80.64±4.6	6.6±0.6	2.3±0.04
0.2*	20	7-10	90.21±3.2	8.2±0.4	3.1±0.1
0.5	20	10-12	65.26±2.6	4.4±0.02	1.7±0.07
1.0	20	10-12	50.24±1.8	3.0±0.05	1.4±0.06
2.0	20	-	-	-	-

The airstrike mark in the table mentioned best result in the current study. Data were presented as Mean±Standard deviation, n=3

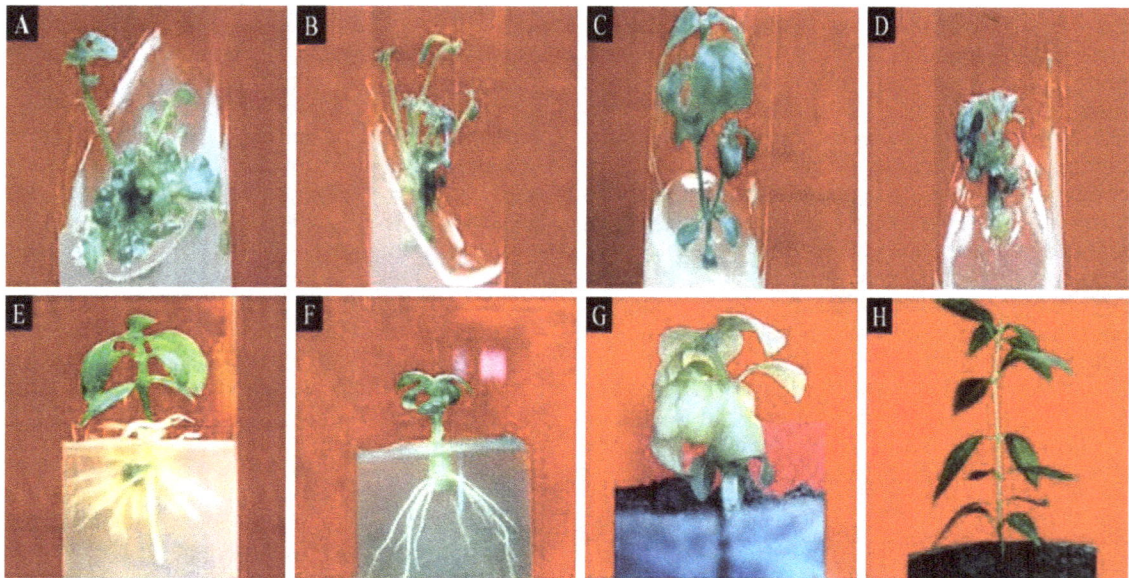

Fig. 1. Shoot regeneration and root induction with subsequent acclimatization from nodal explants and shoot tip. (A) Multiple shoot proliferation from the nodal explants on medium MS + 0.5 mg/l BAP. (B) Shoot proliferation from the shoot tips explants on medium MS + 0.5 mg/l BAP. (C) Shoot proliferation from the nodal explants on medium MS + 0.5 mg/l BAP + 0.1 mg/l NAA. (D) Multiple shoot proliferation from the shoot tips explants on medium MS + 0.5 mg/l BAP + 0.1 mg/l NAA. (E) Root formation in media with MS + 0.2 mg/l IBA. (F) Root induction in media with MS + 0.2 mg/l NAA. (G) Hardening of *in vitro* cultured plant. (H) *In vitro* cultured plant under natural condition after 1 month

3.2 Antibacterial Screening Asssy

The antibacterial activity of crude protein extracts from young leaf of kalmegh against five pathogenic bacteria was presented in Table 5 and showing various degrees of dose and species dependent antagonoistic activitiy. The crude protein exhibited strong antimicrobial activity against all the test organism by showing inhibition zone ranging between 7.9-17.5 mm. Among the test organism *E. coli* showed highest sensitive to the extracts and presented highest 17.5 mm inhibition zone and *P. Aeruginosa* produced 15.01 mm at the same concentration, indicating comparatively resistant strain among the test organism used in the present study. However, all the test species were subjected to considerable inhibition in their growth comparing with the standard drug Gentamicin (30 µg/ disc).

The observed antimicrobial activity of crude protein extracts of *A. paniculata* was mainly attributed to the interaction of some important phytochemical (andrographolide) as well as potent antibacterial polypeptide "arabinogalactan protein" present in the cell wall, playing a significant biological function. *A. paniculata* possess a range of bioactive secondary metabolites (Andrographolide, echiodinin) responsible for inhibitory action againsta rang of infectious microorganism. The results of the current study were in agreement with the findings reported by Singh et al. [41] which demonstrated that aqueous extracts from the leaves of kalmegh containing arabinogalactan proteins exhibited strong activity against a number of bacteria. Among the extraction techniques, methanolic extracts from leaves showed highest antibacterial potentiality against a number of pathogenic

bacteria [20]. The methanolic extract (75%) from the leaves of *Andrographis paniculata*at dose of 3 mg/disk produced 26 mm inhibition zone [20] whereas crude protein extract in the current study showed 16 mm zone at dose of 4 mg/disk against *Staphylococcus aureus*. The higher antimicrobial potential of methanolic extract probably due to existence of higher andrographolide compound then crude protein extract. Test microorganisms were used in the present study, all are pathogenic and associated with a range of infectious disease by targeting multiple organ of human body [42,43]. Both types of test organisms (gram positive and gram negative) were subjected to inhibition because of the inimical action of potential bioactive compound including along with inimical polypeptide which probably capable of disrupting the cell membrane by interfering with lipid molecule on the cell surface [44]. The molecules of antimicrobial peptides interfere with bacterial cell membrane leading to the disruption of transmembrane protein (probably, an ion channel) resulting the reduction of the membrane potential and subsequent cytolysis [45]. The fluctuations of antibacterial activity among the test organisms were attributed to difference in morphological structure of the cell membrane components of test organism, extraction method and dose of bioactive components [46]. All the extraction method along with crude protein extract may contain all the bioactive compounds but the quantity depending upon extraction technique itself. However, considering the antibacterial activity of *A. paniculata* based on previously reported extraction techniques, the present study has strongly supported for crude protein extract of kalmegh as valuable natural raw material against tested bacterial isolates.

Table 5. Inhibition zone (mm) of crude protein extracts of *Andrographis paniculata* measured on five human pathogenic bacteria

Test organisms	Inhibition zone (mm)				Gentamicine (30 µg/ disc)
	0.5mg/disc	1 mg/disc	2 mg/disc	4 mg/disc	
Escheria coli	10.82±0.22	12.42±0.1	15.6±0.8	17.5±0.4	22.6±1.08
Staphylococcus aureus	8.88±0.41	9.32±0.25	12.1±0.40	16.01±0.56	21.6±0.82
Pseudomonas aeruginosa	7.91± 0.33	9.01±0.23	12.2±0.81	15.01±0.55	20.3±1.4
Bacillus subtilis	9.22±0.66	11.21±0.66	14.01±0.1	17.02±0.91	22.1±1.2
Mycobacterium smegmatis	9.01±0.88	10.56±0.91	14.02±0.66	16.56±1.02	16.8±0.55

Data were presented as Mean±Standard deviation, n=3

4. CONCLUSION

In conclusion, the present study describes an efficient, cost effective and successful tissue culture system from shoot tip and nodal explants of *Androgra phispaniculata* with great potentiality for use in the pharmaceutical industry for large scale *in vitro* propagation and acclimatization in field condition. Additionally, rigorous study needs to be carried out to isolate the potent antimicrobial polypeptide along with other inimical bioactive compound from the mixture of different samples with subsequent development of novel drugs to treat of infectious diseases with more safety.

COMPETING INTERESTS

Authors have declared that no competing interests exist.

REFERENCE

1. Dzomba P, Muchanyereyi N. Potential Antimicrobial Plant Extract Based therapeutics from Temnocalyx Obovatus Roots. European J Med Plants. 2012; 2(3):209-215.
2. Odeh Chic I, Tor-Anyiin T. Amom. Phytochemical and Antimicrobial Evaluation of Leaf-extracts of *Pterocarpus santalinoides*. European J Med Plants. 2014;4(1):105-115.
3. Tadeg H, Mohammed E, Asres K, Gebre-Mariam T. Antimicrobial activities of some selected traditional Ethiopian medicinal plants used in the treatment of skin disorders. J Ethnopharmacol. 2005;100: 168–175.
4. Saxena RC, *et al*. A randomized double blind placebo controlled clinical evaluation of extract of *Andrographis paniculata* (KalmCold) in patients with uncomplicated upper respiratory tract infection. Phytomedicine. 2010;17(3-4):178-85.
5. Panossian A, et al. Effect of and rographolide and Kan Jang fixed combination of extract SHA-10 and extract SHE-3 on proliferation of human lymphocytes, production of cytokines and immune activation markers in whole blood cell culture. Phytomedicine 2002;9:598-605.
6. Xu C, Chou GX, Wang CH, Wang ZT. Rare noriridoids from the roots of *Andrographis paniculata*. Phytochemistry. 2012;77:275–279.
7. Zhou J, Zhang S, Ong CN, Shen HM. Critical role of pro-apoptotic Bcl-2 family members in andrographolide-induced apoptosis in human cancer cells. Biochem. Pharmacol. 2006;72(2):132-144.
8. Nugroho AE, Andrie M, Warditiani NK, Siswanto E, Pramono S, Lukitaningsih E. Antidiabetic and antihiperlipidemic effect of and *Rographis paniculata* (Burm. f.) Nees and andrographolide in high-fructose-fat-fed rats. Indian J Pharmacol. 2012;44(3): 377–381.
9. Widharna RM, Ferawati, Wahyu Dewi Tamayanti, Lucia Hendriati, Iwan Sahrial Hamid and Elisabeth Catherina Widjajakusuma. Antidiabetic Effect of the Aqueous Extract Mixture of *Andrographis paniculata* and *Syzygium polyanthum* Leaf. European J Med Plants. 2015;6(2):82-91.
10. Levita J, Nawawi A, Mutalib A, Ibrahim S. Andrographolide: A review of its anti-inflammatory activity via inhibition of NF-kappaB activation from computational chemistry aspects. Int J Pharmacol. 2010; 6:569–576.
11. Neogy S, Das S, Mahapatra SK, Mandal N, Roy S. Amelioratory effect of *Andrographis paniculata*Nees on liver, kidney, heart, lung and spleen during nicotine induced oxidative stress. Environ Toxicol Pharmacol. 2008;25:321–328.
12. Reddy VL, et al. A new bis-andrographolide ether from *Andrographis paniculata* nees and evaluation of anti-HIV activity. Nat Prod Res. 2005;19(3):223-230.
13. Kapil A, Koul IB, Banerjee SK, Gupta BD. Antihepatotoxic effects of major diterpenoid constituents of *Andrographis paniculata*. Biochem. Pharmacol. 1993; 46(1):182-185.
14. Yoopan N, et al. Cardiovascular effects of 14-deoxy-11,12-didehydroandrographolide and *Andrographis paniculata* extracts. Planta Med. 2007;73(6):503-11.
15. Dua VK, Oha VP, Biswas S, Valecha N, Singh N, Sharma VP. Antimalarial activity of different fractions isolated from the leaves of *Andrographis paniculata*. J Med Aromat Plant Sci. 1999;21:1069–1073.
16. Govindarajan M. Evaluation of *Andrographis paniculata* Burm. f. (Family: Acanthaceae) extracts against *Culex quinquefasciatus* (Say) and *Aedesa egypti* (Linn). Asian Pac J Trop Med. 2011;4:176–181.

17. Radhika P, Annapurna A, Nageswara Rao S. Immunostimulant, cerebro protective & nootropic activities of *Andrographis paniculata* leaves extract in normal & type 2 diabetic rats. Indian J Med Res. 2012;135:636–641.

18. Mohmmed Arifullah, Nima Dandu Namsa, Manabendra Mandal, Kishore Kumar Chiruvella, Paritala Vikrama, Ghanta Rama Gopal. Evaluation of anti-bacterial and anti-oxidant potential of andrographolide and echiodinin isolated from callus culture of *Andrographis paniculata* Nees. Asian Pac J Trop Biomed. 2013;3(8):604–610.

19. Mishra US, Mishra A, Kumari R, Murthy PN, Naik BS. Antibacterial Activity of Ethanol Extract of *Andrographis paniculata*. Indian J Pharm Sci. 2009; 71(4):436–438.

20. Pushpendra Kumar Mishra, et al. Antibacterial activity of *Andrographis paniculata* (Burm. f.) Wall ex Nees leaves against clinical pathogens. Jphar Res. 2013;7:459-462.

21. Ameh SJ, Nnekalbekwe, Aminu Ambi, Obiageri Obodozie, Mujtaba Abubakar, MagajiGarba, Herbert Cocker, Karniyus S. Gamaniel, et al. Standardization of *Andrographis paniculata*, Mitracarpusscaber and Nauclealatifolia Herbal Preparations as per European and Nigerian Drug Regulations. European J Med Plants. 2014;4(4):413-443.

22. Pooja Patel, Rajani Nadgauda. Development of Simple, Cost Effective Protocol for Micropropagation of *Tylophoraindica* (Burm f.) Merill. an Important Medicinal Plant European. J Med Plants. 2014;4(11):1356-1366.

23. Shiwali Sharma, Anwar Shahzad. Efficient Micro-propagation of *Spilanthes acmella* (L.) Murr: A Threatened Medicinal Herb. British Biotech J. 2013;3(3):405-415.

24. Pandey V, Agrawal V. Efficient micro-propagation protocol of *Spilanthes acmella* L. possessing strong antimalarial activity. *In vitro* Cell DevBiol-Plant. 2009;45:491-99.

25. Chandra S, Sharma HP, Chandra R, Jha S. Medicinal herbs-*Spilanthes* species: A review. Pharmbit. 2007;15:17-22.

26. Pandey NK, Tewari KC, Tewari RN, Joshi GC, Pandey VN, Pandey G. Medicinal plants of Komaon Himalaya, strategies for conservation. In: Dhar U (eds) Himalayan biodiversity conservation strategies. 1993; 3:293–302.

27. Murashige T, Skoog F. A revised medium for rapid growth and bioassays with tobacco tissue culture. Physiol Plantarum. 1962;15:473–497.

28. Zeng G, Li C, Zhang X, Teng Y, Dong W. Efficient protein extraction method from apple leaves for apple proteomic analysis using two-dimensional electrophoresis analysis. Se Pu. 2009;27(4):484-488.

29. Bagamboula CF, Uyttendaele M, Debevere J. Antibacterial effect of spices and herbs on Shigellasonnei and Shigellaflexneri. J food prot.2003;66:668-673.

30. Das UR, Sayed H, Sarker RH. Somatic embryogenesis and regeneration of plants from immature embryos of maize (*Zea mays* L.) plant tissue culture. 2001; 11(1):65-75.

31. Fatima N, Anis M. Role of growth regulators on *in vitro* regeneration and histological analysis in Indian ginseng (*Withania somnifera* L.) Dunal. Physiol Mol Biol Plants. 2012;18(1):59–67.

32. Fethi Ahmet Ozdemir, Mehmet Ugur Yildirim, Mahsa Pourali Kahriz. Efficient Micropropagation of Highly Economic, Medicinal and Ornamental Plant *Lallemantia iberica* (Bieb.) Fisch. and C. A. Mey. Biomed Res Int. 2014;2014:1-5.

33. Ahmad N, Anis M. *In vitro* mass propagation of *Cucumis sativus* L. from nodal segments. Turk J Bot. 2005;29:237–240.

34. Hiregoudar LV, Murthy HN, Hema BP, Hahn EJ, Paek KY. Multiple shoot induction and plant regeneration of *Feronia limonia* (L.) Swingle Sci Hort. 2003;98:357-364.

35. Patnaik J, Debata BK. Micropropagation of *Hemidesmus indicus* (L.) R. Br. through axillary bud culture. Plant Cell Reports. 1996;15(6):427–430.

36. Smolenskaya SE, Ibragimova SS. Restorative morphogenesis in vitro in the annual medic in the presence of benzylaminopurine. Russian J Develop Biol. 2002;33(6):349–354.

37. Tiwari KN, Sharma NC, Tiwari V, Singh BD. Micropropagation of *Centellaasiaticah*-avaluable medicinal herb. Plant Cell Tissue Organ Cult. 2000;63:179–185.

38. Panigrahi J, Mishra RR, Behera M. *In vitro* multiplication of *Asteracantha longifolia* L. Nees- a medicinal herb. Indian J Biotechnol. 2006;5:562–564.

39. Vijayalaxmi Dandin S, Hosakatte Niranjana Murthy. Regeneration of *Andrographis*

paniculata Nees: Analysis of genetic fidelity and andrographolide content in micropropagated plants. African J Biotech. 2012;11(61):12464-12471.

40. Sivanesan I, Jeong BR. Direct shoot regeneration from nodal explants of *Sida cordifolia Linn*. In Vitro Cell Develop Biol Plant. 2007;43(5):436–441.

41. Singh PK, Roy S, Dey S. Antimicrobial activity of *Andrographis paniculata*. Fitoterapia. 2003;74:692–694.

42. Adams MR, Moss MO. Food microbiology, Cambridge. The Royal Society of Chemistry. 1999;181-203.

43. Yetkin G, Otlu B, Cicek A, Kuzucu C, Durmaz R. Clinical, microbiologic, and epidemiologic characteristics of *Pseudomonas aeruginosa* infection in a University Hospital, Malatya, Turkey. Am J Infect Control. 2006;34:188-192.

44. Shai Y. Mode of action of membrane active antimicrobial peptides. Pept Sci. 2002;66(4):236 –248.

45. Taran SA, Esikova TZ, Mustaeva LG, Baru MB, Alakhov Yu B. Synthesis and Antibacterial Activity of Analogues of the N-Terminal Fragment of the Sarcotoxin IA Antimicrobial Peptide. Russain J Bioorganic Chem. 2002;28(5):357–362.

46. Zhao WH, Hu ZO, Okubo S, Hara Y, Shimamura T. Mechanism of synergy between epigallocatechin gallate and lactams against methicillin-resistant *Staphylococcus aureus*. Antimicrob Agents Chemother. 2001;45:1737-1742.

4

Ex vivo and In vivo Antioxidant Related Effects of Zingiber officinale Roscoe (Ginger) Extracts in Humans

Yousif Y. Bilto[1*] and Nessrin G. Alabdallat[2]

[1]Department of Biological Sciences, The University of Jordan, Amman, Jordan.
[2]College of Applied Medical Sciences, Majmaah University, Majmaah, Saudi Arabia.

Authors' contributions

This work was carried out in collaboration between both authors. Author YYB designed the study, wrote the protocol, the literature searches and wrote the first draft of the manuscript. Author NGA managed the analyses of the study, performed the statistical analysis and helped in literature searches. Both authors read and approved the final manuscript.

Editor(s):
(1) Ghalem Bachir Raho, Biology department, Sidi Bel Abbes University, Algeria.
(2) Marcello Iriti, Department of Agricultural and Environmental Sciences, Milan State University, Italy.
Reviewers:
(1) Arvind Kumar Tripathi, Centre for Biotechnology, APS University, Rewa, MP, India.
(2) Anthony Cemaluk C. Egbuonu, Department of Biochemistry, Michael Okpara University of Agriculture Umudike, Nigeria.

ABSTRACT

Aims: To investigate antioxidant related effects of Zingiber officinale Roscoe (ginger) in humans.
Study Design: Venous blood from healthy volunteers was used to conduct ex vivo experiments. For in vivo study, nine healthy volunteers, each received orally 250 ml of aqueous extract of ginger daily for 5 days. Venous bloods were taken before and one hour after the first dose of aqueous extract (sample I and II respectively) and then one day after the last dose of day five (i.e. day 6, sample III). The first blood taken before the first dose (i.e. sample I), served as control for the next samples of II and III.
Methodology: The following assays were performed: Erythrocyte reduced glutathione (GSH), Malonyldialdehyde (MDA), Protein carbonyl (PC), superoxide dismutase (SOD), Percentage hemolysis, serum total antioxidant status (TAS) and selected biochemical tests.
Results: Pre-incubation of erythrocytes ex vivo with methanolic extract of ginger then exposed to H_2O_2 decreased significantly MDA production (i.e. anti-lipid-peroxidant), PC production (i.e. anti-

protein-oxidant) and oxidant hemolysis (i.e. anti-hemolytic) in a concentration dependent manner. Ginger extract had no effect on GSH of *ex vivo* incubated erythrocytes. Oral administration of aqueous extracts of ginger to healthy volunteers, for 5 days, increased significantly serum TAS (from 1.08 to 1.24 mmol/l = 15% increase), erythrocyte GSH (from 0.74 to 1.53 mg/g Hb = 107% increase) and SOD (from 1005.4 to 1374.5 U/gHb = 37% increase), decreased significantly erythrocyte MDA (from 23.7 to 15.5 nmol//g Hb = 35% decrease), and also caused a significant small decrease within the reference range in serum potassium (K) (from 4.3 to 4.0 mmol/L), and serum urea nitrogen (BUN) (from 17.9 to 13.5 mg/dL) and an increase in serum creatinine phosphokinase (CPK) (from 63.1 to 82.7 U/L), with no effect on other serum biochemical tests for kidney, liver, cardiac and pancrease, compared to 0 time administration.
Conclusion: The study indicates that ginger can improve the base line of the defense mechanisms against possible oxidative stress and possibly inhibit pathological conditions related to oxidative stress.

Keywords: Zingiber officinale extracts; antioxidant related effects; Ex vivo and In vivo studies.

1. INTRODUCTION

Zingiber officinale Roscoe is the botanical name for ginger, a tropical herbal plant found in abundance in Asia. It belongs to the family of *Zingiberaceae*. Generally it is widely used as a spice in traditional and modern cookings [1]. Biochemically, the main active components in ginger are gingerol, shogaol and zingiberene, of which 6-Shogaol having the most potent antioxidant and anti-inflammatory properties [2]. Ginger extract has been extensively studied for its pharmacological and biological activities such as anti-emetic, anti-inflammatory, anti-bacterial, anti-convulsion, analgesic, anti-ulcer, anti-tumour, anti-fungal, Anti-thrombotic, anti-diabetes, peripheral circulatory stimulant, promotive secretion of saliva and gastric juices, increase tone of and peristalsis in intestines, and anti-allergen [3-11].

The anti-oxidant properties of ginger and its components have been studied in various *in vitro* and *in vivo* models. *In vitro* models showed that ginger extracts and gingerols (the components of ginger) have free radical scavenging and anti-lipid peroxidant activities by various *in vitro* antioxidant assays [2,11-14]. Animal *in vivo* models showed that ginger significantly lowered induced lipid peroxidation and raised the levels of reduced glutathione (GSH), and the GSH-dependent enzymes of glutathione peroxidase (GPx), glutathione reductase (GR), and glutathione S-transferase (GST) and superoxide dismutase (SOD) [11,15-17].

Free radicals and reactive oxygen species are continuously produced in the human body. These oxygen species are the cause of cell damage and the progression of chronic diseases.

Therefore, body tissues must be protected from oxidative injury through lines of defense that includes intracellular (reduced glutathione (GSH), superoxide dismutase (SOD), glutathione peroxidase (GPx), glutathione reductase (GR), glutathione S-transferase (GST) and catalase) and extracellular (vitamins, micronutrients, carotenoids, polyphenolics and other bioactive compounds,) antioxidants [18,19].

Despite the large number of *ex vivo* and *in vivo* animal studies performed on ginger extracts, surprisingly few clinical studies are available on humans. However, although this plant is widely used by the public across the world in everyday life as food supplement, no studies exist on testing the effect of ginger on normal healthy humans. This could also be true for most herbal extracts. The present study focused therefore on the antioxidant related effects of ginger on normal human volunteers after oral administration of aqueous extract for 5 days. To compare the in vivo effects with that of *ex vivo* effects, we first tested the effect of methanolic extract of ginger on human erythrocytes exposed to H_2O_2 by *ex vivo* experiments. The following assays were employed in these *ex vivo* and *in vivo* studies: serum TAS, erythrocyte MDA, PC, GSH and SOD and selected serum biochemical tests.

2. MATERIALS AND METHODS

2.1 *Ex vivo* Study Design

Ex vivo experiments were performed on washed erythrocyte suspensions prepared from heparinized venous blood from 28 healthy university student volunteers of either sex, aging 19-30 years. Washed erythrocyte suspensions were prepared by centrifugation of whole blood to remove the buffy cout layer and then washing the packed cells three times with cold phosphate buffered saline.

2.1.1 Preparation of methanolic extract of ginger

Ginger (dried rhizomes), was purchased from a local herbal store in madaba, south of Jordan in June 2013. The dried rhizome was grounded in a blender with a particular size to ensure the powder in identical size, and then 100 g of the powder was soaked for 5-7 days with 1000 ml of 80% methanol at 25°C. After filtration, the filtrate was evaporated with a rotary evaporator to remove the methanol under reduced pressure at 50°C. The dry crude extract of ginger was stored in refrigerator in dark glass bottle until use. A stock solution of 1mg/ml from the crude extract was prepared by dissolving 0.1 g of dry crude extract / standard and diluted in 100 ml of 98% methanol. This stock solution was stored in refrigerator until use for the *ex vivo* study.

2.1.2 Exposure of erythrocytes to H_2O_2 (10 mM)

Washed erythrocyte suspensions with or without pre-incubation with plant extract were exposed to H_2O_2 for 1 hr at 37°C as described previously [20]. After incubation, the suspensions were used to measure erythrocytes MDA, PC, GSH and percentage hemolysis. The final concentrations of giner extract were 0.2 mg/ml, 0.4 mg/ml, 0.6 mg/ml and 0.8 mg/ml.

2.1.3 Determination of erythrocyte MDA

Erythrocyte MDA was determined as a measure of lipid peroxidation according to Stocks and Dormandy's method (1971) using thiobarbituric acid (TBA) as modified by Srour et al. [21]. All MDA concentrations were expressed as nmol/gHb.

2.1.4 Determination of erythrocyte protein carbonyl (PC)

Erythrocyte PC was determined as a measure of protein oxidation using cayman's protein carbonyl assay kit [22]. This assay is based on the reaction between 2, 4-dinitrophenylhydrazine (DNPH) and protein carbonyls in hemolysates of cell suspension (PCV=5%) in a convenient 96-well format. DNPH react with protein carbonyls, forming protein-hydrozone, which can be quantified spectrophotometrically at an absorbance between 385-405 nm. All Protein carbonyl concentrations were expressed as nmol/g Hb.

2.1.5 Determination of erythrocyte reduced glutathione (GSH)

Erythrocyte reduced glutathione was determined using Ellman's method (1951) [23] with slight modification. Briefly, to 1 ml hemolysate, 2 ml of precipitating solution was added, mixed and allowed to stand 5 min at room temperature. Then, the mixture was centrifuged at 4200 xg. To 1.0 ml of the supernatant, 2 ml of phosphate solution (0.3M of Na_2HPO_4) and 0.5 ml of DTNB (40 mg/dl) were added the assay mixture was mixed by inversion 3 times and its absorbance was read within 4 min at 412 nm against blank. Standard GSH dissolved in distilled water (5-20 mg/dl) was assayed as above, omitting the filtration step, and used for construction of a standard curve. All GSH concentrations were expressed in mg/g Hb.

2.1.6 Determination of erythrocyte percentage hemolysis

To induce complete hemolysis, 0.1 ml from each cell suspension was diluted and mixed with 2.9 ml distilled water. All samples before and after dilution with water were then centrifuged at 1200 x for 5 min. and hemoglobin concentration of supernatants was determined spectrophotometrically at 450 nm. Percentage hemolysis was calculated from the ratio of the absorbance of pre- to post- diluted samples.

2.2 *In vivo* Study Design

Nine healthy volunteers (3 men and 6 women) with a mean age of 41.8±7.6 years were recruited in the study after they signed an informed consent according to the Ethics Committee requirements of the University of Jordan. Each volunteer received orally 250 ml of aqueous extract of ginger daily for 5 days. Venous blood samples were taken before and one hour after the first dose of aqueous extract (sample I and II respectively) and then one day after the last dose of day five (i.e. day 6, sample III). The first blood sample taken before the first dose (i.e. sample I), served as control for the next samples of II and III.

2.2.1 Preparation of aqueous extract of ginger

This was prepared as usually used by the Jordanian public in dealing with this plant. Dried ginger rhizome was purchased from the local herbal store in madaba, Jordan. 50 g of this rhizome was boiled with 2.5 L water for 10-15 min, and then left covered soaking for 3-4 hrs at room temperature, then 250 ml of soaked aqueous extract was given orally to each individual daily for 5 days.

2.2.2 Blood samples

Three blood samples were collected in gell clot activator tubes from each healthy volunteer (sample I before drinking the aqueous extract, sample II after one hour of the first dose (drinking aqueous extract) on day one and sample III at day 6 (i.e. one day following the last dose of day five). Gell tubes were centrifuged for 10 min at 3000 x g at room temperature to separate and collect serum. Then 2 ml of distilled water added to the cells under the gell in tubes and the tubes were centrifuged for 5 min at 3000 x g and the supernatant (hemolysate) was collected. All samples (serum and hemolysate) were stored frozen at -20°C until analysis.

2.2.3 Determination of serum total antioxidant status (TAS)

Serum total antioxidant status measured by TAS kit from Randox, in which 2.2'- Azino-di [3-ethylbenzthiazoline sulphonate (ABTS) is incubated with peroxidase (metmyoglibin) and H_2O_2 to produce the radical ABTS^{+}. This has a relatively stable blue-green colour, which is measured at 600 nm. Antioxidants in the added sample cause suppression of this colour production to a degree which is proportional to their concentration.

2.2.4 Determination of erythrocyte superoxide dismutas (SOD) activity

Erythrocyte Superoxide Dismutas (SOD) was measured using kit from Randox. The assay kit [24] employed xanthine and xanthine oxidase (XOD) to generate superoxide radicals which react with 2-(4-iodophenyl)-3-(4-nitrophenol)-5-phenyltetrazolium chloride (I.N.T.) to form a red formazan dye. The superoxide dismutase activity is then measured by the degree of inhibition of this reaction. One unit of SOD is that which causes a 50% inhibition of the rate of reduction of I.N.T. under the conditions of the assay.

2.2.5 Determination of serum biochemical parameters

The kits for determination of serum biochemical parameters were purchased commercially from

Roche and 902 Hitachi analyzer used to perform the following biochemical parameters: serum sodium (Na), potassium (K), urea nitrogen (BUN), creatinine (CREA), uric acid (UA), albumin (ALB), total protein (TP), lactate dehydrogenase (LDH), alanine transaminase (ALT), aspartate transaminase (AST), alkaline phosphatase (ALP), creatinine phosphokinase (CPK) and amylase (AMYL).

2.3 Statistical Analysis

All data are reported as the mean±S.D., statistical analysis was performed using SPSS statistics 17. The results were compared by paired t-test. The results with a value of $P \leq 0.05$ were considered significant.

3. RESULTS

3.1 *Ex vivo* Study

As shown in Figs. 1, 2, 3, exposure of human erythrocytes *ex vivo* to 10 mM H_2O_2 caused a significant increase in MDA (from 14.5 to 300), protein carbonyl (from 510 to 1420) and hemolysis (from 1.7 to 13.8%). Pre-incubation of erythrocytes with methanolic extract of ginger at concentrations of 0.2, 0.4, 0.6 and 0.8 mg/ml *and then exposed to* H_2O_2 decreased significantly MDA production (i.e. anti-lipid-peroxidant), PC production (i.e. anti-protein-oxidant) and oxidant hemolysis (i.e. anti-hemolytic) compared to H_2O_2 alone, in a concentration dependent manner at all concentrations. Whereas, ginger extract had no significant effect on GSH before or after exposure to H_2O_2 (Fig. 4).

3.2 *In vivo* Study

The results of the *in vivo* study are shown in Table 1. As shown in Table 1, oral administration of aqueous extracts of ginger to healthy volunteers for 5 days increased significantly serum total antioxidant status (TAS) (from 1.08 to 1.24 mmol/l = 15% increase), erythrocyte reduced glutathione (GSH) (from 0.74 to 1.53 mg/g Hb = 107% increase), erythrocyte superoxide dismutase (SOD) (from 1005.4 to 1374.5 U/gHb = 37% increase) and decreased significantly erythrocyte Malonyldialdehyde (MDA) (from 23.7 to 15.5 nmol//g Hb = 35% decrease) at day 6 (i.e. one day following the last dose of day five) of administration, compared to 0 time administration. Ginger also decreased significantly serum potassium (K) (from 4.3 to 4.0

mmol/L), serum urea nitrogen (BUN) (from 17.9 to 13.5 mg/dL) and increased significantly serum creatinine phosphokinase (CPK) (from 63.1 to 82.7 U/L) at day 6 (i.e. one day following the last dose of day five) of administration, compared to 0 time administration. However, the decrease in serum K and BUN and the increase in CPK were still within the reference ranges for normal adults (Table 1).

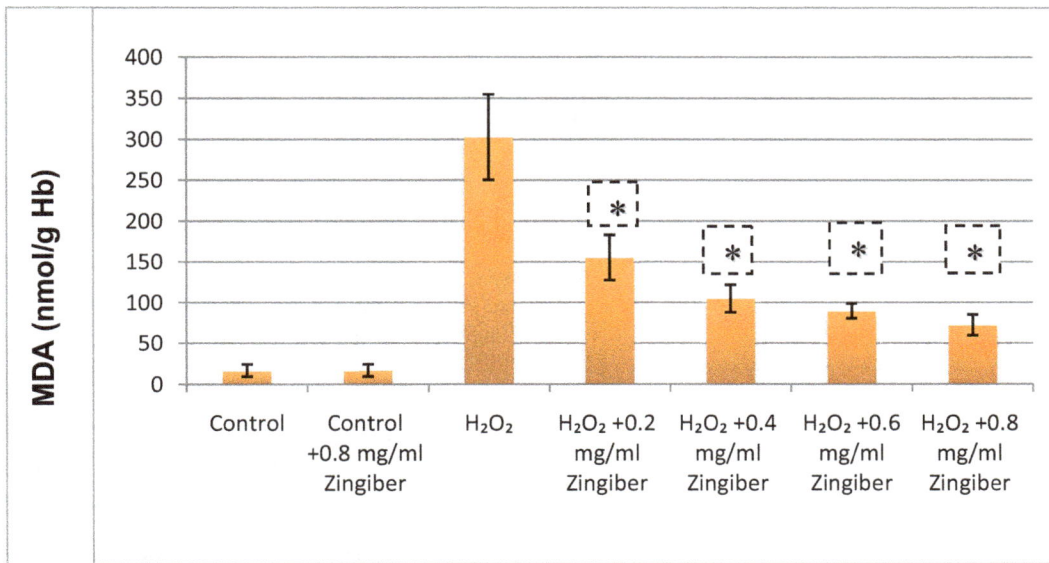

Fig. 1. MDA concentration of normal erythrocytes when incubated at 37°C for 60 min in the absence or in the presence of 10 mM H_2O_2, or in the presence of 10 mM H_2O_2 plus different concentrations of ginger methanolic extract. Each column represents the mean value and bars represent the S.D. (n = 7). *P ≤ 0.05, compared to treatment with H_2O_2 alone

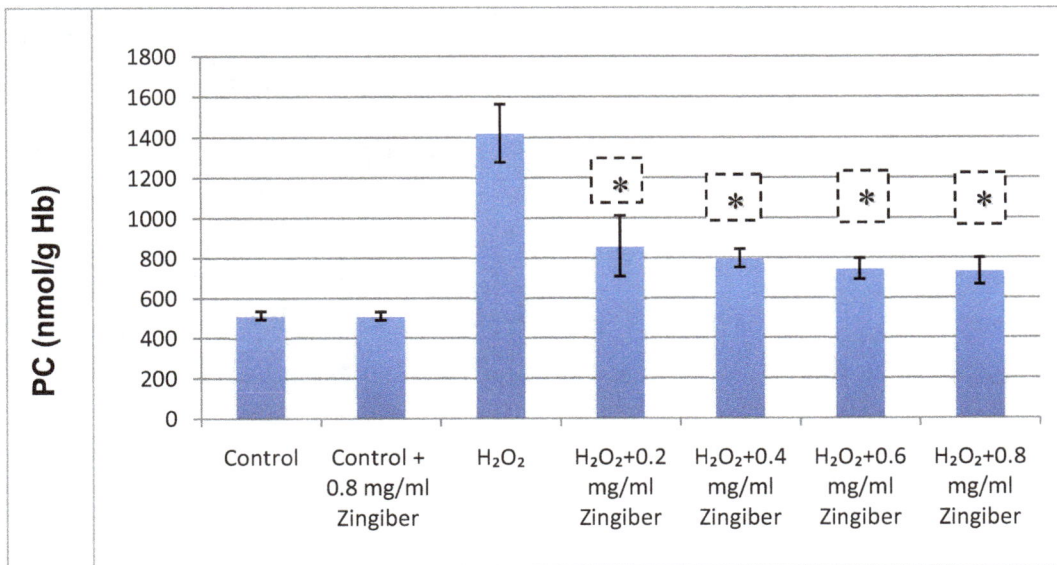

Fig. 2. Protein Carbonyl (PC) concentration of normal erythrocytes when incubated at 37°C for 60 min in the absence or in the presence of 10 mM H_2O_2, or in the presence of 10 mM H_2O_2 plus different concentrations of ginger methanolic extract. Each column represents the mean value and bars represent the S.D. (n = 7). *P ≤ 0.05, compared to treatment with H_2O_2 alone

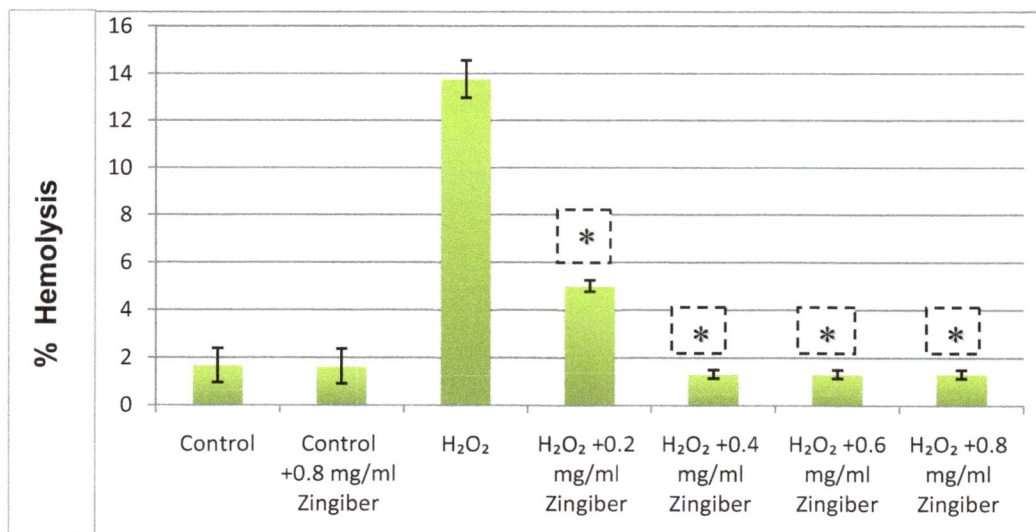

Fig. 3. Percentage hemolysis of normal erythrocytes when incubated at 37°C for 60 min in the absence or in the presence of 10 mM H_2O_2, or in the presence of 10 mM H_2O_2 plus different concentrations of ginger methanolic extract. Each column represents the mean value and bars represent the S.D. (n = 7). *P ≤ 0.05, compared to treatment with H_2O_2 alone

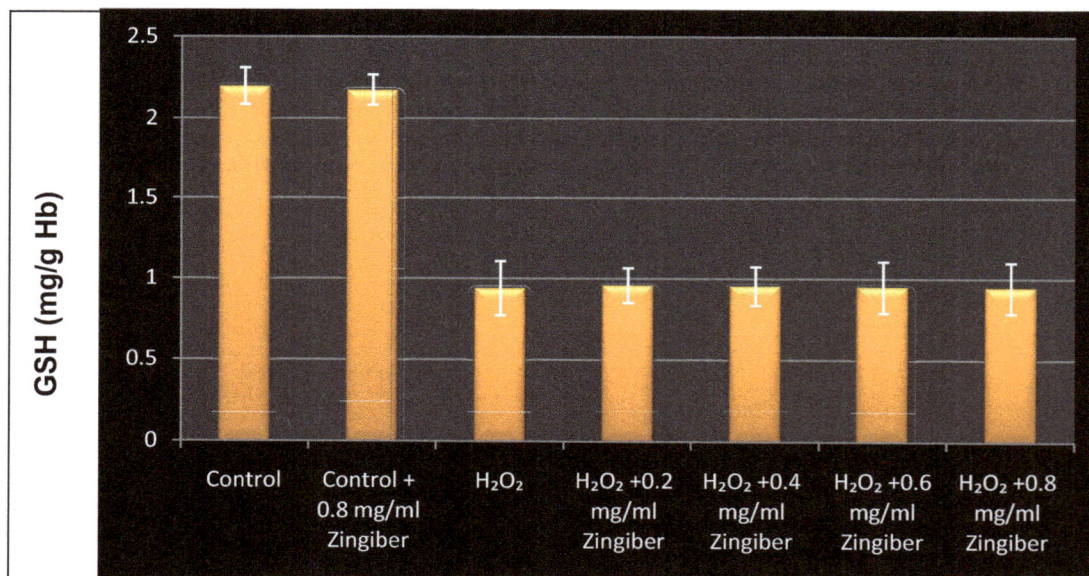

Fig. 4. Reduced Glutathione (GSH) concentration of normal erythrocytes when incubated at 37°C for 60 min in the absence or in the presence of 10 mM H_2O_2, or in the presence of 10 mM H_2O_2 plus different concentrations of ginger methanolic extract. Each column represents the mean value and bars represent the S.D. (n = 7)

Ginger had no significant effect on any of the following serum parameters (sodium, creatinine, uric acid, albumin, total protein, alkaline phosphatase, lactate dehydrogenase, alanine transaminase, aspartate transaminase, amylase) that have been measured at 0 time, 1 hour after the first dose of day 1, or at day 6 (i.e. one day following the last dose of day five) (data not shown).

Table 1. Results of the *In vivo* study of oral administration of ginger aqueous extract to healthy volunteers. Each value represents the mean value ± S.D., (n =9), *P value ≤ 0.05, compared to 0 time administration. NM indicates not measured

Measured parameter	Sample I (0 time)	Sample II (1 hr)	Sample III (day 6)
Serum TAS (mmol/l)	1.08±0.16	1.20±0.10	1.24*±0.12
Erythrocyte GSH (mg/g Hb)	0.74±0.31	NM	1.53*±0.37
Erythrocyte SOD (U/gHb)	1005.4±298.0	NM	1374.5*±160.1
Erythrocyte MDA (nmol//g Hb)	23.7±3.9	NM	15.5*±3.8
Serum K (Ref value = 3.7- 5.2 mmol/L)	4.3±0.47	4.3±0.53	4.0*±0.26
Serum BUN (Ref value = 6 - 20 mg/dL)	17.9±4.5	16.6*±4.5	13.5*±3.6
Serum CPK (Ref value = 38-176 U/L)	63.1±23.9	67.6*±22.6	82.7*±32.5

4. DISCUSSION

The present *ex vivo* study on normal human erythrocytes showed that pre-incubation of erythrocytes with methanolic extract of ginger and then exposed to H_2O_2 decreased significantly MDA production (i.e. anti-lipid-peroxidant), PC production (i.e. anti-protein-oxidant) and oxidant hemolysis (i.e. anti-hemolytic) that were caused by H_2O_2, in a concentration dependent manner (Figs 1, 2, 3). To our knowledge, the anti-protein-oxidant and anti-hemolytic activities of ginger (Figs. 2, 3) have not been reported before, whereas the anti-lipid-peroxidant activity (Fig. 1) has been reported before [6-10,14,15].

The present *in vivo* study on humans showed that oral administration for 5 days of aqueous extracts of ginger increased significantly the serum total antioxidant status (TAS), erythrocyte reduced glutathione (GSH), erythrocyte superoxide dismutase (SOD), and decreased significantly erythrocyte Malonyldialdehyde (MDA). These results coincide with the findings of other researchers in animals exposed to oxidative stress with various means [6-8,10,15-17]. As the present findings are obtained in healthy humans with no oxidative stress induction, this indicates that ginger can improve the base line of the defense mechanisms against possible oxidative stress, thus decreasing susceptibility to diseases related to oxidative stress. However, we could not find in the literature any similar study dealt with the effects of ginger on healthy humans to compare our results.

The present *ex vivo* study showed that ginger extract had no effect on GSH of incubated erythrocytes before or after exposure to H_2O_2 (Fig. 4). This is in contrary to the *in vivo* study of

humans (Table 1), indicate that the *ex vivo* antioxidant activity of the tested extract is not mediated through increasing erythrocyte GSH, probably, because the *ex vivo* experimental condition, which lacks the nutrients, is supposed to be not suitable for the reproduction of GSH.

Absence of ginger effect on serum LDH of healthy volunteers may indicate *in vivo* anti-hemolytic activity for this plant and / or absence of adverse *in vivo* hemolytic activity.

Absence of the effect of oral administration of aqueous extract of ginger on serum biochemical tests for kidney function (BUN,CREA), liver function enzymes and tests (ALT, AST, ALP, Albumin, Total Protein), cardiac enzymes (CPK, LDH, AST) and pancreatic amylase, indicates absence of adverse effects on these organs, this result confirms a similar finding by others in animals exposed to oxidative stress [16,25] and also coincides with others [6] who showed that aqueous extract of ginger given to rats fed on high-fat diet for 6 weeks significantly reduced the high serum levels of liver enzymes of AST, ALT and GGT that have been increased by the high-fat diet . However, the importance of the present *in vivo* study on healthy humans also related to the lifestyle factors such as diet, physical activity, alcohol consumption, cigarette smoking and others, that have been suggested to seriously influence the oxidative stress response in humans, tipping the balance of oxidative burden/antioxidant response to one side or the other, thus a diet rich in vegetables and in natural antioxidants, favoring the antioxidant side, has been found to be preferred by long-lived healthy individuals [26,27].

The decreased level of serum BUN with no effect on creatinine confirms a similar result by others on mice given ginger extract [28], thus indicating a possible beneficial effect for removal of urea from plasma in uremic patients. However, the increase in serum CPK in the present *in vivo* study could be due to the increased cardiac activity by the gingerols contained in ginger, as was shown by others [3,29], that gingerol analogues stimulate sarcoplasmic reticulum Ca2+ - ATpase.

Measurement of various biochemical laboratory tests in serum after oral intake of ginger was also important, to see whether a given plant extract affects laboratory analysis, as many patients may go to the clinical laboratory for analysis after drinking herbal extracts that have become a common habit in public, as there are no published studies showing their might be effects on laboratory tests.

As the present study could not tell the mechanism by which ginger increased cellular GSH in vivo and failed it *ex vivo* and increased activity of SOD, one can speculate that either the increase in GSH triggers the increase in the enzymes dependent on it, or ginger causes the induction of these enzymes independent of GSH. Therefore, further studies are required to gain more insight in to the possible mechanisms of action. Also, the present study could not tell which component(s) of the crude extract was responsible for the observed effects. Ginger extract has been shown to contain several bioactive compounds such as gingerol, shogaol, zingiberene, β-bisabolene, α-farnesene, β-sesquiphellandrene and α-curcumene [2,4,7,12,13], of which 6-Shogaol was found to be the most potent antioxidant and anti-inflammatory, that was attributed to the presence of alpha, beta-unsaturated ketone moiety in its structure [2], and also, Zingerone (a degradation Product of gingerols) was found to scavenge O^{2-} and OH and suppress lipid peroxidation *in vitro* [14]. Therefore, further studies should be conducted to determine which of these components are responsible for the observed effects of ginger. It is expected that the multiple components in ginger may lead to multiple effects on metabolic pathways and to involve multiple mechanisms affecting various aspects of metabolic disorders.

To our knowledge the design of the present *in vivo* study regarding the antioxidant related effects of ginger on healthy volunteers has not been reported before. It should be pointed out that the present study is meant to be a preliminary study involving a small number of participants. However, in order to validate the results of the present *in vivo* study, a larger, more comprehensive long-term study should be carried out to establish the various effects of ginger on humans.

5. CONCLUSION

The antioxidant related effects of ginger on healthy humans that have been obtained by the present in vivo study are comparable with that reported in animals exposed to oxidative stress. *Ex vivo* experimental effects although using cellular systems are shortcoming, compared to in vivo studies. Ginger have efficient antioxidant related effects on humans with no adverse effects, indicating that this plant might be helpful in preventing the occurrence or progress of pathological conditions related to oxidative stress.

CONSENT

All authors declare that they have read the manuscript, and all healthy volunteers were recruited in the study after they signed an informed consent for publication of this study.

ACKNOWLEDGMENTS

We are grateful to the deanship of scientific research, The University of Jordan for the financial support to conduct this study.

COMPETING INTERESTS

Authors have declared that no competing interests exist.

REFERENCES

1. Kemper KJ 1999. Ginger (*Zingiber officinale*). The logwood herbal task force. Available:http://www.mep.edu/herbal/ginger.pdf (16 September 2003).
2. Dugasani, S, Pichika, MR, Nadarajah, VD, Balijepalli, MK, Tandra, S, Korlakunta, JN. Comparative antioxidant and anti-inflammatory effects of [6]-gingerol, [8]-gingerol, [10]-gingerol and [6]-shogaol. J Ethnopharmacol. 2010;127:515–20.
3. Suthar, AC, Banavalikekar MM, Biyani MK. A review on ginger (*Zingiber officinale*): Pre-clinical and clinical trials. Indian J of Traditional Knowledge. 2003;2(1):51-61.

4. Hasan HA, Rasheed Raauf AM, Abd Razik BM, Rasool Hassan BA. Chemical composition and antimicrobial activity of the crude extracts isolated from *Zingiber officinale* by Different Solvents. Pharmaceut Anal Acta. 2012;3(9):184.

5. Gull, I, Saeed, M, Shaukat, H, Aslam, ShM, Samra, ZQ, Athar, AM. Inhibitory effect of *Allium sativum* and *Zingiber officinale* extracts on clinically important drug resistant pathogenic bacteria. Annals of Clinical Microbiology and Antimicrobials. 2012;11:8.

6. Ismail NS. Protective effects of aqueous extracts of cinnamon and ginger herbs against obesity and diabetes in obese diabetic rat. World Journal of Dairy & Food Sciences. 2014;9(2):145-53.

7. Roufogalis, BD. *Review Article: Zingiber officinale* (Ginger): A Future Outlook on Its Potential in Prevention and Treatment of Diabetes and Prediabetic States. New Journal of Science. Article ID 674684. 2014;15.

8. Li Y, Tran VH, Duke CC, Roufogalis BD. Preventive and protective properties of *Zingiber officinale* (Ginger) in diabetes mellitus, diabetic complications, and associated lipid and other metabolic disorders: A brief review. Evidence-Based Complementary and Alternative Medicine. Article ID 516870. 2012;10.

9. Committee on herbal medicinal products (HMPC). Assessment report on *Zingiber officinale* Roscoe, rhizome. European Medicines Agency. United Kingdom; 2011. Available: www.ema.europa.eu

10. Ghosh AK, Banerjee S, Mullick HI, Banerjee J. *Zingiber officinale*: A natural gold. International Journal of Pharma and Bio Sciences. 2011;2(1):283-294.

11. Mashhadi NSh, Ghiasvand R, Askari Gh, Hariri M, Darvishi L, Mofid MR. Anti-oxidative and anti-inflammatory effects of ginger in health and physical activity: Review of current evidence. Int J Prev Med. 2013;4(Suppl 1):36–42.

12. Shirin Adel PR, Prakash J. Chemical composition and antioxidant properties of ginger root (*Zingiber officinale*). Journal of Medicinal Plants Research. 2010;4(24): 2674-79.

13. Eleazu CO, Amadi CO, Iwo G, Nwosu P and Ironua CF. Chemical Composition and Free Radical Scavenging Activities of 10 Elite Accessions of Ginger (*Zingiber officinale* Roscoe). J Clinic Toxicol. 2013;3(1):155.

14. Aeschbach R, Loliger J, Scott BC, Murcia A, Butler B, Halliwell B, Aruoma OI. Antioxidant actions of thymol, carbacrol, 6-gingerol, zingerone and hydroxytyrosol. Food Chem. Toxicol. 1994;32:31-36.

15. Satheesh Kumar D, Kottai Muthuand A, Manavalan R. In-vivo antioxidant and lipid peroxidation effect of whole plant of *Ionidium suffruticosum* (ging.) In rats fed with high fat diet. Asian J Pharm Clin Res. 2012; 5(2):132-135.

16. Al-Kushi AG, El-Boshy MEl, ElSawy NA, Shaikh Omar OA, Header EA. Pathological Comparative Studies on Aqueous and Ethanolic Extracts of *Zingiber officinale* on Antioxidants and Hypolipdemic Effects in Rats. Life Sci J. 2013;10(2):2393-403.

17. Otunola GA, Oloyede OB, Oladiji AT, Afolayan AJ. Selected spices and their combination modulate hypercholestero-lemia-induced oxidative stress in experimental rats. Biol. Res. 2014;47. Santiago.

18. Packer L, Colman C. The Antioxidant Miracle. Canada. John Wiley & Sons Inc. Pub; 1999.

19. Valko M, Leibfritz D, Moncol J, Cronin MT, Mazur M, Telser J. Free radicals and antioxidants in normal physiological functions and human disease. Int. J. Biochem. Cell Biol. 2007;39:44-84.

20. Suboh SM, Bilto YY, Aburjai TA. Protective effects of selected medicinal plants against protein degradation, lipid peroxidation and deformability loss of oxidatively stressed human erythrocytes. Phytotherapy Research. 2004;18:280-84.

21. Srour MA, Bilto YY, Juma M. Evaluation of different methods used to measure malonyldialdehyde in human erythrocytes. Clin. Hemorheol. Microcirc. 2000;23:23-30.

22. Reznick A, Packer L. Oxidative damage to proteins: Spectrophotometric method for carbonyl assay. Methods in Enzymology. 1994;233:357-63.

23. Ellman GL. Tissue Sulfhydryl (-SH) Groups. Archive of Biochemistry and Biophysiology. 1951;82:70-77.

24. Arthur JR, Boyne R. Superoxide dismutase and glutathione peroxidase activities in neutrophilis from selenium deficient and copper deficient cattle. Life Sci. 1985;36:1569-75.

25. Wigler I, Grotto I, Caspi D, Yaron M. The effects of Zintona EC (a ginger extract) on

symptomatic gonarthritis. Osteoarthritis Cartilage. 2003;11:783-89.

26. Dato S, Crocco P, D'Aquila P, de Rango F, Bellizzi D, Rose G, Passarino G. Review: Exploring the role of genetic variability and lifestyle in oxidative stress response for healthy aging and longevity. Int. J. Mol. Sci. 2013;14:16443-72.

27. Aseervatham GSB, Sivasudha T, Jeyadevi R, Arul Ananth D. Environmental factors and unhealthy lifestyle influence oxidative stress in humans—An overview.

Environmental Science and Pollution Research. 2013;20(7):4356-69.

28. Mehrdad M, Messripour M, Ghobadipour M. The effect of ginger extract on blood urea nitrogen and creatinine in mice. Pakistan J. of Biol. Scie. 2007;10(17):2968-71.

29. Ohizumi Y, Sasaki S, Shibusawa K, Ishikawa K, Ikemto F. Stimulation of sarcoplasmic reticulum Ca2+ - ATpase by gingerol analogues. Biol Pharm Bull. 1996;19:1377.

5

Antimicrobial and Antioxidant Potentials, and Chemical Constituents of the Leaf Extracts of the Nigerian *Piliostigma thonningii* (Caesalpiniaceae) Schum

Okwute Simon Koma[1*] and Yakubu Rufa'i[1]

[1]*Department of Chemistry, University of Abuja, P.M.B. 117, Gwagwalada, Federal Capital Territory, Abuja, Nigeria.*

Authors' contributions

This work was carried out in collaboration between both authors. The bench work was done by author YR as a M.Sc. student under author OSK who designed and supervised the project. Author YR also drafted the report while author OSK did the final moderation of the manuscript for publication. Both authors read and approved the final manuscript.

Editor(s):
(1) Thomas Efferth, Department of Pharmaceutical Biology, Institute of Pharmacy and Biochemistry Johannes Gutenberg University, Germany.
(2) Marcello Iriti, Department of Agricultural and Environmental Sciences, Milan State University, Italy.
Reviewers:
(1) Anonymous, Greece.
(2) Anonymous, Algeria.
(3) Anonymous, Egypt.
(4) Anonymous, China.
(5) Anonymous, México.

ABSTRACT

Aims: In this work the 95% ethanol extract of the Nigerian *Piliostigma thonningii* known traditionally to possess a number of medicinal properties was screened for antimicrobial and antioxidant potentials as well as identified its chemical constituents. It was to confirm its traditional medicinal uses.
Study Design: The various local sources of the plant were identified for the collection of the leaves. The plant was authenticated by a taxonomist and a voucher specimen kept for future reference. The plant sample was extracted using 95% ethanol and the crude extract screened for phytochemicals and fractionated. The crude extract and fractions were screened for antimicrobial

*Corresponding author: E-mail: profokwute@yahoo.com

and antioxidant potentials. The antimicrobial hexane fraction was subjected to chromatographic separation to isolate the chemical constituents. Also, the fresh leaves were hydrodistilled to obtain the volatile components. The column isolates and volatile components were identified using GC-MS analysis.

Place and Duration of Study: The study was undertaken between October 2011 and April, 2013, in the Department of Chemistry, University of Abuja, Nigeria and the Advanced Chemistry Laboratory, Sheda Science and Technology Complex, Sheda, Abuja, Nigeria.

Methodology: The air-dried leaves powder of *P. thonningii* was extracted with 95% ethanol to obtain the crude extract. The fresh leaves were also hydrodistilled to obtain the volatile oils. The crude extract was fractionated into acidic, basic, non-polar neutral and polar neutral fractions. It was screened for phytochemicals using standard procedures. Both the crude extract and fractions were screened against some pathogens, including *Escherichia coli, Staphylococcus aureus, Bacillus subtilis, Pseudomonas aeruginosa, Streptococuss* spp. *and Salmonella* spp. The antioxidant potential of the crude extract was also determined using standard procedures. The antimicrobial hexane fraction was subjected to Flash column chromatography. The isolates and the volatile oil were analyzed for their constituents using GC-MS.

Results: The crude extract showed the presence of sterols, phenolics, alkaloids, flavonoids, glycosides, triterpenes, and tannins, but no carbohydrates. The crude extract and fractions and the hydrodistillate showed potential activity against the test organisms including, *Escherichia coli, Staphylococcus aureus, Bacillus subtilis, Pseudomonas aeruginosa, Streptococuss* spp. *and Salmonella spp.* The crude extract equally showed antioxidant potential in DPPH. Column chromatography of the hexane fraction followed by GC-MS analysis led to the identification of lupeol and lup-20(29)-en-3-one. GC-MS analysis of the volatile oil from hydrodistillation of the fresh leaf revealed the presence of 2,5-octadecadiynoic acid, cholestan-3-ol, 2-methylene, isoaromendrene, trans-Z-α-bisabolene epoxide,1-methyl-6-(3-methybuta-3-dienyl)-7-oxabicylo [4.1.0] heptane and aromadendrene oxide.

Conclusion: The crude 95% ethanol extract has demonstrated reasonable antioxidant potential. Also, the crude extract, fractions and the volatile oil have shown antimicrobial activity. Lupeol, lupenone and some volatile components have been identified from the leaves. The presence of these compounds may contribute to the bioactivities of the leaf extracts.

Keywords: Piliostigma thonningii; leaf extracts; antimicrobial; antioxidant; potentials; chemical constituents.

1. INTRODUCTION

Among the plants belonging to the genus Piliostigma the two African species, *P. reticulatum* (DC) Hochst and *P. thonningii* (Schum) Milne-Redhead, inhabit dry and moist savannahs, respectively [1-4]. Various parts of *P. thonningii* were found to be used in the management of ailments in phytomedicines. The bark is used in the management of cough, stomach infections, malaria, leprosy, sore throat and various forms of inflammation. The roots and twigs are used in treating fever, dysentery, snake bites, hookworms and skin infections, while the leaves decoctions are used as laxatives for children and for dressing wounds [5].

The results of a number of pharmacological investigations have revealed that *P. thonningii* has some bioactivities such as antimalarial [6,7],antibacterial [8,9], anthelmintic [10,11], antioxidant [12] and sub-acute toxicity [13,14].

Chemical studies by some researchers showed that the genus *Piliostigma* contains some flavonoids [15], polyphenols [16] and essential oils [17,18]. The presence of griffonilide and some unidentified sterols in the stem bark of the Nigerian *P. thonningii* has been previously reported [19]. Since then there have been several reports on the pharmacological properties, but reports on the chemical constituents have been scarce. In this paper we wish to report on the antimicrobial and antioxidant potentials and in particular on the chemical constituents of the leaf extracts of the Nigerian *P. thonningii*.

2. MATERIALS AND METHODS

2.1 General

All solvents and reagents used in this work were of standard grade and were purified by re-distillation before use.

For the antimicrobial screening, stock solutions of the extracts (crude, acidic, basic, non-polar and polar neutrals and hydrodistillate) were at concentration of 100 μg/ml; the petri-dish, micro-pipette, autoclave, incubator, bunsen flame, loop and dimethylsulphoxide as the solvent were used. The test organisms were *Escherichia coli, Staphylococcus aurues, Bacillus subtilis, Pseudomonas aeruginosa, Streptococcus* spp *and Salmonella* spp. from Gwagwalada Teaching Hospital in Mueller Hinton broth culture made by Beaker Company and kept in a refrigerator at 4°C.

Open flash column chromatography was performed using silica gel Merck 0.063-0.200 mm mesh, 60 G. Thin Layer Chromatography(TLC) analyses of extracts, fractions and isolates were carried out using silica 60 F_{254} precoated glass baked plates (0.25 mm, 20 X 20 cm; Merck Darmstadt, Germany). Spots were detected on TLC plates under short ($λ=254$ nm) and long ($λ=366$ nm) UV light as well as visualized by spraying with 2% (w/v) vanillin in sulphuric acid and in iodine vapour.

2.2 Plant Material

The fresh leaves of *Piliostigma thonningii* were collected from the Medicinal Plant Reserve Garden of Sheda Science and Technology Complex (SHESTCO), Abuja, Nigeria, in September 2011. It was authenticated at the National Institute for Pharmaceutical Research and Development (NIPRD), Idu, Abuja, Nigeria, and a voucher specimen was kept at the Ahmadu Bello University, Zaria, Herbarium (No.171). The leaves were air-dried and ground into fine powder and kept in a non-absorptive nylon bag for subsequent use.

2.3 Extraction and Fractionation Procedure

The ground plant material (1000 g) was extracted using a Soxhlet extractor with 50% aqueous ethanol for six hours. After filtering the extract the solvent was removed using a rotary evaporator to dryness on a water bath. The crude residue (32.0 g) was fractionated into acidic (1.9 g), basic (1.2 g), polar neutral (3.0 g), and non-polar neutral (11.0 g) extracts according to a standard procedure [20].

2.4 Hydrodistillation of fresh leaves

The freshly collected leaves of *P. thonningii* were subjected to hydrodistillation. The hydrodistillate was extracted with diethyl ether and the extract was evaporated to dryness to give an oily residue (2.6 g).

2.5 Phytochemical Screening

Phytochemical screening was carried out on the crude ethanol extract using standard methods [21].

2.6 Determination of Antioxidant Activity of Crude Extract

The antioxidant property of the crude extract was determined according to a standard method using the DPPH radical [22]. The crude extract (0.1 g) was weighed into a test tube and dissolved in 10 ml of methanol, then 5 ml, 2 ml, and 1 ml portions were taken into three separate test tubes labeled A, B, and C, respectively. Further, diluted concentrations were made from A, B, and C test tubes into five tubes D, E, F, G, and H (0.5, 0.1, 0.05, 0.02 and 0.01 mg/ml). From each of these test tubes 1ml was taken into another test tube and 3 ml of methanol and 0.5 ml of DPPH solution were added to prepare a standard test sample. This was allowed to stand for 15 mins. The same procedure was applied to the sample of Vitamin C. The samples were subjected to UV/Visible double beam spectrophotometer with the light set at 517 nm. A reference was also prepared by mixing 3ml of methanol with 0.5 ml of DPPH solution.

The percentage inhibition (I %) of free-radical DPPH was calculated using the standard equation[133]:

$$I\% = 100 \times (A_{Control} - A_{Sample}) / A_{Control}$$

Where $A_{Control}$ is the absorbance of the control reaction (containing all reagents except the test compound), and A_{Sample} is the absorbance of the test compound.

2.7 Antimicrobial Activity Screening of Crude Extract and Fractions

Antimicrobial sensitivity tests were carried out on the 95% ethanol crude extract, the acidic, basic, non polar and polar neutral fractions, and the steam distillate using the Disc Diffusion Method [23]. A stock solution of each extract at concentration of100 μg/ml was screened against the six test organisms. The test organisms were maintained on nutrient agar slants and kept at 4°C until required. Sterile paper discs of 6 mm in diameter prepared from Whatman No.1 filter paper were impregnated with 100 µg/ml of the crude extract and fractions. The paper discs were kept in an incubator at 37°C for 24 hours to evaporate the solvent. 100 µl of the suspension of the organism (0.5 McFarland standard turbidity), containing 10^8 CFU/ml of bacteria was prepared from an overnight Mueller Hinton broth culture. The discs were arranged and firmly pressed on the agar surface of each seeded plate. The plates, after staying at 4°C for 2 hours, were incubated aerobically at 37°C for 24 hours for the organisms to grow. The negative control was also prepared using the same solvent employed to dissolve the plant extract. Antimicrobial activity was evaluated by measuring the zone of inhibition against the test organism. All tests were carried out in triplicates and the average values were taken.

2.8 Column Chromatographic Separation of Hexane Fraction

The neutral non-polar hexane fraction (5 g) was chromatographed on a column of silica gel by eluting with mixtures of n-hexane and ethyl acetate in increasing polarity. Aliquots of 10 ml portion each were collected and the degree of purity of each was monitored by TLC using mixtures of hexane and ethyl acetate. Similar fractions were then combined, evaporated to dryness and weighed. Hexane eluted a fraction which on further purification gave the isolate, PT. H-d (0.4 g).

2.9 IR and GC-MS Analyses

The IR spectrum (neat) of the isolate PT.H-d was then obtained on FTIR 8400S Shimadzu Fourier Transform Spectrophotometer and the absorption values were recorded in wave numbers (cm^{-1}).

The isolate PT. H-d from the non-polar neutral hexane fraction of the crude 95% ethanol extract and the volatile oil (PT. STM-E) from the hydrodistillation of the fresh leaves were subjected to GC-MS analysis.

Thermo-Scientific Trace GC ULTRA system equipped with an AS 3000 auto sampler and a split/split-lessinjector was employed for the GC analysis. The column used was an DB-5 (optima-5), 30 m × 0.25 mm i. d., 0.25 µm d.f., coated with 5% diphenyl-95% polydimethylsiloxane, operated with the following oven temperature programme: 50°C, held for 1min, rising at 3°C/min to 250°C, held for 5 min,

rising at 2°C/min to 280°C, held for 3 min; injection temperature and volume, 250°C and 1.0 µl, respectively ; injection mode, split ratio, 30:1; carrier gas was nitrogen at 30 cm/s linear velocity and inlet pressure 99.8 KPa; detector temperature, 280°C; hydrogen flow rate, 50 ml/min; air flow rate, 400 ml/min; make-up (H$_2$/air). Data were acquired by means of GC solution software (Thermo scientific). Thermo scientific Trace GC ULTRA AS 3000 auto sampler was interfaced with VG analytical 70-250, double- focusing mass spectrometer and the MS operating conditions were ionization: voltage 70eV with ion source of 250°C

3. RESULTS AND DISCUSSION

The results of qualitative phytochemical analysis of the crude extract of the leaf showed the presence of alkaloids, tannins, glycosides, saponins, flavonoids, phenols, triterpenes and sterols, but no carbohydrates. This is consistent with previous reports on some species of the genus [15,19,24], but only in few cases were the chemical constituents isolated and characterised [15,19].

The crude extract was subjected to antioxidant activity test and the results showed that the free radical scavenging activity of P. thonningii leaves crude extract using Vitamin C as standard was reasonably good, increasing with increasing concentration particularly at lower concentrations (Fig. 1). However, some workers have observed that DPPH scavenging activity may not be related to the concentration of the sample, but has a relationship with the time of reaction and that the composition of may have an impact on the antioxidant activity due to the presence of some constituents [25]. The antioxidant potential may be attributed to the presence of phenols and tannins. Previous workers had recorded the antioxidant activity of P. thonningii leaves using carbon tetrachloride-induced hepatic and oxidative damage in rat which showed that P. thonningii leaves protect liver against hepatic and oxidative damage by carbon tetrachloride possibly by acting as an in-vivo free radical scavenger through induction of antioxidant enzymes or drug detoxifying enzymes and by prevention of excessive stimulation of antioxidant enzyme and lipid peroxidation [12]. Thus, the results obtained in this work further support the antioxidant potential of P. thonningii leaves.

The results of antimicrobial activity screening of crude extract, fractions and hydrodistillate with streptomycin as standard and measured as zones of inhibition (mm) are shown in Table 1. The crude extract and the non-polar neutral fraction when compared to the standard antibiotic, streptomycin, were found to be reasonably active against *E. coli, S. aureus, B. subtilis, P. aeruginosa, Streptococcus* spp *and Salmonella* spp at 100 µg/ml. The polar neutral fraction and steam distillate were active against all the test organisms except *B. subtilis*. The acidic fraction was not active against *S. aureus, P. aeruginosa, and Salmonella* spp at the same concentration (Table 1).

Thus, the antimicrobial and antioxidant activitivities of these extracts may be attributable to the phytochemicals found in the crude extract. Hence, it was very necessary to identify the chemical constituents of the fractions, particularly the hexane fraction, as well as the hydrodistillate through column chromatography and GC-MS analysis.

The biologically active n-hexane fraction was separated by column chromatography, eluting with mixtures of hexane and ethyl acetate. The hexane fractions 1-3 from the column were combined and purified to give an antimicrobial isolate PT.H-d (Table 2).

The bioactive column isolate, PT. H-d was subjected to IR analysis and gave the following absorption bands: 3347 supportive of OH group, 1732 which is suggestive of a ketone or ester carbonyl group and 1466 and 1375 for C-H bending vibrations. The GC of PT. H-d (Fig. 2) showed two important peaks at RT. 25.54 min for component PT. H-d-1 and at RT. 29.69 min for component PT.H-d-2. Direct comparison with standard computer library MS data and literature [25,26] were suggestive of lupeol, 1, and lup-20(29)-en-3-one 2. The presence of these components in PT.H-d is supported by the presence of OH and carbonyl CO absorptions in the IR spectrum, the molecular ion (M^+) m/z 426 for lupeol, the molecular ion (M^+) m/z 424 for lupenone and the characteristic MS fragment ions at m/z 218 (base peak), 207 and 189 for lupeol and lup-20(29)-en-3-one [26,27].

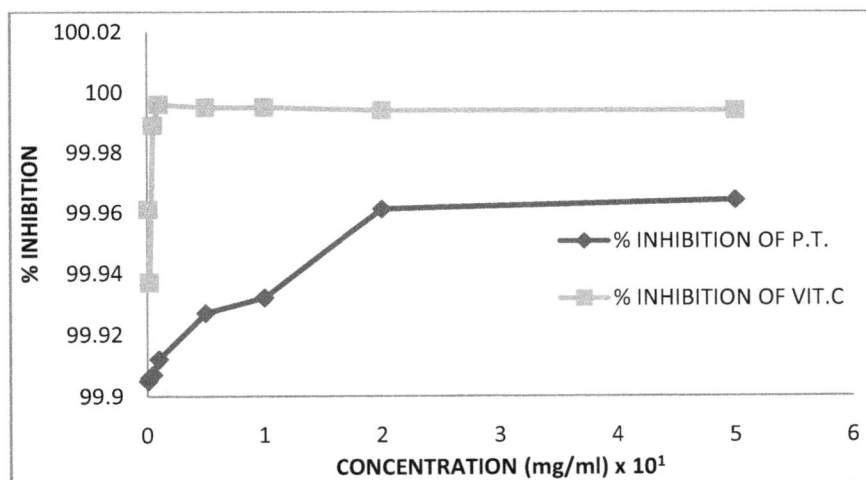

Fig. 1. Comparative percentage inhibitions of *Piliostigma thonningii* and vitamin C

Table 1. Screening of the antimicrobial potential of crude extract and fractions of leaves P. thonningi at 100 µg/mL (mm)

Sample	Sa	Ec	Bs	Ss	Pa	Sm
Crude extract	16.00±0.00	13.83±0.50	9.83±0.17	15.17±0.50	14.00±0.00	12.33±0.67
Non-polar	15.17±0.50	13.17±0.17	9.17±0.17	13.03± 0.03	13.00±0.67	10.07±0.07
Polar	14.17±0.50	10.10±0.57	-	12.23±0.10	12.10±0.57	12.00±0.00
Acidic	14.23±0.43	11.54±0.33	-	10.17±0.50	11.17±0.17	-
Basic	-	-	-	9.00±0.00	9.33±0.33	9.17±0.50
Hydrodistillate	10.10±0.67	10.17±0.50	-	11.00±0.67	12.07±0.07	11.83±0.50
Streptomycin	27.83±0.10	29.10±0.67	26.23±0.13	21.83±0.50	23.90±0.23	27.23±0.13

Values are means of triplicates, Sa= Staphylococcus aureus; Ec=Escherichia coli ; Bs = Bacillus substilis; Ss= Streptococcus spp; Pa= Pseudomonas aeruginosa; Sm=Salmonella spp

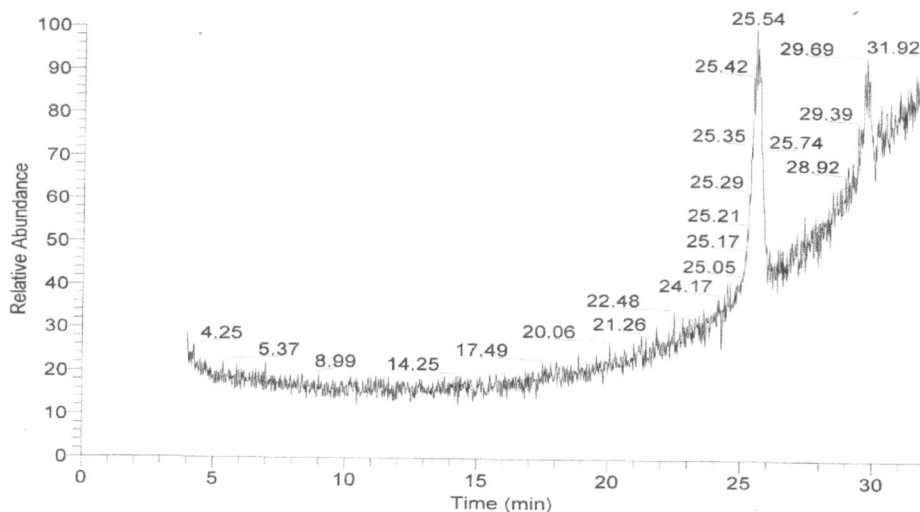

Fig. 2. Gas chromatogram of PT. H-d

The co-occurrence of lupeol, **1** and lup-20 (29)–en-3-one, **2** is not unusual as the ketone is actually a biogenetic oxidation product of the corresponding alcohol.

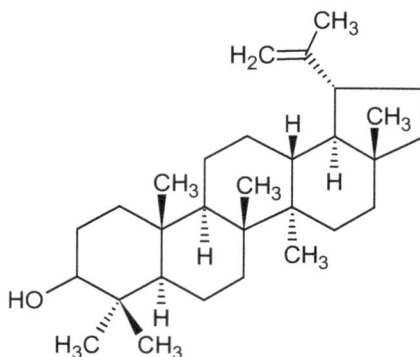

1. lupeol

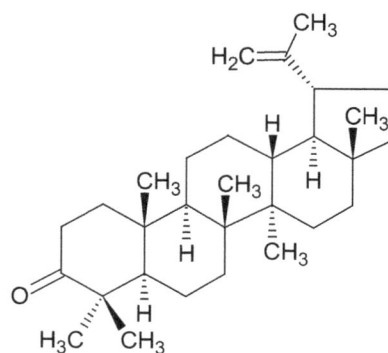

2. lup- 20(29)-en-3-one

Table 2. Screening of antimicrobial potential of isolates from column chromatography of hexane fraction

Sample	Concentration/ Inhibition (mm)	
	5µg/ml	10µg/ml
PT. H-a	13.30±0.33	14.50±0.33
PT. H-b	14.67±0.33	18.50±0.33
PT. H-c	14.05±0.33	18.67±0.33
PT. H-d	15.00±0.00	19.50±0.33
PT. H-e	12.00±.00	14.00.±0.67

Values are means of triplicates, PT.H-a to PT. H-e = column chromatographic isolates from non –polar (hexane) fraction

The fresh leaves were hydrodistilled to give an antimicrobial oily residue, PT.STM-E (Table 1). The GC (Fig. 3) of PT.STM-E showed about six major components which on the basis of their Retention Times(RT), MS characteristics and by comparison with the NIST/EPA/NIH Mass Spectral Library data and literature were tentatively identified as a long chain acetylenic ester, 2,5–octadecadiynoic acid methyl ester [28], 1-methyl-6-3(methylbuta-1,3-dienyl)-7-oxa-bicyclo [4.1.0] heptane, trans-Z-a-bisabolene epoxide [29], cholestan-3-ol, 2-methylene-(3a,5a) [30], aromadendrene oxide-(2) [31] and isoaromadendrene epoxide [32]. The results of GC-MS analysis of PT.STM-E are summarized in Table 3.

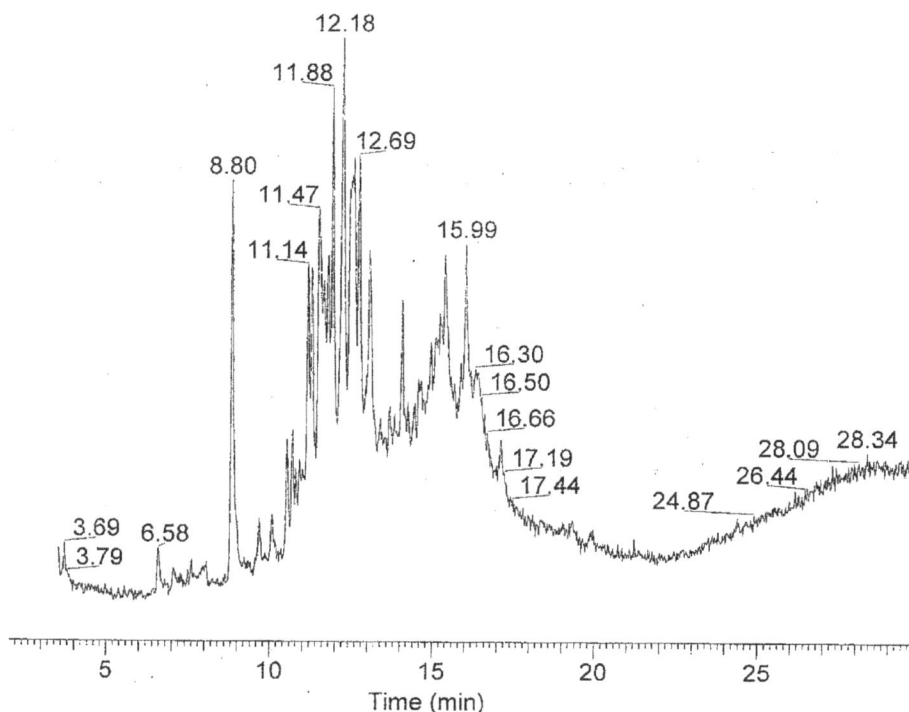

Fig. 3. Gas chromatogram of hydrodistillate PT.STM-E

Table 3. GC-MS of Volatile oil from hydrodistillation of fresh leaves of *P. thonningii*

S/N	Compounds	Retention time(mins)	Mol. Weight	Formula
1.	2, 5-octadiynoic acd methyl ester	8.82	290	$C_{19}H_{30}O_2$
2.	1-Methyl6-(3-methylbuta-1,3-dienyl)-7-oxabicyclo-[4.1.0]heptane	11.47	178	$C_{12}H_{18}O$
3.	Trans-Z- a-bisabolene epoxide	12.49	220	$C_{15}H_{24}O$
4.	Cholestan-3-ol, 2-methylene-(3a, 5a)	14.04	400	$C_{28}H_{48}O$
5.	Aromadendrene oxide-(2),	15.36	220	$C_{15}H_{24}O$
6.	Isoaromadendrene epoxide	15.95	220	$C_{15}H_{24}O$

4. CONCLUSION

The result of this study on the Nigerian *P. thonningii* has lent support to the antiinfective and antioxidant potentials of *P. thonningii* leaf irrespective of geographical location. Qualitative phytochemical screening results showed the presence of alkaloids, tannins, glycosides, triterpenes and phenolics in the 95% crude extract of the leaves. Two lupine triterpenoids known to possess antibacterial activity were identified from the bioactive n-hexane fraction of the *P. thonningii* leaf. The work also identified some volatile components in the leaf of *P. thonningii*. This is the first time these compounds have been identified from *P. thonningii* leaf. This work lends strong support to the traditional medicinal uses of the leaf of *P. thonningii* as an antiinfective agent in Nigeria.

CONSENT

It is not applicable.

ETHICAL APPROVAL

It is not applicable.

ACKNOWLEDGEMENT

The authors offer their appreciation to Sheda Science and Technology Complex (SHESTCO), Sheda, Abuja, Nigeria, for granting laboratory facilities to Mr. Yakubu Rufai' and for the antimicrobial screening and GC-MS analysis of the samples.

COMPETING INTERESTS

Authors have declared that no competing interests exist.

REFERENCES

1.   Allen ON, Allen EK. The leguminosae: A source book of characteristics, Uses and Nodulation. The University of Wisconsin Press, USA.1981;52:9-23.
2.   Schultes RE, Hofmann A. The botany and chemistry of hallucinogens, Charles C, Thomas, Spring Fields III. 1973;267.
3.   Burkill HM. The useful Plants of west Tropical Africa. Edition2. 3, Families J – L. Royal botanic Gardens, Kew. 1995;144-150.
4.   Index kewense. Supplementum 11. 1953;188:1941-1950.
5.   Crepet WL,Taylor DW. Primitive mimosoid flowers from the Paleocene-Eocene and their systematic and evolutionary implications. American Journal of Botany. 1986;73:548-563.
6.   Kwaji A, Bassi PU, Aoill1 M, Nneji CM, Ademowo G. Preliminary studies on *Piliostigma thonningii* Schum leaf extract: Phytochemical screening and *in vitro* antimalarial activity. African Journal of Microbiological Research. 2010;4(9):735-739.
7.   Madara AA, Ajayi JA, Salawu OA, Tijani AY. Anti-malarial activity of ethanolic leaf extract of *Piliostigma thonningii Schum.* (Caesalpiniacea) in mice infected with *Plasmodium berghei berghei.* African Journal of Biotechnology. 2010;9(23): 3475-3480.
8.   Daniyan SY, Galadima M, Ijah UJJ, Odama LE, Yusuf AY, Jigam AA, Abbas Y. Evaluation of antibacterial activity of *Piliostigma thonningii* (crude extract) and fractions 1-3, 4, 5, 6 and 7 against Methicillin-resistant *Staphylococcus aureus* (MRSA*).* Research Journal of Pharmaceutical, Biological and Chemical Sciences. 2011;1(4):173.
9.   Akinpelu DA, Obuotor EM. Antibacterial activity of *Piliostigma thonningii* stems bark. Fitoterapia. 2000;71:442-443.
10. Asuzu IU, Onu UO, Anthelmintic activities of the ethanolic extract of *Piliostigma*

thonningii bark in *Ascaridia galli* infected chickens. Fitoterapia. 1994;65(4):291-297.
11. Asuzu IU, Gray AI, Waterman PG. The anthelmintic activity of D-3-O-methylchiroinositol isolated from *Piliostigma thonningii* stem bark. Fitoterapia. 1999;70:77-79.
12. Taofeek OA. *In vivo* antioxidant potentials of *Piliostigma thonningii (Schum) leaves*: Studies on hepatic marker enzyme, antioxidant system, drug detoxifying enzyme and lipid peroxidation. Human Experimental Toxicology. 2011;30(1):55-62.
13. Daniyan SY, Galadima M, Ijah UJJ, Odama LE. Short term acute and sub acute toxicity studies on *Piliostigma thonningii* leaf extract in rats. International Journal of Research in Ayurveda and Pharmacy. 2011;2(2):481-483.
14. Asuzu IU, Onu OU. The *in vitro* acute toxicity of *Piliostigma thonningii* barks ethanolic extract on selected strongly larvae of cattle. Fitoterapia. 1993; 64(6):524-528.
15. Bombardelli E, Gabetta B, Mustich G. Plants of Mozambique I. Flavonoids of *Piliostigma thonningii.* Fitoterapia. 1973;44(2):85-87.
16. Bombardelli E. Chemical and biological characterisation of *Piliostigma thonningii* polyphenols. Fitoterapia. 1994;65(6):493-501.
17. Tira-Picos V, Nogueira JM, Gbolade AA. Comparative analysis of leaf essential oil constituents of *Piliostigma thonningii* and *Piliostigma reticulatum.* International Journal of Green Pharmacy. 2010;4:67-70.
18. Mustapha AT, Fanna I, Abdulrahman SW, Buba GI, Mala J, Akan BMA, Abubakar SA. Chemical and proximate contents of methanolic leaf extract of *Piliostigma thonningii schum* (camel foot). Journal of Chemical and Pharmaceutical Research. 2012;4(5):2409-2414.
19. Okwute SK, Ndukwe GI, Watanabe K, Ohno N. Isolation of griffonilide from the steam bark of *Bauhinia thonining.* Journal of Natural Products. 1986;49:716-717.
20. Mitscher AL, Drake S, Gollapudi SR, Okwute SK. A modern look at folkloric use of anti-infective agents. Journal of Natural Products. 1987;50(6):1025-1045.
21. Prashant T, Bimlesh K, Mandeep K, Gurpreet K, Harleen K. Phytochemical screening and extraction: A Review.

Internationale Pharmaceutica Sciencia. 2011;1(1).

22. Hatano T, Kagawa H, Yasuhara T, Okuda T. Two new flavonoids and other constituents in licorice root: their relative astringency and radical scavenging effects. Chemical and Pharmaceutical Bulletin. 1988;36:1090-7.

23. Saliu BK, Usman LA, Sani A, Muhammad NO, Akolade JO. Chemical composition and anti bacterial (oral isolates) activitiy of leaf essential oil of *Ocimum gratissimum* grown in north central Nigeria. International Journal of Current Research. 2011;33(3):022-028.

24. Ferreria MA, Prista LN, Alves AC. Chemical study of bark of *Bauhinia thonningii*. Garcia Orta. 1963;11(1):97-105.

25. Zhao C, Zhang M, He J, Ding Y, Li B. Chemical composition and antioxidant activity of the essential oil from the flowers of *Artemisia austio-yunnanensis*. Journal of Chemical and Pharmaceutical Research. 2014;6(7):1583-1587.

26. Maruthupandian A, Mohan VR. GC-MS analysis of some bioactive constituents of *Pterocarpus marsupium* Roxb. Int. J. Chem. Tech. Res. 2011;3(3):1652-1657.

27. Gabriel AF, Okwute SK. Isolation and characterisation of lup-20(29(-en-3-one and diisononyl phthalate from *Pterocarpus erinaceus* (Poir) stem bark. Journal of Chemical Society of Nigeria. 2009; 34(2):156-161.

28. Sadashiva CT, Sharanappa P, Naidoo Y, Balachandran I. Chemical composition of essential oil from the leaves of *Premma coriacea* Clarke. African Journal of Biotechnology. 2013;12(20): 2914-2916.

29. Blassioli-Moraes MC, Laumann RA, Oliveira MWM, Woodcock MP, Hooper A, Pickett JA, Birkett MA, Borges M. Sex pheromone communication in two sympatric neotropical stink bug species *Chinavia ubica* and *Chinavia impicticornis*. Journal of Chemical Ecology. 2012;38(7): 836-845.

30. Thanga KKS, Muthukumarasamy S, Mohan VR. GC-MS determination of bioactive components of *Canscora perfoliata* Lam (Gentianaceae). Journal of Applied Pharmaceutical Science. 2012; 02(08):210-2014.

31. Hossain MA, Shah MD, Sakari M. Gas chromatography-mass spectrometry analysis of various organic extracts of *Morremia borneensis* from Sabah. Asian Pacific Journal of Tropical Medicine. 2011;637-641.

32. Aboutubi EA, El-Tantawy EM, Sharma MM. Chemical constituents and antimicrobial activity of volatile constituents from the roots, leaves and seeds of *Arctium lappa* L. (Asteraceae) grown in Egypt. Egyptian Pharmacy Journal. 2013;12(2):173-176.

In vitro Antioxidant Activities and Phytochemical Analysis of Methanol Extracts of Leaves and Stems of *Lumnitzera racemosa*

Firdaus Mukhtar Quraishi[1], B. L. Jadhav[1*] and Neeti Kumar[1]

[1]*Department of Life Sciences, University of Mumbai, Vidyanagari Campus, Santacruz (E), 400 098, Mumbai, India.*

Authors' contributions

This work was carried out in collaboration between all authors. Authors FMQ and BLJ designed the study, performed the statistical analysis, wrote the protocol and wrote the first draft of the manuscript. Author NK managed the analyses of the study and the literature searches. All authors read and approved the final manuscript.

Editor(s):
(1) Paola Angelini, Department of Applied Biology, University of Perugia, Italy.
(2) Marcello Iriti, Faculty of Plant Biology and Pathology, Department of Agricultural and Environmental Sciences, Milan State University, Italy.
Reviewers:
(1) Anonymous, Egypt.
(2) Mondher Boulaaba, Centre de Biotechnologie de Borj-Cédria, Laboratoire des Plantes Extremophiles, Tunisie.
(3) Amit Roy, Department of Biotechnology, Visva-Bharati University, India.
(4) Anonymous, Spain.
(5) Anonymous, Malaysia.

ABSTRACT

Aim: To study antiradical and the reducing power activities in the leaves and stems methanol extracts of *Lumnitzera racemosa* mangrove species.
Design: Soxhlet extraction of leaves and stems using methanol for *in vitro* antioxidant assay.
Place and Duration of Study: Department of Life Sciences, University of Mumbai, Vidyanagari Campus, Santacruz (East), Mumbai, India, April, 2014 to December, 2014
Methodology: The plant branches were collected in the month of May, identified by an expert taxonomist. The leaves and stems were separated, washed, shed dried, powdered and Soxhlet methanol extracts were prepared to study antioxidant properties using DPPH (1, 1-diphenyl-2-picrylhydrazyl) Scavenging and Reducing power assay.

Corresponding author: E-mail: drbljadhav@gmail.com

Results: Both DPPH test and reducing power assay showed better antioxidant activity in leaves than stems. The scavenging activity in the leaves was (23.31 µg/mL) while in stems (111.5 µg/mL) as compared to ascorbic acid (14.98 µg/mL)

Conclusion: Overall *L. racemosa* has shown antioxidant properties in which leaves were more potent than stems.

Keywords: Lumnitzera racemosa; antioxidant; DPPH; reducing power; scavenging activity.

1. INTRODUCTION

Mangroves are halophytic (salt loving) and salt resistant marine tidal forest comprising trees, shrubs, palms etc. found in tropical climate. Several mangrove species are used as folklore medicine to treat various diseases like infectious diseases, diabetes and asthma [1]. Recent research have shown that Indian mangroves contain antimicrobial [2-5] and antiviral activities [6]. *C. tagal* [7] and *K. candel* [8] mangrove species have shown mild to strong antioxidant properties. The *L. racemosa* mangrove is used for antifertility, herpes, treatment of asthma, diabetes, and snake bite and for skin disorder. [9] This species was also tested for antibacterial [10], hepatoprotective, antioxidant [11,12] and cytotoxic activities [12].

2. MATERIALS AND METHODS

2.1 Plant Material

Mangrove plant *L. racemosa was* collected in the month of May from Ratnagiri coast Maharashtra, India and identified by an expert taxonomist. Leaves and stems were separated, washed thoroughly under running tap water to free them from dust and other contaminants, oven dried at 40ºC to remove the moisture content, grinded, resultant powder was individually sieved through a muslin cloth and used for the study.

2.2 Extract Preparation

20 g sample powder were extracted by Soxhlet with 80% aqueous methanol .The extract solvent was completely evaporated by rotary evaporator to obtain sticky gummy residue. In 1g residue 10mL aqueous methanol (10%, v/v) was added and analyzed for free radical scavenging activity and reducing power. Antioxidant assays were carried out in triplicate for each sample.

2.3 DPPH Radical Scavenging Activity

The antioxidant activity of the extracts was measured on the basis of the free radical scavenging activity by as follows [13]. Aliquots of 25 to 500 µg/mL of the test samples were placed in test tubes and added to 3.9 mL freshly prepared DPPH (25 mg/L) solution in methanol, mixed thoroughly and after 30 min absorbance was measured at 517 nm. Standard Ascorbic acid was used as a positive control. The percentage of radical scavenging activity was calculated as:

% Scavenging activity=

$$\frac{Absorbance\ of\ Control - Absorbance\ of\ Sample}{Absorbance\ of\ Control} \times 100$$

Where,

Absorbance of Control= DPPH
Absorbance of Sample = Leaves and stems extracts of plant.

The inhibition curve was plotted and the IC_{50} values were determined in µg/mL

2.4 Reducing Power Assay

The reducing power of the extracts was determined [14] as follows. Various concentration from 0 to 525 µg/mL with regular interval of 75 were prepared in 1 mL distilled water and mixed with phosphate buffer (2.5 mL, 0.2M, pH6.6) and potassium ferricyanide $K_3[Fe(CN)_6]$ (2.5 mL, 1%). The mixture was incubated at 50°C for 20min then 2.5 ml 10% trichloroacetic acid was added to the mixture and centrifuged at 3000 rpm for 10 min. 2.5 mL upper layer of the solution were mixed with 2.5 mL, distilled water and 0.5 ml $FeCl_3$ (0.1%) then absorbance was measured at 700 nm. Increased absorbance of the reaction mixture indicated increased reducing power. Ascorbic acid was used as a positive control.

2.5 Phytochemical Analysis

2.5.1 HPTLC analysis

Quantitative phytochemical analysis was carried out by HPTLC (High Performance Thin layer Chromatography) Linomat V supplied by CAMAG in Anchrom, R & D laboratory, Mulund, Mumbai [15]. Details of solvent system, extract preparation, detecting reagent and visualization of flavonoids, anthraglycosides, bitter principles, essential oil, saponins, coumarin triterpenes, phenol carboxylic acid and alkaloids are shown in Table 1.

2.5.2 Chromatographic condition

Each extract was loaded on readymade fluorescent pre coated silica gel G aluminum plate (Supplied by MERCK) and developed using appropriate solvent systems. The resultant chromatograms were illuminated for the characteristic quenching or fluorescence respectively for the particular class of bioactive compounds. The plates were derivatized and heated if necessary on a HPTLC heater for the detection of compounds.

3. RESULTS AND DISCUSSION

Various abiotic stresses lead to the over production of reactive oxygen species (ROS) in plants which are highly reactive and toxic and cause damage to proteins, lipids, carbohydrates and DNA which ultimately results in oxidative stress. Phenolics are often produced and accumulated in the subepidermal layers of plant tissues exposed to stress and pathogen attack. Recent researches have shown that antioxidants of plant origin with free radical scavenging property could have great importance as therapeutic agents in management of oxidative stress. Antioxidants are important in the prevention of human diseases. Naturally occurring antioxidants in leafy vegetables and seeds, such as ascorbic acid, vitamin E and Phenolic compounds possess ability to reduce the oxidative damage associated with many diseases, inducing cancer, cardiovascular disease, cataracts, atherosclerosis, diabetes, arthritis, immune deficiency diseases and aging [16]. Therefore, it is important to evaluate antioxidant activity of the plants either to elucidate the mechanism of their pharmacological action or to provide information on antioxidant activity [17].

Mangroves grow under stressful conditions such as violent environment, high concentration of moisture, high and low tides of water and abundant living microorganisms and insects. Therefore may have ability to produce variety of secondary metabolites.

Polar solvents are used for the extraction of antioxidants due to their polar nature. Soxhlet method extracts large amount of drug with much smaller quantity of solvent. Therefore Soxhlet extracts are used for the evaluation of antioxidant activities.

3.1 DPPH Radical Scavenging Activity Assay

DPPH radical was used as a substrate to evaluate free radical scavenging activities of extract. It involves reaction of specific antioxidant with stable free radical 1,1 –diphenyl-2-picryl-hydrazyl(DPPH). As a result, there is reduction of DPPH concentration by antioxidant, which decreases the optical absorbance of DPPH; this is detected by spectrophotometer at 517 nm. Ascorbic acid was used as standard [18]. The free radical scavenging activity of the extracts was evaluated based on the ability to scavenge the synthetic DPPH. This assay provided useful information on the reactivity of the compounds with stable free radical, because of odd number of electrons. The leaves extracts have shown better free radical scavenging activity 23.31 µg/mL than stems 111.5 µg/mL. The antioxidant activities of many traditional medicinal plants have not been systematically studied due to lack of popularity.

3.2 Reducing Power Assay

The reduction capacity of a compound may serve as a significant indicator of its potential antioxidant activity [19]. The reductive capabilities of the extracts were compared with ascorbic acid. A higher absorbance indicates a higher ferric reducing power. The reducing properties are generally associated with the presence of reductones, which have been shown to exert antioxidant action by breaking the free radical chain by donating hydrogen atom [20].

The reducing activity of ascorbic acid and both the parts of the selected mangrove species was found to be directly proportional to concentration of samples (Table 2; Fig. 1). As concentration increased reducing activity increased. At 525 µg/mL maximum absorbance of the leaves and stem extracts were 1.67 and 0.793 as against ascorbic acid 2.5 and 2.05 respectively. Absorbance of the sample increased linearly with concentration. The colour of the test solution changes from yellow to green when Fe^{3+} reduced to Fe^{2+}. This initiates the compounds to exert an antioxidant response [21]. Coumarin, bitter principle, essential oil, terpenes, flavonoids, anthraglycosides and saponins compounds are capable of donating hydrogen ions thereby exert antioxidant response. These phytochemicals are recorded in the leaves and stems extracts of L. racemosa which may be responsible for high reducing ability of the plant.

Table 1. Solvent system, extract preparation, detecting reagent and Visualization for HPTLC

Classes	Solvent system	Extract preparation	Reagent	Visualization wavelength	Color
Flavonoids	Ethyl acetate: formic acid: glacial acetic acid: Water(10:0.5:0.5:1.3)	Powdered drug(1 gm) in 5 ml methanol was extracted by heating on water bath for 10 min	Anisaldehyde sulphuric acid	365	Blue
Anthraglycosides	Ethyl acetate: methanol :water(100:13.5:10)	Powdered drug(1 gm) in 5 ml methanol was extracted by heating on water bath for 10 min	10% KOH	Visible	Red, yellow
Bitter principle	Ethyl acetate: methanol: water (100:13.5:10)	Powdered drug(1 gm) in 5 ml methanol was extracted by heating on water bath for 10 min	Vanillin sulphuric acid	Visible	Red, violet, yellow, blue, brown, green
Saponin	Chloroform: acetic acid :methanol: water (6.4:3.2:1.2:0.8)	Above extract prepared , filtered and evaporated to 1 ml, mixed with 0.5 ml water and extracted with 3 ml n-butanol	Vanillin sulphuric acid	Visible	Blue, blue violet, red, yellow,brown
Triterpenes	Chloroform: methanol (9.5:0.5)	Powdered drug (1 gm) was extracted by heating under reflux for 15 min with 10 ml dichloromethane. Filtrate was evaporated and residue was dissolved in 0.5 ml toluene	Anisaldehyde sulphuric acid	Visible	Blue violet, red to red violet
Phenol carboxylic acid	n-butanol:acetic acid: water(4:1:1)	Powdered drug (1gm) was extracted by heating under reflux for 15 min with 10 ml dichloromethane. Filtrate was evaporated and residue was dissolved in 0.5 ml toluene	FeCl$_3$	Visible	Brown grey or black
coumarin	Toluene: ethyl acetate (93:7)	Powdered drug (1 gm) was extracted by heating under reflux for 15 min with 10 ml dichloromethane. Filtrate was evaporated and residue was dissolved in 0.5 ml toluene	10% KOH	365	Light blue, brown
Essential oil	Toluene: ethyl acetate (93:7)	Powdered drug (1 gm) was extracted in 5 ml dichloromethane. The suspension was filtered and	Vanillin sulphuric acid	Visible	Red, yellow, blue, brown, green

Classes	Solvent system	Extract preparation	Reagent	Visualization wavelength	Color
		clear filtrate was evaporated to dryness. The residue was dissolved in 1ml toluene.			
Alkaloids	Toluene :ethyl acetate: diethylamine (7:2:1)	Powder drug (1 gm) was moistened with 1 ml, 10% ammonia solution on water bath.	Dragendroff reagent	Visible	Orange brown

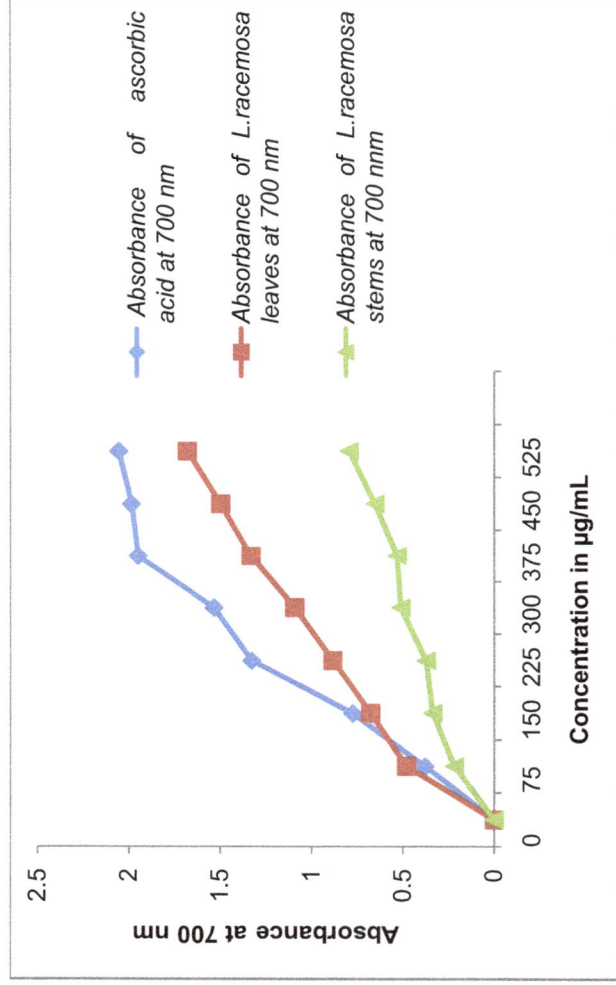

Fig. 1. Reducing power of *L. racemosa* leaves and stems

Table 2. IC_{50} for free radical scavenging by DPPH radical

Sample	Parts	IC_{50}µg/mL
Ascorbic acid	-	14.99 µg/mL
L. racemosa	Leaves	23.31 µg/mL
	Stems	111.5 µg/mL

3.3 Phytochemical Analysis

3.3.1 HPTLC analysis

Plant produces various classes of secondary metabolites like alkaloids, flavonoids, phenol, terpenes, steroids and quinines. The medicinal properties of plant depend upon quality and quantity of these phytochemicals.

Different composition of solvent systems for HPTLC analysis was studied to obtain high resolution and reproducible peaks of various classes of secondary metabolites. The aim was to determine number of compounds in each class of secondary metabolites. The leaves have shown 4 different types of coumarins with 4 different Rf (Retention factor) values between 0.22 to 0.62 while stem showed 3 types with Rf values 0.22, 0.38 and 0.82. Among these coumarin 1 and 3 of leaves has similar Rf value to that of coumarin 1 and 2 of stem indicating they were same compounds. This suggests leaves and stem contain all together 5 different types of coumarins (Table 9; Fig 2, supplementary). Beside this leaves recorded 4 different types of bitter principles with 4 different

Rf values from 0.15 to 0.40 while stem showed 3 different types with Rf values between 0.12 to 0.74. All the Rf values of bitter principles in leaves and stem were different from each other, indicating 7 types of bitter principles in the plant (Table 4; Fig. 4 supplementary).

The leaves and stem contain 3 different types of essential oils in each with different Rf values, indicating 6 types of essential oils in the plant (Table 7; Fig. 3 supplementary).

Leaves and stem recorded 3 different types of terpenes in each with different Rf values. Among these one Rf value 0.57 was common in both the parts. This shows presence of 5 types of terpenes in the plant (Table 8; Fig. 8 supplementary). 2 types of saponins were seen in leaves with Rf values 0.33 and 0.45 (Table 10; Fig. 6 supplementary). Similarly 3 different types of flavonoids with Rf values 0.29, 0.74, 0.87 were recorded in stem (Table 6; Fig. 5 supplementary) while 2 different types of anthraglycosides with 2 Rf 0.47, 0.52 were seen in leaves (Table 5; Fig. 7 supplementary).

The overall results of phytochemical studies have confirmed the presence of several types of bitter principle, anthraglycosides, flavonoids, essential oils, terpenes, coumarins and saponins in leaves and stem (Table. 3). Among these flavonoids, saponins, terpenes and other phenolic compounds are reported to have antioxidant activity [22]. The antioxidant properties in the *L. racemosa* leaves and stem can be related to the presence of these classes of compounds.

Table 3. Number of constituents in various classes of secondary metabolites in mangrove plant

Secondary metabolites	No of constituents (Leaves)	No of constituents (Stems)
Bitter principle	04	03
Anthraglycosides	02	-
Flavonoids	-	03
Essential oil	03	03
Terpenes	03	03
Coumarin	04	03
Saponins	02	-
Phenol carboxylic acid	—	—
Alkaloids	—	—

Table 4. Bitter principle profile of methanol extracts of leaves and stem of *L. racemosa*

	Peak	Retention factor (Rf)	Height	Area	Assigned substance
	1	0.05	10.3	89.3	unknown
	2	0.11	14.4	155.0	unknown
	3	0.15	22.1	312.9	Bitter principle 1
	4	0.19	56.7	950.6	Bitter principle 2
	5	0.21	53.3	879.0	unknown
Leaves	6	0.32	44.6	904.1	unknown
	7	0.36	88.4	2339.0	Bitter principle 3
	8	0.40	89.6	2001.4	Bitter principle 4
	9	0.45	27.5	622.9	unknown
	10	0.65	42.6	1613.8	unknown
	11	0.73	136.2	6267.9	unknown
	12	0.81	162.9	5931.3	unknown
	1	0.08	12.3	130.1	unknown
	2	0.09	13.2	120.4	unknown
	3	0.12	14.2	156.1	Bitter principle 1
Stems	4	0.14	13.7	172.7	Bitter principle 2
	5	0.41	51.5	863.4	unknown
	6	0.65	23.3	854.1	unknown
	7	0.74	81.5	3610.4	Bitter principle 3
	8	0.81	61.5	2534.0	unknown
	9	0.89	11.7	280.2	unknown

Table 5. Anthraglycosides profile of methanol extracts of leaves of *L. racemosa*

	Peak	Retention factor (Rf)	Height	Area	Assigned substance
	1	0.09	205.5	2615.2	unknown
	2	0.18	11.3	111.1	unknown
	3	0.23	40.9	957.4	unknown
	4	0.30	91.7	4441.6	unknown
	5	0.36	57.3	861.8	unknown
	6	0.39	62.4	1029.1	unknown
Leaves	7	0.47	174.9	7616.6	Anthraglycosides 1
	8	0.52	152.1	3822.9	Anthraglycosides 2
	9	0.60	44.5	1113.3	unknown
	10	0.83	26.3	947.3	unknown

Table 6. Flavonoids profile of methanol extracts of stems of *L. racemosa*

	Peak	Retention factor (Rf)	Height	Area	Assigned substance
	1	0.15	13.1	454.5	unknown
	2	0.29	64.8	2678.4	Flavonoids 1
Stem	3	0.74	16.7	468.1	Flavonoids 2
	4	0.82	97.9	1902.7	unknown
	5	0.87	10.2	103.8	Flavonoids 3
	6	0.91	39.7	543.0	unknown

Table 7. Essential oil profile of methanol extracts of leaves and stem of *L.racemosa*

	Peak	Retention factor (Rf)	Height	Area	Assigned substance
	1	0.06	16.2	228.2	unknown
Leaves	2	0.09	10.9	117.1	unknown
	3	0.20	96.8	2224.7	Essential oil 1

	Peak	Retention factor (Rf)	Height	Area	Assigned substance
	4	0.30	141.5	4192.1	unknown
	5	0.33	73.9	1335.4	unknown
	6	0.50	129.7	19665.6	Essential oil 2
	7	0.77	198.9	11574.9	unknown
	8	0.88	342.8	13749.0	Essential oil 3
Stem	1	0.09	19.3	249.5	unknown
	2	0.15	22.2	403.4	Ess.oil 1
	3	0.20	75.6	1574.8	unknown
	4	0.30	88.6	2106.5	Essential oil 2
	5	0.50	26.5	1476.6	unknown
	6	0.78	80.4	5580.9	Essential oil 3
	7	0.90	18.6	350.1	unknown

Table 8. Terpenes profile of methanol extracts of leaves of *L. racemosa*

	Peak	Retention factor (Rf)	Height	Area	Assigned substance
Leaves	1	0.31	27.7	1037.8	Terpenes 1
	2	0.47	76.6	3153.0	unknown
	3	0.57	119.6	5152.4	Terpenes 2
	4	0.75	220.5	14354.1	Terpenes 3
	5	0.84	199.4	8756.6	unknown
	6	0.88	230.9	6094.6	unknown
	7	0.90	278.3	3901.4	unknown
Stems	1	0.33	17.0	797.1	Terpenes 1
	2	0.41	32.6	1287.1	unknown
	3	0.48	55.0	2045.2	Terpenes 2
	4	0.57	53.2	2587.0	Terpenes 3
	5	0.69	45.3	1663.9	unknown
	6	0.75	61.6	3315.4	unknown
	7	0.83	37.8	986.4	unknown
	8	0.88	68.6	1356.7	Unknown
	9	0.90	48.4	533.5	unknown

Table 9. Coumarin profile of methanol extracts of leaves and stem of *L. racemosa*

	Peak	Retention factor (Rf)	Height	Area	Assigned substance
Leaves	1	0.22	736.8	16148.9	Coumarin 1
	2	0.32	43.6	896.1	Coumarin 2
	3	0.38	634.1	20357.9	Coumarin 3
	4	0.46	32.3	670.1	unknown
	5	0.62	28.7	1030.6	Coumarin 4
Stem	1	0.22	85.2	1728.8	Coumarin 1
	2	0.38	42.3	1067.1	Coumarin 2
	3	0.56	13.8	534.3	unknown
	4	0.72	16.6	864.7	Coumarin 3
	5	0.82	11.5	338.8	unknown

Table 10. Saponins profile of methanol extracts of leaves of *L. racemosa*

	Peak	Retention factor (Rf)	Height	Area	Assigned substance
Leaves	1	0.10	23.0	321.5	unknown
	2	0.33	14.3	473.2	Saponin1
	3	0.45	19.6	839.1	Saponin 2
	4	0.56	85.6	3475.6	unknown

4. CONCLUSION

In the present study, antioxidant activities of the methanol extract of leaves and stems obtained from *L. racemosa* were investigated. The extract demonstrated effective antioxidant properties, as determined by the scavenging assay and reducing power assay, the leaves were more potent than stems. The phytochemical analysis indicated that leaves and stems contain bitter principle, essential oil, terpenes, and coumarin. Therefore, it can be inferred that the phenolics present in the *L. racemosa* plant might be responsible for its antioxidant properties presenting meaningful information for the collection and application of *L. racemosa* in both healthcare and food industry.

CONSENT

It is not applicable.

ETHICAL APPROVAL

It is not applicable.

ACKNOWLEDGEMENTS

We thank University Grant Commission, India for providing Non NET and RGNF Fellowship and funding for this research.

COMPETING INTERESTS

Authors have declared that no competing interests exist.

REFERENCES

1. Bandaranayake WM. Bioactive compounds and chemical constituents of mangrove plants. AIMS Report. 2002;35:1-75.
2. Mitter CS, Jadhav BL. Bactericidal and bioactivity guided fractionation studies of mangrove species *Derris indica* and *D. trifoliata*. Research Journal of Biotechnology. 2011;6(4):57–61.
3. Suraiya NN, Jadhav BL. Screening of the antimicrobial properties of *Acanthus illicifolius and Ex. agallocha* spp of the Mumbai coast. Trends in Life Sciences. 2000;15(2):59-65.
4. Mukesh Pimpliskar, Pramod Shinde, Vijay Savakare, Vaishali Jadhav, Jadhav BL. Comparative performance of activity of antimicrobial principles of Mangroves *Rhizophora* species along Mumbai coast. Indo - Global Research Journal of Pharmaceutical Sciences. 2012;2(4):426-429.
5. Jaimini D, Sarkar Aftab AS, Jadhav BL. Evaluation of antibacterial properties of mangrove plant *Sonneratia apetala* (Buch. Ham) leaf. World Applied Sciences Journal. 2011;14(11):1683–1686.
6. Premanathan M, Chandre K, Bajpai SK, Kathiresan K. Antiviral activity of marine plants against New castle disease virus. Tropical Biomedicine. 1994;10:31-33.
7. Jadhav BL, Quraishi FM, Pagare BG. Evaluation of Antioxidant Properties and Phytochemical analysis in the stem and leaves of *Ceriops tagal* mangroves. Research journal of Biotechnology. 2013; 8(9):28-31.
8. Wei SD, Zhou HC, Lin YM. Antioxidant activities of extract and fractions from the hypocotyls of the mangrove plant *Kandelia candel*. Int. J. Mol. Sci. 2010;11:4080-4093. DOI:10.3390/ijms11104080.
9. Bandarnayake WM. Traditional and medicinal uses of mangroves. Mangroves and salt Marshes. 1998;2(3):133-148.
10. D'souza L, Wahidulla S, Prabhadevi. Antibacterial phenolics from the mangrove *Lumnitzera racemosa*. Indian Journal of Geo- Marine Sciences. 2010;39(2):294-298.
11. Ravikumar S, Gnanadesigan M. Hepatoprotective and antioxidant activity of a mangrove plant *Lumnitzera racemosa*. Asian Pacific Journal Tropical Biomedicine. 2011;1(5):348–352.
12. Thao NP, Luyen BTT, Diep CN, Tai BH, Kim EJ, Kang HK, et al. *In vitro* evaluation of the antioxidant and cytotoxic activities of constituents of the mangrove *Lumnitzera racemosa* Willd. Arch. Pharm. Res; 2014. DOI: 10.1007/s 12272-014-0429-y
13. Braca A, Tommasi ND, Bari LD, Pizza C, Politi M, Morelli I. Antioxidant principles from *Bauhinia terapotensis*. Journal of Natural Products. 2001;64:892-895.
14. Oyaizu M. Studies on product of browning reaction prepared from glucose amine. Japanese Journal of Nutrition. 1986;44(6): 307-315.
15. Wagner H, Bladt S. Plant drug analysis: A Thin layer chromatography, Atlas, 2Springer-Verlag, Berlin. 1996;349-364.
16. Basniwal PK, Suthar M, Rathore GS, Gupta R, Kumar V, Pareek A, Jain D. *In vitro* antioxidant activity of hot aqueous

extract of *Helieteres isora* Linn. Fruits. Nat Prod Radi. 2009;8(5):483-487.

17. Molan AL, Faraj AM, Mahdy A. Antioxidant activity and phenolic content of some medicinal plants traditionally used in Northern Iraq. J Phytopharmacol. 2012; 2(2):224-233.

18. Kaushik D, Khokra SL, Kaushik P, Sherma C, Aneja KR. Evaluation of antioxidant and antimicrobial activity of *Abutilon indicum*. Pharmacology. Online. 2010;1:102-108.

19. Nikhat F, Satynarayana D, Subhramanyam EVS. Isolation, characterization and screening of antioxidant activity of the roots of *Syzygium cuminii (L)* Skeel. Asian Journal of Research Chemistry. 2009; 2(2):218-221.

20. Duh PD, Tu, YY, Yen, GC. Antioxidant activity of water extract of harn jyur (Chyrsanthemu morifolium Ramat). Lebensmittel- Wissenschaft und-. Technologie - Food Science and Technology. 1999;32:269–277.

21. Hatano T, Edamatsu R, Hiramatsu M, Mori A, Fujita Y. Effects of the interaction of tannins with co-existing substances. VI: Effects of tannins and related polyphenols on superoxide anion radical and on 1, 1-diphenyl-2-picrylhydrazyl radical. Chem Pharm Bull. 1989;37(8):2016-2021.

22. Shie yin NG, Abdullah S, Phin CK. phytochemical constituents from leaves of *Elaeis guineensis* and their antioxidant and antimicrobial activities. International Journal of Pharmacy and Pharmaceutical Sciences. 2013;(5):137-140.

7

HPLC Profiling and Antioxidant Properties of the Ethanol Extract of *Hibiscus tiliaceus* Leaf Available in Bangladesh

Hemayet Hossain[1*], Proity Nayeeb Akbar[1], Shaikh Emdadur Rahman[2], Sabina Yeasmin[2], Tanzir Ahmed Khan[3], Md. Mahfuzur Rahman[3] and Ismet Ara Jahan[1]

[1]*BCSIR Laboratories, Bangladesh Council of Scientific and Industrial Research, Dhaka, Dr. Qudrat-E-Khuda Road, Dhaka-1205, Bangladesh.*
[2]*Pharmacy Discipline, Life Science School, Khulna University, Khulna-9208, Bangladesh.*
[3]*Institute of Food Science and Technology, Bangladesh Council of Scientific and Industrial Research, Dhaka, Dr. Qudrat-E-Khuda Road, Dhaka-1205, Bangladesh.*

Authors' contributions

This work was carried out in collaboration between all authors. Authors HH, PNA, SER, TAK and IAJ designed the study, performed the statistical analysis, wrote the protocol and wrote the first draft of the manuscript. Authors MMR and SY managed the analyses of the study and the literature searches. All authors read and approved the final manuscript.

Editor(s):
(1) Thomas Efferth, Department of Pharmaceutical Biology, Institute of Pharmacy and Biochemistry, Johannes Gutenberg University, Germany.
(2) Marcello Iriti, Department of Agricultural and Environmental Sciences, Milan State University, Italy.
Reviewers:
(1) Asaduzzaman Khan, The Research Center for Preclinical Medicine, Luzhou Medical College, Sichuan, China.
(2) Anonymous, Taiwan.
(3) Slobodan Jankovic, Pharmacology and toxicology department, Faculty of Med. Sciences, University of Kragujevac, Serbia.
(4) Nicola Caporaso, Department of Agriculture, University of Naples Federico II, Italy.
(5) Anonymous, Egypt.

ABSTRACT

The aim of this research was to investigate the antioxidant activity and HPLC fingerprinting profiles of the ethanolic leaf extract of *Hibiscus tiliaceus* growing in Bangladesh. Catechin, rutin hydrate, ellagic acid and quercetin contents were quantified in the sample by HPLC-DAD (99.00 ± 1.88, 79.20 ± 1.59, 59.40 ± 1.36 and 69.30 ± 1.47 mg/100 g of dry extract), respectively. The antioxidant

Corresponding author: E-mail: hemayethossain02@yahoo.com

potential by 2,2-azino-bis(3-ethylbenzthiazoline-6-sulphonic acid (ABTS) radical scavenging activity, reducing power, total antioxidant capacity and total phenolic and flavonoid content were determined. In all the methods, the extract exhibited potent antioxidant activity. The IC_{50} value of the extract on ABTS radical was found to be 6.25 ± 0.15 µg/ml, and at 250 µg/ml, maximum absorbance of reducing power was obtained 0.6475 ± 0.021. The total antioxidant capacity, total phenolic and flavonoid contents were found in considerable amount (595.2 ± 3.61 mg of ascorbic acid/g, 298.07 ± 2.01 mg/g of gallic acid, and 13.69 ± 0.06 mg/g of quercetin equivalent), respectively. Substantial amounts of phenols and flavonoids were noticed and thus, justify the free radical scavenging and antioxidant characteristics of the extract.

Keywords: Hibiscus tiliaceus, antioxidant, HPLC, rutin hydrate, ellagic acid, quercetin, ABTS, reducing power.

1. INTRODUCTION

Hibiscus tiliaceus L. (*H. tiliaceus*) is a coastal plant belonging to the Malvaceae family. They also go by other names like beach hibiscus, sea hibiscus, Indian hibiscus and wild cotton tree. In Bangladesh, however, *H. tiliaceus* is locally known as Bhola. These plants are aboriginal to the shorelines of the Indian and Pacific oceans and grow mainly as an ornamental tree to a height of 3-6 m.

Plants of Malyaceae family are used in a wide range of areas. They are sources of natural fibres. They are used as treatment for the irritation of mucous membranes, gargle for mouth, throat ulcers and gastric ulcers [1]. Woods, leaves, barks and flowers of *H. tiliaceus* have many medicinal purposes. Traditionally, the flower is broadly used for birth control in Asian and African countries. In Malaysia and Indonesia, the flowers are used to treat fever [2]. The flower bud and bark of *H. tiliaceus* contain a slimy, juicy sap, which when soaked can be used as medicine for congested chests, fevers, coughs, dysentery, ear infections, abscesses and as laxative [3,4]. The buds can also be chewed and eaten to treat dry-throat. An infusion of the dried wood of *H. tiliaceus* is usually used to expel the placenta and to combat post-parturition disorders [5]. An aqueous extract of wood and fresh flowers have also been reported to be useful in treating skin diseases [6,7].

Previous phytochemical investigations revealed the potential role of the plants of *Hibiscus* genus. They are a valuable source of triterpene derivatives, phytosteroids and antioxidants [8]. Flowers and leaves of *H. tiliaceus* contain stigmasterol, stigmastadienol, stigmastadienone, vanillic acid, syringic acid, n-trans-feruloyltiramine, n-cis-feruloyltyramine and beta-sitostenone. A new coumarin, hibiscusin, and a new amide, hibiscusamide along with p-hydroxybenzoic acid, scopoletin and p-hydroxybenzaldehyde were also isolated from the stem wood of *H. tiliaceus* [9].

The methanol wood extract of *H. tiliaceus* showed significant anti-inflammatory and anti-depressant activity [10] in addition to strongly inhibiting the mutagenic action of tert-butyl-hydroperoxide [11]. The extract showed antioxidant activity against oxidative DNA damage [12]. *In vivo* antioxidant properties and antimutagenic effects of the flower extract were also evaluated. The antinociceptive and anti-inflammatory activity of leaf when tested exhibited significant activity results. Other than that, *H. tiliaceus* showed selective cytotoxicity against breast cancer cells [13] and against three strains of bacteria: *S. aureus*, *E. coli* and *S. paratyphi* [14]. The plant also revealed antipyretic and antiulcer properties [15]. No antifungal activity was demonstrated [16].

In the present investigation, we attempted to determine the antioxidant properties of the ethanol leaf extract of *H. tiliaceus* growing in Bangladesh, and quantify the major bioactive polyphenolic compounds through HPLC.

2. MATERIALS AND METHODS

2.1 Plant Material

Leaves of *H. tiliaceus* were collected from Khulna, Bangladesh during January 2013 (Accession no: DACB 36722). All plant materials were properly washed, shade dried, ground, and submitted to extraction with ethanol.

2.2 Extraction

Powdered leaf sample was extracted in an orbital shaker with 95% ethanol. Ethanol extract was obtained by continuous stirring at room temperature for 1 week. The extract was then filtered first with a cotton plug to get rid of plant debris, and afterwards through Whatman filter paper no. 1 and concentrated using a vacuum rotary evaporator (R-215, Buchi, Switzerland) at 60°C.

2.3 Chemicals

Vanillic acid (VA), (+)-catechin hydrate (CH), caffeic acid (CA), gallic acid (GA), (-)-epicatechin (EC), rutin hydrate (RH), p-coumaric acid (PCA), ellagic acid (EA), quercetin (QU), 2,2-azino-bis(3-ethylbenzthiazoline-6-sulphonic acid (ABTS), ascorbic acid, folin-ciocalteu's phenol reagent were purchased from Sigma–Aldrich (St. Louis, MO, USA). Methanol (HPLC), acetonitrile (HPLC), ethanol, acetic acid (HPLC), phosphate buffer (pH 6.6), potassium ferricyanide $[K_3Fe(CN)_6]$, trichloroacetic acid (TCA), ferric chloride $(FeCl_3)$, EDTA, sodium phosphate, ammonium molybdate and sodium carbonate were purchased analytical grade from Merck (Darmstadt, Germany).

2.4 HPLC Analysis

2.4.1 Instrumentation

Chromatographic analysis was performed on an HPLC system model Thermo Scientific Dionex UltiMate 3000 Rapid Separation LC systems (RSLC) from Thermo Fisher Scientific Inc., MA, USA. They were equipped with a diode array detector (DAD: 3000RS), quaternary pump system (LPG: 3400RS) and Ultimate 3000RS autosampler (WPS: 3000). The system was controlled by Version 6.80 RS 10 Dionix Chromeleon software. Acclaim® C18 (4.6 x 250 mm; 5 µm) column from Dionix, USA was used for the chromatographic separation of polyphenols that was maintained at 30°C using a column compartment (TCC:3000).

2.4.2 Chromatographic conditions

A solution of H. tiliaceus was prepared at a concentration of 5 mg/ml in ethanol by mixing for 30 min. The solutions were allowed to stand at 5°C in the dark. These were then spiked to recognize the individual polyphenols. The sample solutions were next filtered through 0.2 µm nylon syringe filter (Sartorius, Germany) before being degassed for 15 min in an ultrasonic bath (Hwashin, Korea). Finally, the compounds were isolated with reverse-phased HPLC and their

respective chromatograms were obtained [17,18].

Acetonitrile (solvent A), pH 3.0 acetic acid solution (solvent B) and methanol (solvent C) were used for the mobile phase. The gradient program consisted of a 0 min run at 5%A/95%B, a 10 min run at 10%A/80%B/10%C, a 20 min run at 20%A/60%B/20%C and a 35min run at 100%A before the column was washed and reconditioned. A flow rate of 1 ml/min was maintained throughout the analytical run, and the sample injection volume was 20 µl. The detection wavelength was: λ 280 nm held for 18.0 min, changed to λ 320 nm and held for 6 min, and finally changed to λ 380 nm and held for the rest of the analysis and the diode array detector was controlled at a wavelength of 200 nm to 700 nm.

Individual phenolic compounds were identified by comparing their retention time and UV spectrum with those obtained by injecting standards in the same HPLC conditions. The detection and quantification of CH, GA, VA, EC and CA were carried out at 280 nm, while PCA, EA, and RH were read at 320 nm, and QU at 380 nm, respectively. Analyses were performed in triplicate.

2.4.3 Standard and sample preparation

Ethanol stock solutions (100 µg/ml) containing phenolic compounds were prepared and diluted to appropriate concentrations to make standard solutions of 20 µg/ml for all the polyphenolic compounds except for caffeic acid, which was prepared to 8 µg/ml, and quercetin to 6 µg/ml. The reaction mixtures were afterwards stored in a dark place at 5°C. The calibration curves were constructed by plotting the peak under the curve area versus the concentration of the analytes.

2.5 Antioxidant Activities

2.5.1 ABTS radical scavenging test

The ABTS radical cation scavenging activity was performed with slight modifications described by Fan et al. [19]. $ABTS^+$ radical cations were formed during the reaction of 7 mM ABTS in water and 2.45 mM potassium persulfate, stored in a dark place at rtp for 12-16 h. Right before use, the ABTS solution was diluted with pH 7.4 phosphate buffered saline (PBS) solution to an absorbance of 0.70±0.02 and read at 734 nm. Free radical scavenging activity was assessed by mixing 1 ml of the test sample with 1 ml of ABTS working standard. The reaction was allowed to reach completion by letting it stand at room temperature for 6 min before reading the absorbance at 734 nm. The percentage scavenging activity was calculated with the formula:

Percentage inhibition (%) = (A_o – A_s / A_o) x 100, Where, A_o=absorbance of blank; A_s=absorbance of sample

2.5.2 Reducing power assay

Reducing power assay of the leaf extract of *H. tiliaceus* was evaluated using the process of Hemayet et al. and Dehpour et al. [20,21]. The extract at different concentration (2.5 ml) was mixed with ethanol (1 ml), 0.2 M phosphate buffer pH 6.6 (2.5 ml) and 1% potassium ferricyanide (2.5 ml). The reaction mixtures were incubated for 20 min at 50°C and centrifuged for 10 min at 5000 rmp after the addition of 10% solution of trichloroacetic acid (2.5 ml). 2.5 ml of the supernatant was mixed with de-ionized water (2.5 ml) and 0.1% ferric chloride (0.5 ml). Absorbance of the samples was read in triplicates at 700 nm.

2.5.3 Total antioxidant capacity

Total antioxidant capacity of the leaf extract of *H. tiliaceus* was evaluated by the process of Prieto et al. [22]. The extract was prepared in ethanol and mixed with the reagent solution (1 ml). The reaction solution included 0.6 M sulphuric acid, 28 mM sodium phosphate and 4 mM ammonium molybdate mixture. These were then incubated at 95ºC for an hour and half. The mixture was cooled to rtp and their absorbance was measured at 695 nm. Ascorbic acid was used as the standard and its equivalents were calculated using the calibration curve. All values were read in triplicates.

2.5.4 Total phenolic content

Total phenolic content of the *H. tiliaceus* ethanol extract was calculated using the process of Folin-Ciocaltu [23,24] with slight alterations to it. 0.5 ml of extract (1 mg/ml) was reacted to 5 ml Folin-Ciocaltu reagent, which was prepared in the ratio 1:10 v/v with distilled water, and 4 ml (75 g/l) sodium carbonate. The solutions were left standing for the next 30 min at 40ºC for the color to develop. The absorbance was measured at a wavelength of 765 nm against a blank sample. The total phenolic content is expressed as mg per gram of gallic acid equivalents (GAE) with the equation, y = 6.993x+0.0379, R^2 = 0.9995.

2.5.5 Total flavonoid content

The total flavonoid content was calculated by the aluminium chloride colorimetric method with slight alterations to it [25,26]. Absorbance of the mixture was read with an UV spectrophotometer (Model 205, Jena, Germany) at 430 nm. Standard curve was calibrated using quercetin with the equation, y = 6.2548x+0.0925; R^2 = 0.998 and expressed as mg per gram of quercetin equivalent.

2.6 Statistical Analysis

All calculations and results were carried out in triplicates and demonstrated as mean ± standard deviation (S.D).

3. RESULTS AND DISCUSSION

3.1 HPLC Assay of *H. tiliaceus*

Phenolic compounds in the leaf extract of *H. tiliaceus* were analyzed by HPLC-DAD. As demonstrated in Fig. 1, the retention times and the standard peaks were compared and four phenolic compounds were detected: (+) catechin, rutin hydrate, ellagic acid and quercetin, respectively. The most abundant polyphenol noted in the extract of *H. tiliaceus* was (+) catechin (99.00±1.88 mg/100 g dry extract), which was followed by rutin hydrate (79.20±1.59 mg/100 g dry extract). Ellagic acid and quercetin were also detected in moderate quantities (59.40±1.36 and 69.30±1.47 mg/100 g dry extract, respectively). The HPLC chromatogram and the bioactive polyphenolic compounds in the ethanol extract of *H. tiliaceus* are presented in Fig. 1 & Table 1, respectively.

Phenolic compounds have strong antioxidant activities associated with their abilities to scavenge free radicals, donate hydrogen ions, chelate metals and break radical chain reactions *in vitro* and *in vivo* [27]. As is observed in Table 1, *H. tiliaceus* showed a rich content of these active components, and thus could be used as powerful antioxidants for industries and health care centres.

3.2 Antioxidant Activities

The antioxidant characteristics of the extract of *H. tiliaceus* were evaluated for by different *in vitro* antioxidant assays such as ABTS radical scavenging activity, reducing power assay, total phenolic and flavonoid content and total antioxidant capacity.

3.2.1 ABTS radical scavenging activity

The ABTS scavenging ability was determined based on the percentage inhibition of the ABTS cation by hydrogen donating and chain-breaking antioxidants in the sample (Fig. 2, Table 2). The sample effectively neutralised the radical cation $ABTS^+$. The activity was found to increase in a dose-dependent manner at a concentration of 10 to 250 µg/ml. At minimum concentration (10 µg/ml), the highest activity obtained by the leaf extract of *H. tiliaceus* was 80.86±0.15% inhibition value exceeding that of ascorbic acid (48.60±0.17%). The leaf extract exhibited an IC_{50} value of 6.25±0.15 µg/ml, which was similar to that of the ascorbic acid (12.34±0.12 µg/ml). Therefore, *H. tiliaceus* leaf extract can be said to possess strong free radical scavenging ability [28].

3.2.2 Reducing power assay

The reducing power assay is related to its electron donating ability was evaluated based on its relative maximum absorbance (Fig. 3). At 250 µg/ml, the maximum absorbance of the extract

was found to be 0.6475±0.021, while ascorbic acid read an absorbance of 1.1115±0.009. Absorbance of the sample increased linearly with concentration. As Fe^{3+} oxidized to Fe^{2+} and donated a hydrogen atom, the free radical chain is interrupted. When this happens, the yellow color of the test solution changes to green and blue depending on the reducing power ability of the extract. This initiates the compounds to exert an antioxidant response [29]. Phenolic compounds are capable of donating hydrogen ions and hence, these phenolic compounds in the extract of *H. tiliaceus* might be a reason behind the high reducing ability of the extract.

3.2.3 Total antioxidant capacity

Total antioxidant capacity of *H. tiliaceus* leaf extract is based on the reduction of phosphomolybdenum, Mo (VI) to green molybdenum (V) by the extract. The total antioxidant capacity observed in the ethanol extract of *H. tiliaceus* was 595.20±3.61 mg of AAE/g of extract (Fig. 4) [30,31,32].

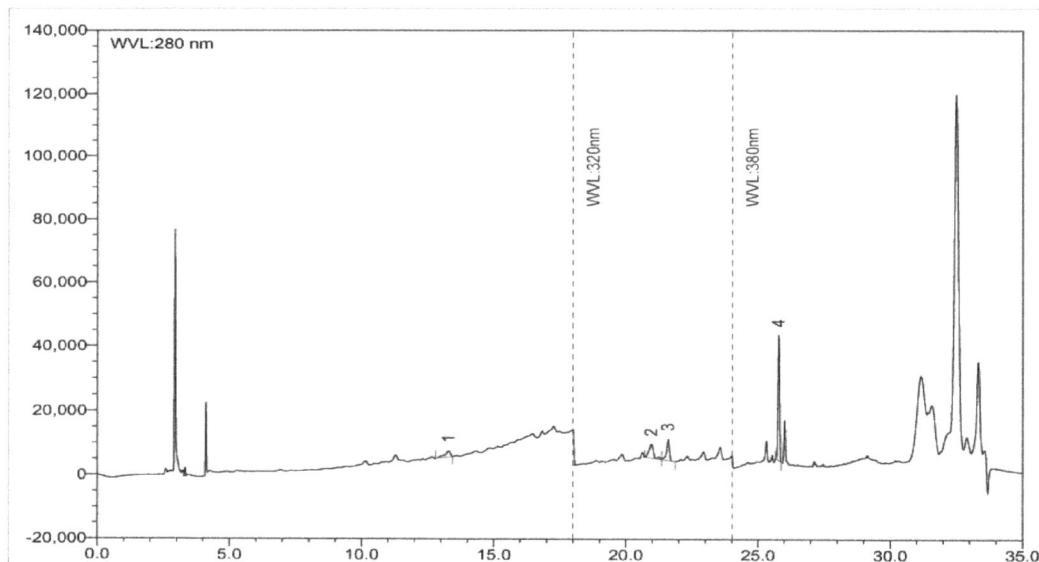

Fig. 1. Chromatogram obtained from HPLC of *H. tiliaceus* ethanol leaf extract. Peaks: 1, (+)-catechin; 2, rutin hydrate; 3, ellagic acid; 4, quercetin

Table 1. Bioactive polyphenols obtained from the ethanol extract of *H. tiliaceus* (n = 3)

Polyphenols	Ethanol extract of *H. tiliaceus* leaf	
	Content (mg/100 g dry extract)	% relative standard deviation (RSD)
Catechin	99.00	1.88
Rutin hydrate	79.20	1.59
Ellagic acid	59.40	1.36
Quercetin	69.30	1.47

3.2.4 Total phenolic and flavonoid content

Fig. 4 gives information on the total phenolic and total flavonoid content of *H. tiliaceus* leaf extract. The total phenolic and flavonoid content of the leaf extract of *H. tiliaceus* were found to be 298.07±2.01 mg per gram of gallic acid equivalent and 13.69±0.06 mg per gram of quercetin equivalent, respectively. Phenolic and flavonoid compounds are effective free radical scavengers and have convincingly demonstrated powerful antioxidant characteristics, hence, making itself useful in the field of medicine [33,34,35,36]. The presence of polyphenols in the *H. tiliaceus* leaf extract is a possible explanation for the high percentage inhibition value obtained. As a result, it can be concluded that the extract of *H. tiliaceus* shows significant antioxidant activity due to these phenolics, flavonoids, etc.

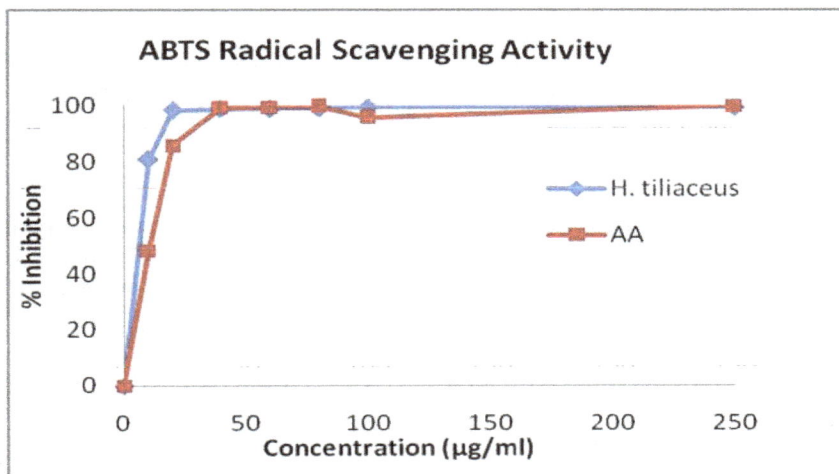

Fig. 2. ABTS radical scavenging activity of *H. tiliaceus* leaf extract with standard ascorbic acid

Table 2. IC$_{50}$ value of *H. tiliaceus* leaf extract and standard ascorbic acid in ABTS radical scavenging activity

	H. tiliaceus leaf extract	Ascorbic acid
IC$_{50}$	6.25±0.15	12.34±0.12

The values are expressed as mean ± standard deviation (n=3).

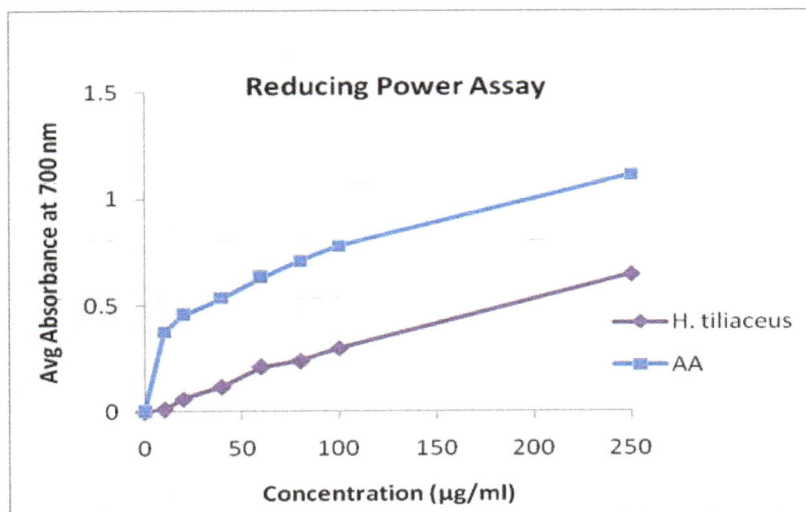

Fig. 3. Reducing power assay of *H. tiliaceus* leaf extract with standard ascorbic acid

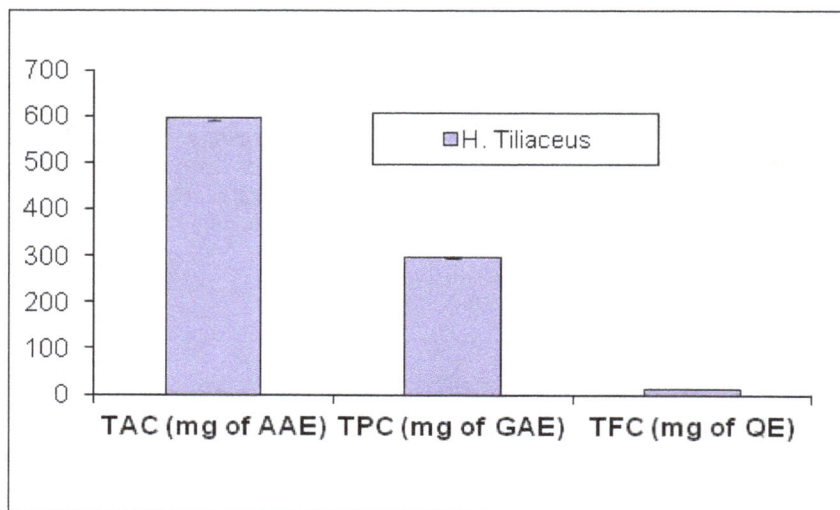

Fig. 4. Total antioxidant capacity (TAC), total phenolic content (TPC) and total flavonoid content (TFC) of *H. tiliaceus* leaf extract with standard ascorbic acid. AAE: Ascorbic Acid Equivalent; GAE: Gallic Acid Equivalent; QE: Quercetin Equivalent

4. CONCLUSION

In the present study, antioxidant activities of the ethanol leaf extract obtained from *H. tiliaceus* were investigated. The extract demonstrated effective antioxidant properties, as determined by the scavenging effect on the $ABTS^+$, reducing power assay, total antioxidant activity and total phenolic and flavonoid content. According to the results, the extract was effective in antioxidant properties. It was also found that the leaf extract contains a substantial amount of phenolic compounds. Therefore, it can be inferred that the phenolics present in the *H. tiliaceus* sample might be responsible for its antioxidant properties presenting meaningful information for the collection and application of *H. tiliaceus* in both healthcare and food industry. Nonetheless, a large, systematic study of *H. tiliaceus* from different sources would be helpful.

CONSENT

It is not applicable.

ETHICAL APPROVAL

It is not applicable.

COMPETING INTERESTS

Authors have declared that no competing interests exist.

REFERENCES

1. John SW. Christy MW. Herbal therapies: The facts and the fiction; Drug topics; 1997.
2. Brondegaard VJ. Contraceptive plant drugs. Planta Med. 1973;23:167-172.
3. Kepler AK. Hawaiian Heritage Plants. 1984;08.
4. Lebler BA. Wildflowers of South-Eastern Queensland. 1977;01.
5. Kobayashi J. Early Hawaiian uses of medicinal plants in pregnancy and childbirth. The J Trop Pediatr Environ Child Health. 1976;22:260-262.
6. Singh YN, Ikahihifo T, Panuve M, Slatter C. Folk medicine in Tonga. A study of the use of herbal medicines for obstetric and gynaecological conditions and disorders. J Ethnopharmacol. 1984;12(3):305-329.
7. Whistler WA. Traditional and herbal medicine in cook islands. J Ethnopharmacol. 1985;13:239-280.
8. Elemar GM, Rafael da Costa Halmenschlagerb, Renato Moreira Rosaa, João Antonio Pegas Henriquesa B, Ana Lígia Lia de Paula Ramosb, Jenifer Saffia,b. Pharmacological evidences for the extracts and secondary metabolites from plants of the genus Hibiscus. Food Chem. 2010;118:1-10.
9. Chen JJ, Huang SY, Duh CY, Chen IS, Wang TC, Fang HY. A new cytotoxic amide from the stem wood of *Hibiscus*

tiliaceus. Planta Med. 2006;72(10):935-938.

10. Borhade PS, Dalal PS, Pachauri AD, Lone KD, Chaudhari NA, Rangari PK. Evaluation of anti-inflammatory activity of *Hibiscus tiliaceus* linn wood extract. Int J Pharm Biomed Sci. 2012;3(3):1246-1250.

11. Cláudia V, Paula B, Sabrina S, Samanta IV, Maria ISM, Elina BC, Ionara RS. Antidepressant-like effects of methanol extract of *Hibiscus tiliaceus* flowers in mice. BMC Complem and Altern Med. 2012;12:41.

12. Rosa RM, Moura DJ, Melecchi MI, dos Santos RS, Richter MF, Camarão EB, Henriques JA, de Paula Ramos AL, Saffi J. Protective effects of *Hibiscus tiliaceus L.* methanolic extract to V79 cells against cytotoxicity and genotoxicity induced by hydrogen peroxide and tert-butyl-hydroperoxide. Toxicol *In Vitro*. 2007;21(8):1442-52.

13. Shaikh JU, Darren GI, Evelin T. Cytotoxic Effects of Bangladeshi Medicinal Plant Extracts. J Evid Based Complementary Altern Med. Article ID 578092. 2011;7.

14. Ramproshad SA, Afrozb T, Mondala B, Haquea A, Araa S, Khana R, Ahmed S. Antioxidant and antimicrobial activities of leaves of medicinal plant *Hibiscus tiliaceus* L. Pharmacologyonline. 2012;3:82–87.

15. Varahalarao V. Absence of anti fungicidal activity of few Indian medicinal plants methanolic extracts. Asian Pac J Trop Dis. 2012;393-395.

16. Li L, Huang X, Sattler I, Fu H, Grabley S, Lin W. Structure elucidation of a new friedelane triterpene from the mangrove plant *Hibiscus tiliaceus*. Magn Reson Chem. 2006;44:624–628.

17. Khirul I, Nripendra NB, Sanjib S, Hemayet H, Ismet AJ, Tanzir AK, Khalijah A, Jamil AS. Antinociceptive and antioxidant activity of *Zanthoxylum budrunga* wall (Rutaceae) seeds. Scientific World Journal; 2014. Available:http://dx.doi.org/10.1155/2014/869537

18. Sarunya C, Sukon P. Method development and determination of phenolic compounds in Broccoli Seeds Samples. Chiang Mai J Sci. 2006;33(1):103-107.

19. Fan YJ, He XJ, Zhou SD, Luo AX, He T, Chun Z. Composition analysis and antioxidant activity of polysaccharide from *Dendrobium denneanum*. Int J Biol Macromol. 2009;45:169-173.

20. Hemayet H, Shaikh ER, Proity NA, Tanzir AK, Mahfuzur MR, Ismet AJ: Determination of antioxidant activity and HPLC profile of *Euphorbia cotinifolia* Linn. leaf exract growing in Bangladesh. World J Pharm Res. 2014;3(7):93-104.

21. Dehpour AA, Ebrahimzadeh MA, Nabavi SF, Nabavi SM. Antioxidant activity of methanol extract of *Ferula assafoetida* and its essential oil composition. Grasas Aceites. 2009;60(4):405-412.

22. Prieto P, Pineda M, Aguilar M. Spectrophotometric quantitation of antioxidant capacity through the formation of a phosphomolybdenum complex: Specific application to the determination of vitamin E. Anal Biochem. 1999;269:337–341.

23. Hemayet H, Shahid-Ud-Daula AFM, Ismet AJ, Tarek A, Subrata B, Utpal K: Antinociceptive and antioxidant potentials of crude ethanol extract of the leaves of *Ageratum conyzoides* grown in Bangladesh. Pharm Biol. 2013;51(7):893-898.

24. Wootton-Beard PC, Moran A, Ryan L. Stability of the total antioxidant capacity and total polyphenol content of 23 commercially available vegetable juices before and after in vitro digestion measured by FRAP, DPPH, ABTS and Folin-Ciocalteu methods. Food Res Int. 2011;44(1):217-224.

25. Hemayet H, Ismet AJ, Sariful IH, Jamil AS, Shubhra KD, Arpona H: Anti-inflammatory and antioxidant activities of ethanolic leaf extract of *Brownlowia tersa* (L.) Kosterm. Orient Pharm Exp Med. 2013;13:181-189.

26. Chang C, Yang M, Wen H, Chern J. Estimation of total flavonoid content in propolis by two complementary colorimetric methods. J Food Drug Anal. 2002;10:178-182.

27. Uddin R, Saha MR, Subhan N, Hossain H, Jahan IA, Akter R, Alam A. HPLC-Analysis of polyphenolic compounds in *Gardenia jasminoides* and determination of antioxidant activity by using free radical scavenging assays. Adv Pharm Bull. 2014;4(3):273-81.

28. Meir S, Kanner J, Akiri B, Hadar SP. Determination and involvement of aqueous reducing compounds in oxidative systems of various senescing leaves. Journal of Agric Food Chem. 1995;43:1813-1817.

29. Hatano T, Edamatsu R, Hiramatsu M, Mori A, Fujita Y. Effects of the interaction of tannins with co-existing substances. VI: Effects of tannins and related polyphenols on superoxide anion radical and on 1, 1-

diphenyl-2-picrylhydrazyl radical. Chem Pharm Bull. 1989;37:2016-2021.

30. Saha MR, Alam A, Akter R, Jahangir R. *In-vitro* free radical scavenging activity of *Ixora coccinea* L, Bangladesh. J Pharm. 2008;3(2):90-96.

31. Abubakar BA, Mohammed AI, Aliyu MM, Aisha OM, Joyce JK, Adebayo OO. Free radical scavenging and total antioxidant capacity of root extracts of *Anchomanes difformis* Engl. (Araceae). Acta Pol Pharm-Drug Res. 2013;70(1):115-121.

32. Heim KE, Tagliaferro AR, Bobilya DJ. Flavonoid antioxidants: Chemistry, metabolism and structure- activity relationships. J Nutr Biochem. 2002;13:572–584.

33. Hemayet Hossain, Shaikh Emdadur Rahman, Proity Nayeeb Akbar, Tanzir Ahmed Khan, Md. Mahfuzur Rahman, Ismet Ara Jahan. Determination of antioxidant activity and HPLC profile of *Euphorbia cotinifolia* linn. leaf extract growing in Bangladesh. World J Pharm Res. 2014:3(7):93-104.

34. Tanaka M, Kuie CW, Nagashima Y, Taguchi T. Application of antioxidative Maillard reaction products from histidine and glucose to sardine products. B Jpn Soc Sci Fish. 1988;54:1409-1414.

35. Takako Y, Cui PC, Erbo D, Takashi T, Gen-Ichiro N, Itsuo N. Study on the Inhibitory Effect of Tannins and Flavonoids against the 1, 1-Diphenyl-2 picrylhydrazyl Radical. Biochem Pharmacol. 1998;56(2):213–222.

36. Mahfuza K, Ekramul I, Rafikul I, Aziz AR, AHM KA, Proma K, Mamunur R, Shahnaj P. Estimation of total phenol and *In vitro* antioxidant capacity of *Albizia procera* leaves. BMC Res Notes. 2013;6:121.

8

Evaluation of Multiple Functions of *Polygonum* Genus Compounds

Antoine H. L. Nkuété[1,2]**, Ludovico Migliolo**[2,3]**, Hippolyte K. Wabo**[1]**, Pierre Tane**[1]
and Octávio L. Franco[2,3*]

[1]*Department of Chemistry, Faculty of Science, University of Dschang, Dschang, Cameroon.*
[2]*Center of Proteomical and Biochemical Analyses, Genomic Sciences and Biotechnology, Catholic University of Brasilia, DF, Brazil.*
[3]*S-Inova, Biotechnology, Catholic University Dom Bosco, Campo Grande, Mato Grosso doSul, Brazil.*

Authors' contributions

This work was carried out in collaboration between all authors. Authors AHLN, LM, HKW, PT and OLF designed and wrote the review. All authors read and approved the final manuscript.

<u>Editor(s):</u>
(1) Marcello Iriti, Faculty of Plant Biology and Pathology, Department of Agricultural and Environmental Sciences, Milan State University, Italy.
<u>Reviewers:</u>
(1) Gyula Oros, PPI HAS, Budapest, Hungary.
(2) Isiaka A. Ogunwande, Natural Product Research Unit, Department of Chemistry, Faculty of Science, Lagos State University, Ojo, Nigeria.

ABSTRACT

For thousands of years, traditional medicinal plants have been used to control several diseases, based on traditional knowledge and experience. Nevertheless, many potential medicinal plants have not attracted attention to their useful pharmacological properties and remain to be discovered. In recent years, a number of plants from various genera, species and families have been scientifically studied for their pharmacological potential. Among them, the genus *Polygonum* contains 300 species worldwide. Many document reported various studies of phytochemical and pharmacological potential of crude extracts and compounds isolated from several *Polygonum* species.

Aims: The present review describes some traditional uses from the *Polygonum* genus, the phytochemistry, the pharmacological effects, the pharmacokinetics, the toxicology and the known potential phytoconstituents of therapeutic importance that have been isolated.

Place and Duration of Study: Department of Chemistry, Faculty of Science, University of

Corresponding author: E-mail: ocfranco@gmail.com

Dschang, Dschang, Cameroon and Centro de Analises Proteômicas e Bioquimicas, Pós-Graduação em Ciencias Genomicas e Biotecnologia, Universidade Catolica de Brasilia, Brasilia, DF, Brazil, between September 2012 and September 2013.

Methodology: A review of literature was carried out using several resources such as scientific papers, classical books, pubmed, Scifinder, Sirus, the web of Science and ethnobotanical information.

Results: Plants from *Polygonum* are widely distributed in the world and used as traditional medicine. Several compounds including phenolic compounds (flavonoids, chalcones, stibenes, coumarins and others) have been isolated and characterized from these plants and some of them are used as the effective pre-clinical to control various diseases in the world.

Conclusion: The present review covers many medicinal properties of some species from the *Polygonum* genus, setting out further mechanism of actions and toxicity yet to be established. Studies on *Polygonum* plant extracts could be targeted to develop novel anticancer, anti allergic agents, potential antiplasmodial and anti-inflammatory drugs, from the active compounds. Apart from this, a new approach could be developed for preparing this herbal product, as well as in combination with other plants. Other pharmacological properties for use in artherosclerosis, neurological disorders, diabetes, hypertension and immunomodulatory effects should be evaluated.

Keywords: Polygonum; Polygonaceae; metabolites; phytoconstituents; pharmacological potential.

1. INTRODUCTION

Traditional medicinal plants have long been used in the cure of several human and animal diseases, based on knowledge and experience. Many of these plants have not been studied scientifically and therefore their active principles are still undiscovered. Even though herbal plants in crude form are available for treatment in folk medicine, their uses and activities have unproven track records. In recent years, a number of medicinal plants from various genera, species and families have been scientifically evaluated. Many active principles have been isolated and evaluated for their role in the prevention, control and treatment of many disease conditions.

The *Polygonum* genus contains 300 species found all over the world. They contain diverse pharmacologically active constituents with various properties [1]. These species are predominantly herbs, found in tropical and temperate regions [2]. Some species are important traditional medicines, as illustrated in Fig. 1. Many of these *Polygonum* species and their active principles have been studied for phytochemical screening, biological and pharmacological purposes. Some of them have shown efficacy in the prevention and treatment of diseases such as cancer, malaria, gastric ulcers, bacterial and fungal infections; their toxic effects have also been evaluated.

The present review focuses on some traditional plants from the *Polygonum* genus, their pharmacological and biological effects, and the

known phytochemicals of potential therapeutic importance that have been isolated.

2. BOTANY

Polygonaceae family contains several genus includes *Polygonum* which is one of most important. *Polygonum* name is from the Greek poly, "many" and gonu, "knee" referring to the swollen-jointed stem. Different species from *Polygonum* genus vary widely from prostrate herbaceous annual plants (4-5 cm high) to herbaceous perennial plants (3–4 m tall). Others are trees or perennial woody vines and grow to around 20–30 m high, or trees. Many species are aquatic and naturally grow in the swampy area as floating plants in the rivers or ponds. The leaves vary in shape between from lanceolate to oval forms. They range from 1 to 30 cm long. The stems are usually red, reddish and sometime red-speckled. Generally, flowers are formed in dense clusters from the leaf joints and the youngest are white, pink or greenish [2].

3. TRADITIONAL USES

In China, "Rèlínqīng Kēlì" is the name of *Polygonum* extract. It's used in the folk medicine to cure urinary tract infections [3]. According to the Chinese Pharmacopoeia, *P. cuspidatum* has been used to relieve joint pain, to treat jaundice caused by a bacterial infection or fungal problems and cough with amenorrheal expectoration. *Polygonum cuspidatum* is also called "Hu Zhang" in China, and is used as a decoction to treat liver diseases or as a cream for topical application in burns, wounds and traumatic injuries [4]. It's currently also used in different forms such as powder, decoction or infusion to cure hepatitis and several other diseases [5]. In Korea, the rhizomes of *P. cuspidatum* are commonly used to maintain oral and dental hygiene [6]. In traditional Chinese medicine, *Polygonum multiflorum* has been used to treat mental and physical signs of aging, malaria, constipation and eczema. In Cameroonian traditional medicine, the raffia wine and aqueous extracts of the leaves of *Polygonum limbatum* are respectively used to cure gastrointestinal disorders, venereal diseases and skin infections [7]. In India, preparations of *Polygonum nepalense* are employed in colds, influenza, swelling, hemorrhoids, diarrhea and rheumatism [8]. The juice extract of the whole plant is taken orally for fetal mal-position and the decoction is also taken orally for juvenile pregnancy in Cameroon [9]. In Argentina, *Polygonum ferrurgineum* is used to heal infected wounds in local medicine, it's also used to control several bacteria and fungi [10]. In Bangladesh *Polygonum lapathifolium* is used as an insecticide [11]. In Brazil, *Polygonum spectabile* is used by indigenous people for the treatment of diarrhea, ulcers, gingivitis, skin infections and rheumatism [12]. *Polygonum hydropiper* is used as spice to flavor foods by Chinese and Malaysian indigenous because this specie possesses strong peppery taste [13]. In Turkey, the roots of *Polygonum amphibium* are very important in folk medicine and are used as an astringent and cleanser for skin [14,15]; they are also eaten raw, or sometimes they are dried, pounded and the infusion is used in the treatment of chest colds [16]. These data show that the *Polygonum* genus is widely distributed around the world and is being used on all continents to control numerous illnesses.

4. PHYTOCHEMISTRY

Several investigations were carried out to determine the possible chemical components from *Polygonum* plants. This genus is also well known for producing a wide variety of secondary metabolites including flavonoids [13], triterpenoids [17], anthraquinones [18], coumarins [19], phenylpropanoids [20], lignans [21], sesquiterpenoids [22], stilbenoids [23], tannins [1], proteins, amino acids and carbohydrates [8], and sucrose phenyl propanoid esters [19]. Amongst them, flavonoids are the most common components found in *Polygonum*

spp. and have been used as chemotaxonomic markers of the genus [22]. Fig. 1. presents some bioactive compounds obtained from the *Polygonum* genus and Table 1. shows the pharmacological effects of some extracts and compounds isolated from some *Polygonum* plants. In summary, the present review focuses on studies of a number of traditional medicinal plants from the *Polygonum* genus, their pharmacological and biological effects, and the known potential phytoconstituents of therapeutic importance isolated so far.

5. PHARMACOLOGICAL EFFECTS

5.1 Anticancer Effects

Recently, Hu and coworkers studied the activities of aqueous *Polygonum cuspidatum* extract on hepatocarcinoma cells (Bel-7402 and Hepa 1-6) in suspension [4]. In this study, the sample (extract) significantly (P<0.05) inhibited the proliferation of these cells in suspension in a dose-dependent and time-dependent manner. This extract also respectively showed the significant inhibition and induction of hepatocarcinoma cells in soft agar and anoikis in human Bel -7402 cells. Previously, crude extracts and compounds such as emodin and resveratrol showed anticancer activities [24,25]. The growth of cancer cells specially Ehrlich's carcinoma was inhibited by aqueous extracts (20 g/kg/day) [25], alternatively the ethanol extract showed an antiproliferative activity against two different cancer cells (human Lung H1650 and A549), in a dose-dependent manner [26]. Resveratrol reduced by using 2.5 and 10 mg.kg^{-1} for 5 days the volume and the weight of Lewis Lung tumor respectively (42%) and (44%). The tumor growth and metastasis in lungs are prevented by resveratrol (56%) [27]. Using resveratrol, several significant anticancer activities have been obtained by different research team. In an experiment on rats with intracerebral gliomas, the molecule (40 mg/kg/day, 150 days) exhibited anticancer activity such as higher and longer rat survival time and slower tumor growth [24]. Resveratrol in other experiments also showed cytotoxicity activities against lymph cancer [28], hepatic cancer [29], MCF-7 cells with IC50 (58.4 µg.mL^{-1}) and adriamycin-resistant MCF-7 cells with IC50 (56.7 µg.mL^{-1}) [30], ovarian cancer [31], human neuroblastomas and uveal melanoma tumors [32], atypical teratoid or rhabdoid tumors [33].

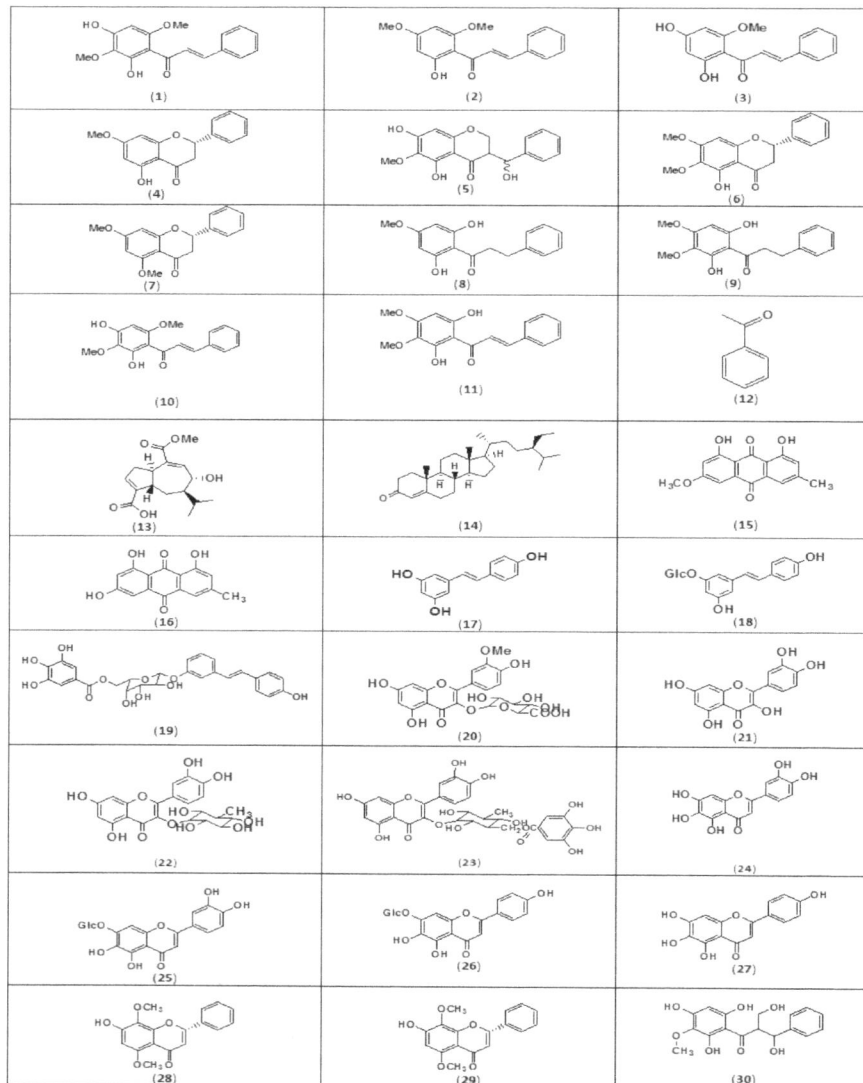

Fig. 1. Some bioactive compounds obtained from the *Polygonum* genus. (1) 2',4'-dihydroxy-3',6'-dimethoxychalcone; (2) 2'-hydroxy-4',6'-dimethoxychalcone; (3)cardamomin; (4)(S)-(-)-pinostrobin; (5) (±)-polygohomoisoflavanone; (6) (2S)-(-)-5-hydroxy-6,7-dimethoxyflavanone; (7) (2S)-(-)-5,7-dimethoxyflavanone; (8) 2',6'-dihydroxy-4'-methoxydihydrochalcone; (9) 2',6'-dihydroxy-3',4'-dimethoxydihydrochalcone; (10) 2',4'-dihydroxy-3',6'-dimethoxychalcone;(11) 2',6'-dihydroxy-3',4'-dimethoxychalcone; (12)acetophenone ; (13)viscozulenic acid ; (14) sitosterone; (15) physcion; (16) emodin; (17) resveratrol; (18) polydatin; (19) resveratrol 4-O-D-(2'-galloyl)-glucopyranoside; (20) quercetin 3-O-β-D-glucuronide; (21) quercetin; (22)quercitrin; (23) galloyl kaempferol 3-glucoside; (24) kaempferol 3-glucoside; (25) 6-Hydroxyluteolin; (26) 6-Hydoxyluteolin 7-O'-D-glucopyranoside; (27) 6-Hydroxyapigenin; (28) scutillarein; (29) 5.8-dimethoxy-7-hydroxyflavanone;(30) homoferrugen-dihydrochalcone

Emodin also exerted cytotoxic effects against human prostate cancer cell LNCaP, glioma cells [33] and human chronic myelocytic leukemia K562 cells [34]. The anticancer activities of the crude extract, fractions and flavonoids isolated from *Polygonum limbatum* were studied [7]. In experiment, the cytotoxicity of samples studied on several cancer cells such as breast carcinoma MCF-7, Leukemia THP-1, prostate carcinoma PC-3, Lung A549, cervical carcinoma HeLa. The results showed that, more than 50% inhibition of the proliferation was observed on above cell lines except Lung A549. Cardamomin and 2',4'-dihydroxy-3',6'-dimethoxychalcone are very active against THP-1 cell with IC_{50} below 4 $\mu g.mL^{-1}$ [7]. Furthermore, the cytotoxicity of crude extracts and compounds from *Polygonum spectabile* were also evaluated [22,35]. The cytotoxicity of crude extracts and compounds such as 2'-hydroxy-4',6'-dimethoxychalcone, 2',4'-dihydroxy-3',6'-dimethoxychalcone and 3-O-β-D-glucosyl-β-sitosterol (500-0.125 $\mu g.mL^{-1}$) to Vero and LLCMK2 cells were evaluated by using MTT assay. Each test was carried out in four replicates with at least four different concentrations. The results revealed that the three compounds isolated from *P. spectabile* showed moderate *in vitro* cytotoxicity activity against Vero and LLCMK2 cells with $CC_{50}<50$ $\mu g.mL^{-1}$ [35].

5.2 Antioxidant and Free Radical Scavenging Effects

The antioxidant effect of *Polygonum chinense* extract was evaluated. In this experiment, the preventive effects of aqueous extract against gastric mucosal injury in rats were determined [36]. The result of study showed that this extract significantly protects gastric mucosal [36]. The anti-ulcer activity of aqueous extract of *Polygonum minus* against gastric ulcer was also investigated. The results revealed that the plant extract induced a marked reduction in edema and conferred gastric protection [37]. Moreover, the toxicity of *P. minus* was studied. The higher dose (5 $g.kg^{-1}$) did not show any toxicological sign in rats [37]. The antioxidant effects of some *Polygonum* species have been examined by Hsu and coworkers. In this experiment, the ethanol extract of the root of *P. cuspidatum* was used as sample and evaluated the antioxidant activities, free radical scavenging, superoxide radical scavenging, lipid peroxidation assays have been used and IC_{50} values have been respectively obtained; 110 $mg.g^{-1}$, 3.2 $mg.g^{-1}$ and 8 $mg.g^{-1}$. Furthermore, the extract of this plant had a DNA-protective activity. The results indicated that *P. cuspidatum* extract had antioxidant activities [38]. In another experiment in 1993, in fact, Jin and coworkers evaluated the antioxidant activity of polydatin (3.2, 6.4, 12.8 and 25.6 $\mu mol.l^{-1}$), a molecule isolated from *P. cuspidatum* extract. Polydatin also showed a strong potential to scavenge oxygen free radicals with IC_{50} = 14.6 $\mu mol.L^{-1}$ for superoxide radicals (O^{2-}), hydroxyl radicals (OH^-) (IC_{50} = 29.6 $\mu mol.l^{-1}$) and hydrogen peroxide (H_2O_2) (IC_{50} = 13.0 $\mu mol.L^{-1}$) [39].

The *in vitro* antioxidant activity of *P. barbatum* extract was investigated by different strategies including hydroxyl radical scavenging assay, DPPH radical scavenging assay, superoxide scavenging assay, nitric oxide scavenging assay and total phenolic content. The IC_{50} (32.62 $\mu g.ml^{-1}$) value found in the DPPH radical scavenging method was higher than with other methods. *P. barbatum* extract contained phenolic compounds, which showed significative antoxidant effects [39]. The *in vitro* studies clearly showed that the ethanolic extract of *P. barbatum* is a new source of natural antioxidants that might prevent and control the process of oxidative stress [39].

5.3 Anti-inflammatory Effects

In 2008, one American research team studied the anti-inflammatory effects of *P. cuspidatum*. In this experiment, the plant material was extract with ethanolic solution and use as sample. The study evaluated the ability of sample to inhibit animal (mouse) ear inflammation. Sample was applied to both ears of animals at different doses 0.075, 0.15, 0.3, 1.25 and 2.5 $mg.ear^{-1}$ 30 min after topical application of 12-*O*-tetradecanoylphorbol-13-acetate administration (2 $\mu g.ear^{-1}$). Comparing to the topical application of 12-*O*-tetradecanoylphorbol-13-acetate as control, sample treatment at different doses siginficantly decreased ear edema. Myeloperoxidase effect was inhibited at *P. cuspidatum* extract doses $\geq$ 1.25 $mg.Kg^{-1}$. Trans-resveratrol also inhibit inflammation at different comparables doses. The development edema is inhibited by the extract of *P.cuspidatum* [40].

5.4 Wound Healing Effects

After wound treatment, a scar often forms, yielding an unpleasant spot. It is therefore necessary to erase the scar to regain the original luster. Based on multiple activities of plants of the genus *Polygonum*, the wound healing activity of *P. barbatum* was evaluated. Ethanol and water were used as solvent to extract the whole plant [41]. Excision and incision were two wound models used to study this effect. The extracts responded significantly ($P<0.001$) in both the wound models tested. Between the two extracts, the aqueous extract was more active than the ethanol extract [41].

5.5 Anti Allergic Effects

The anti allergic activity of *P. cuspidatum* radix extract was investigated by Lim and co-workers [42]. In this experiment, the extract was tested against two different mast cells and the sample showed very potent inhibitory effect with IC_{50} values (62±2.1) $\mu g.ml^{-1}$ for RBL-2H3 and (46±3.2) $\mu g.mL^{-1}$ for bone marrow–derived mast cells by antigen stimulation. The extract also exhibited the ability to supress the expression of interleukin-4 in RBL-2H3 cells and tumor necrosis factor-α. Concerning the *in vivo* animal allergy model, in dose dependent manner, *P.cuspidatum* radix inhibited passive cutaneous anaphylaxis, a local allergic reaction. The same sample also showed significative inhibition to activate phosphorylation of Syk and expressed the ability to suppress the mitogen-activated protein kinases ERK1/2 [42].

5.6 Anti Molluscidal and Antiplasmodial Effects

The anti molluscidal activity of crude aqueous and methanol extracts and compounds from *Polygonum senegalense* was evaluated [43] and the samples showed significative molluscidal effect against two different strains snails (*Biomphalaria pfeifferi* and *Biomphalaria sudanica*). One of compounds namely 2',4'-dihydroxy-3',6'-dimethoxychalcone was very active with 100% lethal to both snails in less tahn six hours. Two other fractions (hydrophobic and hydrophylic) of methanol extract of this plant also showed molluscidal activity on these snails [43]. Furthermore, the *in vitro* antiplasmodial activity of extract and compounds (polygohomo isoflavanone (19.2±0.6) μM for D6 and (18.2±1.8 μM), 2'- hydroxy- 4',6'- dimethoxychalcone (15.7±1.2 μM) for D6 and (11.3±0.2 μM) for W2 and 2',6'- dihydroxy- 3',4'- dimethoxychalcone (3.1±0.8 μM) for D6 and (2.4±0.3 μM) from *P. senegalense* was evaluated against two strains of *Plasmodium falciparum* (D6 and W2). The result showed that compounds isolated from *P. senegalense* are significantly active with IC_{50} between (19.2 to 2.4 μM) against two strains (D6 and W2) malaria parasite [44].

5.7 Antibacterial and Antifungal Effects

Several experiments have documented the antibacterial and antifungal potential of extracts and compounds from the genus *Polygonum*. The extract and compounds isolated from *Polygonum*

spectabile were also evaluated for their effects on 15 bacteria. Hydrophylic extracts of *P. spectabile* were active against *Staphylococcus aureus, Bacillus subtillis, Micrococcus luteus, Micrococcus canis, Trichophyton mentagrophytes* and *Trichophyton rubrum*. The results indicated that the use of *P. spectabile* may act as an antibacterial and antifungal agent [35]. Another antimicrobial screening of ethanol leaf extract of *P. barbatum* was assessed on ten microorganisms which include four Gram-positive, four Gram-negative bacteria and two fungi. The ethanol leaf extract showed considerable activity on both the bacteria and fungi, with inhibition zone diameter ranging from 14.17 to 31.45 mm and the minimum inhibitory concentrations ranging from 12 to 16 $\mu g.mL^{-1}$. These results showed that the ethanol extract of this plant is a broad-spectrum antimicrobial agent which can be used against Gram-positive and -negative bacteria and also against fungi [39].

The antimicrobial activities of *P. cuspidatum* were also investigated [45]. In this experiment, the aqueous extract of *P. cuspidatum* (1.0 $g.mL^{-1}$) showed antibacterial activity against *Staphylococcus aureus, Staphylococcus albus, Escherichia coli, α–Streptococcus, β–Streptococcus, Bacterium typhosum and Pseudomonas aeruginosa*; the inhibition zones were 1.122, 1.113, 1.127, 0.800, 0.929, 0.903,1.112 cm, respectively [46]. The methanol extracts of this plant also exhibited antibacterial activities against *Streptococcus sobrinus* and *Streptococcus mutans* at the minimum inhibitor concentration (MIC) (0.5–4 $mg.mL^{-1}$). This result suggested that the methanol extract could be used to control dental plaque and dental caries formation [6,47]. In another experiment, the crude extract of *P. cuspidatum* was tested against five common foodborne bacteria. The sample exhibited antibacterial activities against *Bacillus cereus, S. aureus* and *Listeria monocytogenes* at the minimum inhibitor concentrations of 312.5, 312.5 and 156.3 $\mu g.mL^{-1}$ respectively, and the bactericidal minimum inhibitor concentrations were 625, 1250 and 312.2 $\mu g.mL^{-1}$ [48]. In 2010, the antibacterial activities of methanol extract and fractions of *P. cuspidatum* on the development of dental caries were re-investigated. The results of the experiment showed that the ethyl acetate fraction, constituted mainly of polydatin, resveratrol, emodin and anthraglycoside B, exhibited significant antibacterial activities against eight different strains of *Streptococcus*, including *Streptococcus sobrinus* KCTC 3388, S.

mutans from different strains (KCTC 3308, KCTC 3307, KCTC 3389, KCTC 3306, KCTC 3300, KCTC 3298) and *Streptococcus cricetus* KCTC 3292, with minimum inhibitor concentrations of 0.5, 1, 0.5, 1, 0.5, 0.5, 0.125 and 0.25 mg.mL^{-1} respectively, and minimum bactericidal concentrations of 2, 4, 2, 2, 2, 1, 2, 0.5 mg.mL^{-1} respectively [49].

5.8 Genotoxicity Effects

Genotoxicity is a destructive effect on a cell's genetic material (DNA, RNA) affecting its integrity. *Polygonum multiflorum* has been designed for its potential to control genotoxicity. In this context, Zhang and coworkers studied genotoxicity in mouse peripheral lymphocyte cells with the use of *Panax ginseng* and *P. multiflorum* and the activity of their combination [50]. They administered them individually or in combination, on mouse peripheral lymphocyte DNA. *P. multiflorum* and its combination with *Panax ginseng* were orally administered to mice at gradient doses (low, medium and high) for seven consecutive days. On the first, third and seventh days, two hours after drug administration, blood samples were collected from the vein cluster behind the eye. *Panax ginseng* (0.43, 1.3 and 3.9 g.kg^{-1}) was found to have no harmful effects on peripheral lymphocyte DNA. *P. multiflorum* (3.9 and 11.7 g.kg^{-1}), on the other hand, had harmful effects on peripheral lymphocyte DNA on the first, third and seventh days. The combination of both plants (5.2 and 15.6 g.kg^{-1}) induced harmful effects on peripheral lymphocyte DNA on the first day, as showed in tail DNA tail length. Nevertheless, these harmful effects decreased on the third and seventh days. The results showed that the combination of these two plants may be used to control potential genotoxic effects and this activity is induced by *P. multiflorum* [50].

5.9 Hepatotoxicity Effects

Several experiments investigated the *in vitro* and *in vivo* hepatoxicity of hot-water-extracts of *P. multiflorum* in mice [51]. After treating primary cultured hepatocytes with *P. multiflorum* extracts at three final concentrations (0.5, 1.0 and 5.0 mg.mL^{-1}) with or without acetaminophen (10 mM) for 24 h, no cytotoxic effects was observed. Cell viability and lactate dehydrogenase leakage were significantly improved at the highest *P. multiflorum* extract dose compared with controls. Mice that received the *P. multiflorum* extracts (20 or 340 mg extracts/mouse x 2) orally

administered twice daily for 10 days indicated no unfavorable effect on the liver function. When the mice sub-chronically received the higher dose of *P. multiflorum* extract (340 mg) before the treatment with a single-bolus dose of acetaminophen (500 mg.kg^{-1}), attenuation of acetaminophen-induced hepatotoxicity was significantly *in vivo* established [51]. The results showed that *P. multiflorum* does not induce any toxicological effect on the liver and may in fact elicit useful but limited beneficial effects on the liver *in vivo* [51].

5.10 Antiviral Effects

An antiviral activity, an important and specific effect of *P. cuspidatum* was extensively investigated. Several experiments have shown that crude extracts or compounds isolated from *P. cuspidatum* have ability to control HIV [26,52,53]. In 1998, Jiang and coworkers evaluated the antiviral effect of water extract of this plant (50 mg/mouse/day, for 1 month); the sample exhibited an antiviral activity in an HIV-infected murine model [52]. Several compounds such as resveratrol, catechin, 5,7-dimethoxyphthalide and emodin 8-*O*-β-D-glycopyranoside isolated from *P. cuspidatum* showed significant antiviral activity against HIV-1; EC$_{50}$ values were 4.37±1.96 μg.ml^{-1}, 14.4±1.34 μg.ml^{-1}, 19.97±5.09 μg.ml^{-1} and 11.29±6.26 μg.ml^{-1} respectively [26]. In addition, resveratrol was also considered as a new molecule for anti-HIV therapeutics [53]. In fact, resveratrol pretreatment dose-dependently increased sirtuins 1 protein expression and intracellular NAD+ level. This compound and the extract of *P. cuspidatum* were used against Epstein-Barr virus (EBV) [54], hepatitis B virus (HPV) [55].

6. PHARMACOKINETICS

Plants from the *Polygonum* genus have many pharmacological effects, including anticancer, antioxidant and free radical scavenging, anti-inflammatory, wound healing, anti allergic, anti molluscidal, antiplasmodial, antibacterial, antifungal, genotoxic, hepatotoxic and antiviral effects. From these biological activities it can be noted that several extracts and pure compounds isolated from *Polygonum* genus plants have a promising future to control, prevent various pathogenics. The preliminary results suggest the viability of future investigations, such as studies involving the mechanisms of action, pharmacokinetics and pharmacodynamics of these pure compounds.

Table 1. Pharmacological effects of some extracts and compounds isolated from some *Polygonum*

Plants	Extracts. compounds	Pharmacological effects	Minimal active concentration.dose	In vivo. in vitro	Reference
Polygonum spectabile	Hexane extract	Anti-Tricophyton mentagrophytes	18.5±0.8 mg.disc^{-1}	In vitro	[35]
		Anti-Tricophyton rubrum	10.5±1.1 mg.disc^{-1}	In vitro	
		Anti-Micrococcus canis	9.5±1.4 mg.disc^{-1}	In vitro	
		Anti-Vero cells	83.6±4.6 µg.ml^{-1}	In vitro	
		Anti- LLCMK$_2$Cells	71.3±3.5µg.ml^{-1}	In vitro	
	Dichloromethane extract	Anti-Tricophyton mentagrophytes	11.5±0.8 mg.disc^{-1}	In vitro	[35]
		Anti-Tricophyton rubrum	10.5±0.5 mg.disc^{-1}	In vitro	
		Anti-Micrococcus canis	8.5±0.9mg.disc^{-1}	In vitro	
		Anti-Vero cells	128.2±6.9µg.ml^{-1}	In vitro	
		Anti- LLCMK$_2$Cells	117.9±7.2µg.ml^{-1}	In vitro	
	Ethyl acetate extract	Anti-Staphylococcus aureus	8.8±0.8 mg.disc^{-1}	In vitro	[35]
		Anti-Tricophyton mentagrophytes	12.0±0.9 mg.disc^{-1}	In vitro	
		Anti-Tricophyton rubrum	9.5±0.6 µg.ml^{-1}	In vitro	
	Ethanol extract	Anti-Staphylococcus aureus	7.5±0.5 µg.ml^{-1}	In vitro	[35]
		Anti-Micrococcus luteus	9.5±0.5 µg.ml^{-1}	In vitro	
		Anti-HHV-1[a]	21.9±1.8µg.ml^{-1}	In vitro	
	2'-hydroxy-4',6'-dimethoxychalcone	Anti-Staphylococcus aureus	15.2±0.9 mm	In vitro	[35]
		Anti-Staphylococcus epidermides	11.3±0.5 mm	In vitro	
		Anti-Bacillus subtillus	12.7±0.8 mm	In vitro	
		Anti-Micrococcus luteus	11.3±0.5 mm	In vitro	
		Anti-Micrococcus canis	14.6 mm	In vitro	
		Anti-Tricophyton mentagrophytes	24.7 mm	In vitro	
		Anti-Tricophyton rubrum	24.3 mm	In vitro	
	2',4'-dihydroxy-3',6'-dimethoxychalcone	Anti-Vero cells	31.5 µg.mL^{-1}	In vitro	[35]
		Anti- LLCMK$_2$Cells	29.6 µg.mL^{-1}	In vitro	
	3-O-β-D-glucosyl-β-sitosterol	Anti-Vero cells	27.2 µg.mL^{-1}	In vitro	[35]
		Anti- LLCMK$_2$Cells	7.8 µg.mL^{-1}	In vitro	
Polygonum limbatum	cardamomin	Anti-THP-1 (Leukemia)	1.8 µg.mL^{-1}	In vitro	[7]
		Anti-Hela (cervix)	17 µg.mL^{-1}	In vitro	
		Anti-PC-3 (prostate)	49 µg.mL^{-1}	In vitro	
		Anti-MCF-7 (breast)	32 µg.mL^{-1}	In vitro	

Plants	Extracts. compounds	Pharmacological effects	Minimal active concentration.dose	In vivo. in vitro	Reference
	(±) Polygohomoisoflavanone	Anti-THP-1 (Leukemia)	32.5 µg.mL^{-1}	In vitro	[7]
		Anti-PC-3 (prostate)	40 µg.mL^{-1}	In vitro	[7]
		Anti-MCF-7 (breast)	36 µg.mL^{-1}	In vitro	[7]
	2',4'-dihydroxy-3',6'-dimethoxychalcone	Anti-THP-1 (Leukemia)	3.5µg.mL^{-1}	In vitro	[7]
		Anti-Hela (cervix)	22 µg.mL^{-1}	In vitro	[7]
	(S)(−)-pinostrobin	Anti-THP-1 (Leukemia)	9 µg.mL^{-1}	In vitro	[7]
		Anti-PC-3 (prostate)	40 µg.ml^{-1}	In vitro	[7]
		Anti-MCF-7 (breast)	36 µg.mL^{-1}	In vitro	[7]
	(2S)-(−)-5-hydroxy-6,7-dimethoxyflavanone	Anti-THP-1 (Leukemia)	25.5 µg.m^{-1}L	In vitro	[7]
		Anti-MCF-7 (breast)	47 µg.mL^{-1}	In vitro	[7]
	(2S)-(−)-5,7-dimethoxyflavanone	Anti-THP-1 (Leukemia)	10 µg.mL^{-1}	In vitro	[7]
		Anti-MCF-7 (breast)	37 µg.mL^{-1}	In vitro	[7]
	Methanol extract	Anti-THP-1 (Leukemia)	10 µg.mL^{-1}	In vitro	[7]
		Anti-PC-3 (prostate)	28 µg.mL^{-1}	In vitro	[7]
		Anti-MCF-7 (breast)	20 µg.mL^{-1}	In vitro	[7]
	n-Butanol extract	Anti-THP-1 (Leukemia)	9 µg.mL^{-1}	In vitro	[7]
		Anti-PC-3 (prostate)	9 µg.mL^{-1}	In vitro	[7]
		Anti-MCF-7 (breast)	18 µg.mL^{-1}	In vitro	[7]
	Ethyl acetate extract	Anti-THP-1 (Leukemia)	8.5 µg.mL^{-1}	In vitro	[7]
		Anti-MCF-7 (breast)	23 µg.mL^{-1}	In vitro	[7]
Polygonum cuspidatum	Ethanol extract	Anti-inflammatory(reduced ear edema induced by TPA)	0.075 mg.ear^{-1}	In vivo	[40]
		Anti-inflammatory(reduced myeloperoxidase activity)	2.5 mg.ear^{-1}	In vivo	[40]
	polydatin	Inhibits the vasoconstrictive effect	1.71 mmol.L^{-1}	In vivo	[60]
		Reduce lipogenesis of rats	50 mg.kg^{-1}	In vivo	[61]
		Enhanced MCF-7 proliferation	20 µmol.L^{-1}	In vitro	[62]
	physcion	Inhibition of melanogenesis effect	10 µmol.L^{-1}	In vitro	[63]
	emodin	Inhibition of melanogenesis effect	10 µmol.L^{-1}	In vitro	[63]
		Anti-HSV-1	4 mg.mL^{-1}	In vivo	[64]
		Anti-human chronic myelocytic leukemia K562 cells	25 µmol.L^{-1}	In vitro	[34]
		Anti-human prostate cancer cells	10 µmol.L^{-1}	In vitro	[65]

Plants	Extracts. compounds	Pharmacological effects	Minimal active concentration.dose	In vivo. in vitro	Reference
		Anti-glioma cells	100 µmol.L^{-1}	In vitro	[66]
	cytreosein	Inhibition of melanogenesis effect	10 µmol.L^{-1}	In vitro	[63]
	anthraglycoside	Inhibition of melanogenesis effect	10 µmol.L^{-1}	In vitro	[63]
	Water extract	Anti-Escherichia coli	1 g.mL^{-1}	In vitro	[46]
		Anti-Bacterium typhosum	1 g.mL^{-1},	In vitro	[46]
		Anti-pseudomonas aeruginosa	1 g.mL^{-1}	In vitro	[46]
		Anti-Staphylococcus aureus	1 g.mL^{-1},	In vitro	[46]
		Anti-Staphylococcus albus	1 g.mL^{-1},	In vitro	[46]
		Anti-α-Streptococcus aureus	1 g.mL^{-1}	In vitro	[46]
		Anti-β-Streptococcus	1 g.mL^{-1}	In vitro	[46]
	resveratrol	Anti-tumor	40 mg.kg^{-1}	In vivo	[24]
		Anti-uveal melanoma tumors	20 mg.tumor.times^{-1}	In vivo	[32]
		Anti-human neuroblastomas	5 mg.tumor.times^{-1}	In vivo	[32]
		Anti-lymph cancer	100 µmM	In vitro	[28]
		Anti-atypical teratoid tumors	150 µM	In vitro	[33]
	resveratrol	Anti-hepatic cancer	12.5 µM	In vivo	[38]
	resveratrol	Anti-EBV	13.8 µM	In vitro	[54]
Polygomun senegalense	2',6'-dihydroxy-4'-methoxydihydrochalcone	Anti-D6 plasmodium falciparum	23.5 µM	In vitro	[44]
		Anti-W2 plasmodium falciparum	22.8 µM	In vitro	[44]
	2',6'-dihydroxy-3',4'-dimethoxydihydrochalcone	Anti-D6 plasmodium falciparum	11.8 µM	In vitro	[44]
		Anti-W2 plasmodium falciparum	12. µM	In vitro	[44]
	2',4'-dihydroxy-3',6'-dimethoxychalcone	Anti-W2 plasmodium falciparum	17.8 µM	In vitro	[44]
		Anti-D6 plasmodium falciparum	16.6 µM	In vitro	[44]
Polygonum Barbatum	Acetophenone	Anti-DPPH	1.8 x 10^{-1} mg.mL^{-1}	in vivo	[67]
	Viscozulenic acid	Anti-DPPH	1.2X10^{-1}mg.mL^{-1}	In vitro	[67]
	Sitosterone	Anti-DPPH	2.1X10^{-1}mg.mL^{-1}	In vitro	[67]
Polygonum hydropiper	Quercetin 3-O-β-D-glucuronide	Antioxidant	5.08 (TEAC value)	In vitro	[13]
	Quercetin	Antioxidant	4.65(TEAC value)	In vitro	[13]
	Quercitrin	Antioxidant	3.46 (TEAC value)	In vitro	[13]
	Galloyl kaempferol 3-glucoside	Antioxidant	2.90 (TEAC value)	In vitro	[13]
	Kaempferol 3-glucoside	Antioxidant	1.39 (TEAC value)	In vitro	[13]
	6-Hydroxyluteolin	Antioxidant	2.33 (TEAC value)	In vitro	[13]
	6-Hydroxyluteolin 7-O'-D-	Antioxidant	2.87 (TEAC value)	In vitro	[13]

Plants	Extracts. compounds	Pharmacological effects	Minimal active concentration.dose	In vivo. in vitro	Reference
	glucopyranoside				
Polygonum ferrugineum	5.8-dimethoxy-7-hydroxyflavanone	Anti-*Trichophyton mentagrophytes* ATCC9972	250 µg.mL^{-1}	*In vitro*	[68]
		Anti-*Trichophyton rubrum* CCC113	250 µg.mL^{-1}	*In vitro*	[68]
		Anti-*Epidermophyton floccosum* CCC114	250 µg.mL^{-1}	*In vitro*	[68]
	Homoferrugen-dihydrochalcone	Anti-*Trichophyton mentagrophytes* ATCC9972	200 µg.mL^{-1}	*In vitro*	[68]
		Anti-*Trichophyton rubrum* CCC113	250 µg.mL^{-1}	*In vitro*	[68]
	Methanol extract	*Microsporum gypseum* CCC 115	125 µg.mL^{-1}	*In vitro*	[68]
		Anti-*Trichophyton rubrum* CCC113	50 µg.mL^{-1}	*In vitro*	[68]
		Anti-*Trichophyton mentagrophytes* ATCC9972	125 µg.mL^{-1}	*In vitro*	[68]
		Anti-*Epidermophyton floccosum* CCC114	50 µg.mL^{-1}	*In vitro*	[68]

Furthermore, a few pharmacokinetic investigations have been done on *Polygonum* plants. In 2008, one pharmacokinetic experiment with rats received the extract of *P. cuspidatum*. After this experiment, methanol was used as polar organic solvent to extracted tissues and solid-phase extraction was used to clean urinary and bilary samples. The secondary metabolites were analyzed and identified in mass spectrometry. The major of the chemical constituents of this extract was resveratrol, which was distributed in the liver, kidney, duodenum and stomach [56]. With this result, other scientists then evaluated different active compounds of *P. cuspidatum*. In particular, emodin was investigated in rats using selective HPLC method. The result of this experiment clearly showed that emodin is quickly absorbed into the blood stream and rapidly transferred into the liver [57]. In 2012, the results of experiments using a HPLC method showed that after oral administration of *Polygonum cuspidatum* extract, glucuronides or sulfates of resveratrol and emodin were the best forms in distribution and organs [58,59].

7. TOXICOLOGY

Plants from the *Polygonum* genus have long been used as an important medicinal plant in the world. Some of these plants are traditionally considered to be toxic, such as *P. cuspidatum*, which according to Chinese folk medicine, the plant induces abortion and for this reason, it's prohibited for pregnant women [5]. The aqueous extract of *Polygonum minus* was administrated orally in rats with 5 g.kg^{-1} (higher dose), the acute toxicity was studied and animals model did not present toxicological signs [37]. It was also reported that LD$_{50}$ of emodin (249.5±34.3 mg.kg^{-1}) and polydatin (1000±57.3 mg.kg^{-1}) were (249.5±34.3 mg.kg^{-1}) administrated orally did not cause death in mice. In one acute toxicity study, rats were treated with the extract of *P. chinense* at a dose of 2 or 5 g.kg^{-1}. Despite the bad health of rats, no signs of toxicity have been observed at these doses. No abnormalities have been observed after biochemical serology and histological indicators of liver and kidney analysis [36].

8. CONCLUSION AND PROSPECTS

The present review covers many medicinal properties of some plants from the *Polygonum* genus, with further mechanism of actions and toxicity yet to be established. Studies on

Polygonum plant extracts could be targeted to develop novel anticancer and anti allergic agents and potential antiplasmodial and anti-inflammatory drugs, from the active compounds [69]. These active principles could be clinically evaluated to develop therapeutic drugs with more safety, efficacy and tolerability. Apart from this, a new approach could be developed for preparing this herbal product, as well as in combination with other plants. Other pharmacological properties for use in artherosclerosis, neurological disorders, diabetes, hypertension and immunomodulatory effects should be evaluated. Moreover, in agriculture, the anti-nematode and anti-insecticidal activities of *Polygonum* plants extracts against potato pathogens will also be evaluated. In summary, data reviewed here clearly show the enormous potential of *Polygonum* plants for the development of new pharmaceuticals, adding this genus to the list of highly promising native compounds to undergo further research.

CONSENT

Not applicable.

ETHICAL APPROVAL

Not applicable.

COMPETING INTERESTS

Authors have declared that no competing interests exist.

REFERENCES

1. Wang KJ, Zhang YJ, Yang CR. Antioxidant phenolic compounds from rhizomes of *Polygonum paleaceum*. Journal of Ethnopharmacology. 2005;96(3):483-487.
2. Hutchinson J, Dalziel JM. Flora of west tropical Africa revised by Keay RWJ. Whitefriars, London. 2nd edition. Crown Agents. London; 1954.
3. Luczaj L. Archival data on wild food plants used in Poland in 1948. Journal of Ethnobiology and Ethnomedicine. 2008;4:4.
4. Hu B, An HM, Shen KP, Song HY, Deng S. *Polygonum cuspidatum* extract induces anoikis in hepatocarcinoma cells associated with generation of reactive oxygen species and downregulation of focal adhesion kinase. Evidence-Based

Complementary and Alternative Medicine, Ecam; 2012. DOI: 1155/2012/607675.

5. State administration of traditional Chinese medicine. 1999;1(1).

6. Song JH, Kim SK, Chang KW, Han SK, Yi HK, Jeon JG. *In vitro* inhibitory effects of *Polygonum cuspidatum* on bacterial viability and virulence factors of *Streptococcus mutans* and *Streptococcus sobrinus*. Archives of Oral Biology. 2006;51(12):1131-1140.

7. Dzoyem JP, Nkuete AH, Kuete V, Tala MF, Wabo HK, Guru SK, Rajput VS, Sharma A, Tane P, Khan IA, Saxena AK, Laatsch H, Tan NH. Cytotoxicity and antimicrobial activity of the methanol extract and compounds from *Polygonum* limbatum. Planta medica. 2012;78(8):787-792.

8. Rakesh KG, Kalra S, Mahadevan NS, Dhar VJ. Pharmacognostic investigation of *Polygonum nepalense*. International Journal of Recent Advances in Pharmaceutical Research. 2011;1:40-44.

9. Focho DA, Newu MC, Anjah MG, Nwana FA, Ambo FB. Ethnobotanical survey of trees in Fundong, Northwest Region, Cameroon. Journal of Ethnobiology and Ethnomedicine. 2009;5:17.

10. Del Vitto LA, Petenatti EM, Petenatti ME, Recursos herbolarios de San Luis (República Argentina). Primeira parte: plantas nativas. Mendoza. 1997;6:49-66

11. Ahmed M, Khaleduzzaman M, Saiful Islam M. Isoflavan-4-ol, dihydrochalcone and chalcone derivatives from *Polygonum lapathifolium*. Phytochemistry. 1990;29:2009-2011.

12. Pio Corrêa M, Dicionário das plantas uteis do Brasil e das exóticas cultivadas. IBDF - Rio de Janeiro: Imprensa Nacional. 1978;6.

13. Peng ZF, Strack D, Baumert A, Subramaniam R, Goh NK, Chia TF, Tan SN, Chia LS, Antioxidant flavonoids from leaves of *Polygonum hydropiper* L. Phytochemistry. 2003;62(2):219-228.

14. Singh G, Kachroo P. Forest Flora of Srinagar and plants of Neighborhood. Bishen Singh Mahendra Pal Singh: Delhi, India. 1976;27-218.

15. Coffey T. The history and folklore of north American wild flowers. Houghton Mifflin: Boston, USA. 1994;36-189.

16. Moerman D. Native American ethnobotany. Timber Press: Portland, Oregon, USA. 1998;42:691.

17. Duwiejua M, Zeitlin IJ, Gray AI, Waterman PG. The anti-inflammatory compounds of *Polygonum bistorta*: Isolation and characterisation. Planta Medica. 1999;65(4):371-374.

18. Matsuda H, Shimoda H, Morikawa T, Yoshikawa M, Phytoestrogens from the roots of *Polygonum cuspidatum* (*Polygonaceae*): Structure-requirement of hydroxyanthraquinones for estrogenic activity. Bioorganic & Medicinal Chemistry Letters. 2001;11(14):1839-1842.

19. Sun X, Sneden AT. Neoflavonoids from *Polygonum perfoliatum*. Planta Medica. 1999;65(7):671-673.

20. Murai Y, Kashimura S, Tamezawa S, Hashimoto T, Takaoka S, Asakawa Y, Kiguchi K, Murai F, Tagawa M. Absolute configuration of (6S,9S)-roseoside from *Polygonum hydropiper*. Planta Medica. 2001;67(5):480-481.

21. Kim HJ, Woo ER, Park H. A novel lignan and flavonoids from *Polygonum aviculare*. Journal of Natural Products. 1994;57:587-596.

22. Datta BK, Datta SK, Rashid MA, Nash RJ, Sarker SD. A sesquiterpene acid and flavonoids from *Polygonum viscosum*. Phytochemistry. 2000;54(2):201-205.

23. Nonaka G, Miwa N, Nishioka I. Stilbene glycoside gallates and proanthocyanidins from *Polygonum multiflorum*. Phytochemistry. 1982;21:429-432.

24. Tseng SH, Lin SM, Chen JC, Su YH, Huang HY, Chen CK, Lin PY, Chen Y. Resveratrol suppresses the angiogenesis and tumor growth of gliomas in rats. Clinical cancer research: An Official journal of the American Association for Cancer Research. 2004;10(6):2190-2202.

25. Zhou LD, Zhou XH, Zhang SC. Inhibitive effect of water extracts of *Polygonum cuspidatum* on Ehrlich's carcinoma. Chinese Journal of Integrated Traditional Western Medicine. 1989;9:111.

26. Lin HW, Sun MX, Wang YH, Yang LM, Yang YR, Huang N, Xuan LJ, Xu YM, Bai DL, Zheng YT, Xiao K. Anti-HIV activities of the compounds isolated from *Polygonum cuspidatum* and *Polygonum multiflorum*. Planta medica. 2010;76(9):889-892.

27. Kimura Y, Okuda H. Resveratrol isolated from *Polygonum cuspidatum* root prevents tumor growth and metastasis to lung and tumor-induced neovascularization in Lewis

lung carcinoma-bearing mice. The Journal of Nutrition. 2001;131(6):1844-1849.

28. Yan Y, Gao YY, Liu BQ, Niu XF, Zhuang Y, Wang HQ. Resveratrol-induced cytotoxicity in human Burkitt's lymphoma cells is coupled to the unfolded protein response. BMC Cancer. 2010;10:445.

29. Hsu CM, Hsu YA, Tsai Y, Shieh FK, Huang SH, Wan L, Tsai FJ. Emodin inhibits the growth of hepatoma cells: Finding the common anti-cancer pathway using Huh7, Hep3B, and HepG2 cells. Biochemical and Biophysical Research Communications. 2010;392(4):473-478.

30. Feng L, Zhang LF, Yan T, Jin J, Tao WY. Studies on active substance of anticancer effect in *Polygonum cuspidatum*. Zhong yao cai = Zhongyaocai = Journal of Chinese Medicinal Materials. 2006;29(7):689-691.

31. Guo L, Peng Y, Yao J, Sui L, Gu A, Wang J. Anticancer activity and molecular mechanism of resveratrol-bovine serum albumin nanoparticles on subcutaneously implanted human primary ovarian carcinoma cells in nude mice. Cancer Biotherapy & Radiopharmaceuticals. 2010;25(4):471-477.

32. van Ginkel PR, Sareen D, Subramanian L, Walker Q, Darjatmoko SR, Lindstrom MJ, Kulkarni A, Albert DM, Polans AS. Resveratrol inhibits tumor growth of human neuroblastoma and mediates apoptosis by directly targeting mitochondria. Clinical Cancer Research: An Official Journal of the American Association for Cancer Research. 2007;13(17):5162-5169.

33. Kao CL, Huang PI, Tsai PH, Tsai ML, Lo JF, Lee YY, Chen YJ, Chen YW, Chiou SH. Resveratrol-induced apoptosis and increased radiosensitivity in CD133-positive cells derived from atypical teratoid/rhabdoid tumor. International Journal of Radiation Oncology, Biology, Physics. 2009;74(1):219-228.

34. Chun-Guang W, Jun-Qing Y, Bei-Zhong L, Dan-Ting J, Chong W, Liang Z, Dan Z, Yan W. Anti-tumor activity of emodin against human chronic myelocytic leukemia K562 cell lines *in vitro* and *in vivo*. European Journal of Pharmacology. 2010;627(1-3):33-41.

35. Brandao GC, Kroon EG, Duarte MG, Braga FC, de Souza Filho JD, de Oliveira AB. Antimicrobial, antiviral and cytotoxic activity of extracts and constituents from *Polygonum spectabile* mart.

Phytomedicine: International Journal of Phytotherapy and Phytopharmacology. 2010;17(12):926-929.

36. Ismail IF, Golbabapour S, Hassandarvish P, Hajrezaie M, Abdul Majid N, Kadir FA, Al-Bayaty F, Awang K, Hazni H, Abdulla MA. Gastroprotective activity of *Polygonum chinense* aqueous leaf extract on ethanol-induced hemorrhagic mucosal lesions in rats. Evidence-Based Complementary and Alternative Medicine: eCAM; 2012.

37. Wasman SQ, Mahmood AA, Zahra AA, Salmah I. Cytoprotective activities of *Polygonum minus* aqueous leaf extract on ethanol-induced gastric ulcer in rats. Journal of Medicinal Plants Research. 2010;4:2658-2665.

38. Hsu CY, Chan YP, Chang J. Antioxidant activity of extract from *Polygonum cuspidatum*. Biological research. 2007;40(1):13-21.

39. Sheela QR, Ramani A. *In vitro* antioxidant activity of *Polygonum barbatum* leaf extract. Asian Journal of Pharmaceutical and Clinical Research. 2011;4:113-115.

40. Bralley EE, Greenspan P, Hargrove JL, Wicker L, Hartle DK. Topical anti-inflammatory activity of *Polygonum cuspidatum* extract in the TPA model of mouse ear inflammation. Journal of Inflammation (Lond). 2008;5:1-7.

41. Kinger KH, Gupta KM. Wound healing activity of *Polygonum barbatum* Linn. (whole plant). Journal of Pharmacy and Pharmaceutical Sciences. 2012;1:1084-1091.

42. Lim BO, Lee JH, Ko NY, Mun SH, Kim JW, Kim do K, Kim JD, Kim BK, Kim HS, Her E, Lee HY, Choi WS. *Polygoni cuspidati* radix inhibits the activation of syk kinase in mast cells for anti allergic activity. Experimental Biology and Medicine (Maywood). 2007;232(11):1425-1431.

43. Maradufu A, Ouma HJ. A new chalcone as a natural molluscide from *Polygonum senegalense*. Phytochemistry. 1978;17.

44. Midiwo JO, Omoto FM, Yenesew A, Akala MH, Wangui J, Liyala P, Wasunna C, Waters CN. The first 9-hydroxy homoisoflavanone, and antiplasmodial chalcones, from the aerial exudates of *Polygonum senegalense*. ARKIVOC. 2007;9:21-27.

45. Wang H, Dong Y, Xiu ZL. Microwave-assisted aqueous two-phase extraction of piceid, resveratrol and emodin from *Polygonum cuspidatum* by

ethanol/ammonium sulphate systems. Biotechnology Letters. 2008;30(12):2079-2084.

46. Wang QL, Li BY, Qiu SC, Li YL, Mi W, Song HY. Study on antibacteria effect *in vitro* of *Polygonum cuspidatum* sieb. Lishizhen Medicine and Material Medica Research. 2006;(17):762-763.

47. Song JH, Yang TC, Chang KW, Han SK, Yi HK, Jeon JG. *In vitro* effects of a fraction separated from *Polygonum cuspidatum* root on the viability, in suspension and biofilms, and biofilm formation of mutans streptococci. Journal of Ethnopharmacology. 2007;112(3):419-425.

48. Shan B, Cai YZ, Brooks JD, Corke H. Antibacterial properties of *Polygonum cuspidatum* roots and their major bioactive constituents. Food Chemistry. 2008;109:530-537.

49. Ban SH, Kwon YR, Pandit S, Lee YS, Yi HK, Jeon JG. Effects of a bio-assay guided fraction from *Polygonum cuspidatum* root on the viability, acid production and glucosyl tranferase of mutans streptococci. Fitoterapia. 2010;81(1):30-34.

50. Zhang Q, Wu C, Duan L, Yang J. Genotoxic studies on panax genseng and *Polygonum multiflorum* and their combination in mouse peripheral lymphocyte cells. Asian Journal of Traditional Medicine. 2007;(2):217-134.

51. Noda T, Yamada T, Ohkubo T, Omura T, Ono T, Adachi T, Awaya T, Tasaki Y, Shimizu K, Matsubara K. Hot-water-extracts of *Polygonum multiflorum* do not induce any toxicity but elicit limited beneficial effects on the liver in mice. Journal of Health Science. 2009;55:720-725.

52. Jiang S, Lin K, Lu M. A conformation-specific monoclonal antibody reacting with fusion-active gp41 from the human immunodeficiency virus type 1 envelope glycoprotein. Journal of Virology. 1998;72(12):10213-10217.

53. Zhang HS, Zhou Y, Wu MR, Zhou HS, Xu F. Resveratrol inhibited Tat-induced HIV-1 LTR transactivation via NAD(+)-dependent SIRT1 activity. Life sciences. 2009;85(13-14):484-489.

54. Yiu CY, Chen SY, Chang LK, Chiu YF, Lin TP. Inhibitory effects of resveratrol on the Epstein-Barr virus lytic cycle. Molecules, 2010;15(10):7115-7124.

55. Chang JS, Liu HW, Wang KC, Chen MC, Chiang LC Hua YC, Lin CC. Ethanol extract of *Polygonum cuspidatum* inhibits hepatitis B virus in a stable HBV-producing cell line. Antiviral Research. 2005;66(1):29-34.

56. Wang DG, Xu YR, Liu BB. Tissue distribution and excretion of resveratrol in rat after oral administration of *Polygonum cuspidatum* extract (PCE). Phytomedicine: International Journal of Phytotherapy and Phytopharmacology. 2011;15:859-866.

57. Peng J, Song ZF, Ma C. Emodin studies on pharmacokinetics and distribution in rat liver after *Polygonum cuspidatum* extract administration. World science and technology medernization of traditional Chinese medicine and Materia Medica. 2008;10:64-67.

58. Lin SP, Chu PM, Tsai SY, Wu MH, Hou YC. Pharmacokinetics and tissue distribution of resveratrol, emodin and their metabolites after intake of *Polygonum cuspidatum* in rats. Journal of Ethnopharmacology. 2012;144(3):671-676.

59. Jin WJ, Chen SY, Qian ZX, Shi XH. Effects of polydatin IV on inhibiting respiratory burst of of PMNs and scanvenging oxygen free radicals. Chinese Pharmacological Bulletin. 1993;355-357.

60. Luo SZ, Zhang PW, Li RS. Dilating action of 3,4,5-trihydroxystibene-3-p-mono-D-glucoside on rabbit's blood vessels. Journal of First Military Medical University. 1992;12:10-13.

61. Arichi H, Kimura Y, Okuda H, Baba K, Kozawa M, Arichi S. Effects of stilbene components of the root of *Polygonum cuspidatum* sieb. Et zucc. On lipid metabolism. Chemical & Pharmaceutical Bulletin. 1980;30:1766-1770.

62. Jeong ET, Jin MY, Kim MS, Chang YH, Park SG. Inhibition of melagenesis by piceid isolated from *Polygonum cuspidatum*. Archives of Phamacology Research. 2010;33:1331-1338.

63. Leu YL, Hwang TL, Hu JW. Anthraquinones from *Polygonum cuspidatum* as tyrosinase inhibitors for dermal use. Phytotherapy Research. 2008;22:552-556.

64. Wang ZH, Huang TN, Guo SF, Wang RH. Effects of emodin extracted from Rhizoma *Polygoni cuspidati* in treating HSV-1 cutaneous infection in guinea pigs. Journal of Anhui Traditional Chinese Medical College. 2003;22:36-39.

65. Yu CX, Zhang XQ, Kang LD, Zhang PJ, Chen WW, Liu WW, Liu QW, Zhang JY.

Emodin induces apoptosis in human prostate cancer cell LNCaP. Asian Journal of Andrology. 2008;10:625-634.

66. Kuo TC, Yang JS, Lin MW, Hsu SC, Lin JJ, Lin HJ, Hsia TC, Liao CL, Yang MD, Fan MJ, Wood WG. Emodin has cytotoxic and protective effects in rat C6 glioma cells: Roles of Mdr1a and nuclear factor Kappa B in cell survival. Journal of Pharmacology and Experimental Therapeutics. 2009;330:736-744.

67. Mazid AM, Datta KB, Nahar L, Bashar KMAS, Bachar CS, Saker SD. Phytochemical studies on *Polygonum barbatum* (L) hara var. barbatua

(Polygonaceae). Records of Natural Products. 2011;5(2):143-146.

68. Lopez SN, Manuel GS, Susana JG, Ricardo LF, Susana AZ. An unusual homoisoflavonone and a structurally-related dihydrochalcone from *Polygonum ferrugineum (Polygonaceae)*. Phytochemistry. 2006;67:2152-2158.

69. Bulbul L, Uddin MJ, Sushanta SM, Roy J. Phytochemical screening, anthelmintic and antiemetic activities of *Polygonum lapathifolium* flower extract. European Journal of Medicinal Plants. 2013;3:333–344.

9

Synergistic Antimicrobial and Antioxidant Activity of Saponins-Rich Extracts from *Paronychia argentea* and *Spergularia marginata*

Malika Ait Sidi Brahim[1], Mariam Fadli[2], Mohamed Markouk[1], Lahcen Hassani[2] and Mustapha Larhsini[1*]

[1]*Laboratory of Biotechnology, Protection and Valorization of Plant Resources; Phytochemistry and Pharmacology of Medicinal Plants Unit, Department of Biology, Faculty of Sciences Semlalia, Cadi Ayyad University, Marrakech, Association CNRST URAC35, Morocco.*
[2]*Laboratory of Biology and Biotechnology of Microorganisms, Department of Biology, Faculty of Science Semlalia, Cadi Ayyad University, Marrakech, Morocco.*

Authors' contributions

This work was carried out in collaboration between all authors. Author MASB performed all extraction, chemical and biological tests and achieved literature searches. Authors MF and LH contributed to the study of antimicrobial experiments and literature searches. Authors MM and ML designed the whole study, managed the literature searches, statistical analysis and revised the final version of the manuscript. All authors read and approved the final manuscript.

Editor(s):
(1) Shanfa Lu, Institute of Medicinal Plant Development, Chinese Academy of Medical Sciences & Peking Union Medical College, China.
(2) Marcello Iriti, Faculty of Plant Biology and Pathology, Department of Agricultural and Environmental Sciences, Milan State University, Italy.
Reviewers:
(1) Anonymous, Serbia.
(2) Sophia Wan-Pyo Hong, Dept. of Biology, Chungbuk National University (CBNU), Cheongju City, South Korea.
(3) M. V. N. L. Chaitanya, Pharmacognosy and Phytopharmacy, JSS College of Pharmacy, India.

ABSTRACT

Aims: The crude saponins extracted from the aerial parts of *Paronychia argentea* and the roots of *Spergularia marginata* were tested for their antioxidant, antimicrobial and synergistic effects with antibiotics.
Methodology: Antioxidant activity was evaluated using the 2,2-diphenyl-1-picryl-hydrazyl (DPPH) free radical, β-carotene-linoleic acid and reducing power assays. However, the antibacterial activity was assessed by the agar disc diffusion method, whereas the MIC determination and the

Corresponding author: E-mail: larhsini@uca.ma

synergistic interaction with antibiotics were evaluated using microdilution method.

Results: Saponins-rich extract from *Paronychia argentea* showed a higher antioxidant activity than that from *Spergularia marginata*. Using DPPH assay, the IC_{50} values for saponins-rich extracts from *P. argentea* and *S. marginata* were 19.08 and 29.65 µg/ml, respectively. For β-carotene-linoleic acid assay, IC_{50} values were 98.24 and 614 µg/ml respectively for *P. argentea* and *S. marginata*. However, for reducing power assays, the IC_{50} values for saponins-rich extracts from *P. argentea* and *S. marginata* were respectively 27.22 and 61.44 µg/ml. The result of MIC assay showed that both saponins-rich extracts was found to be active against the majority of *Candida* strains and Gram-positive bacteria. However, crude saponins extracted from *S. marginata* was more active on microorganisms than that from *P. argentea*. In fact, the *in vitro* association of saponin extracts and some commercial antibiotics showed a synergistic effect. For bacteria strains, 30 combinations were studied, 17 (56.66%) combinations had total synergism, 7 (23.33%) had partial synergism, 4 (13.33%) had no effect and 2 (6.66%) had antagonism effect. For *Candida* strains, 8 combinations of saponins extracts and fluconazol are tested. All of these combinations (100%) exhibited a total synergism with FICi ranging from 0,31 to 0,50.

Conclusion: The results founded suggested that further work should be performed on the isolation and identification of the antioxidative and antimicrobial components of these saponins-rich extracts.

Keywords: Antimicrobial; antioxidant activity; medicinal plants; Paronychia argentea; Spergularia marginata; synergistic activity; saponins.

1. INTRODUCTION

Paronychia argentea and *Spergularia marginata* are two indigenous plants belonging to the family of Caryophyllaceae which includes a large number of species rich in saponins with various pharmacological properties. *P. argentea* is a perennial plant, locally known as "hiddourtRaii". Infusion of *P. argentea* is commonly used in Moroccan popular medicine as aperitif and diuretic [1]. The uses of this plant in folk medicine differ from country to another. In Algeria, the plant is used as diuretic, hypoglycemic and as antiurolithiasis plant [2]. In Portugal, infusion of *P. argentea* is used as gastric analgesic, bladder and prostate ailments, abdominal ailments, and stomach ulcers [3]. In Jordan, it is used as diuretic, in treatment of kidney stones, diabetes and heart pains [4]. *S. marginata* is an annual plant native to Mediterranean area, usually used in traditional medicine for the treatment of female infertility as well as aphrodisiac [1].

Saponins have many pharmacological properties such as haemolytic, molluscicidal, anti-inflammatory, antifungal, antibacterial, antiparasitic and immunostimulant [5-7], anti-cancer [6,8] and antiproliferative [9]. Many studies have been dealing with the antimicrobial and antioxidant activities of saponins extracted from several plants [10,11]. However, no studies have been conducted to investigate the antioxidant and antimicrobial activities of saponins extracted from aerial part of *Paronychia argentea* and root part of *Spergularia marginata*.

The present study was undertaken to evaluate the antioxidant and antimicrobial activities of these saponins-rich extracts. Furthermore, the synergistic interaction using combination between saponin extracts and some usual antibiotics was also evaluated.

2. MATERIALS AND METHODS

2.1 Extraction of Crude Saponins

Aerial parts of *P. argentea* and roots of *S. marginata* were collected respectively from Oukaimeden (near to Marrakech) and Essaouira (Morocco) and identified by Prof. Abbad, Laboratory of Ecology Faculty of Sciences Semlalia, Marrakesh and voucher specimens are deposited at the Herbarium of the Faculty. Plants were dried at room temperature and ground into fine powder. The plant powders were extracted 3 times with methanol-water (v/v) and placed in an orbital shaker, set at 200 rpm for 24 h. The extracts were filtered and evaporated under reduced pressure to yield residues. The residues were suspended in hot water and extracted with water-saturated n-butanol. Crude saponin extracts were obtained by precipitation with Petroleum ether.

2.2 Detection of Saponins in Crude Extracts

2.2.1 Thin layer chromatography

20 µl of samples was applied by capillary on the line marked on silica gel 60 F254 TLC plates.

Then, TLC plate was placed into a separation chamber in presence of small amount of eluent. Subsequently, the plate was sprayed with the Godin reagent. Sprayed TLC plates were then heated at 100°C. Different spots were observed.

2.2.2 Determination of foaming index

2 mg of plants powder was transferred into an Erlenmeyer flask containing 100 ml of water. The mixture was boiled for 30 min, then cooled, filtered and transferred to 100 ml volumetric flask, sufficient water was added to make up the volume. The decoction was poured into the 10 test-tubes. After 15 min, the height of foam was measure [12].

2.3 Antioxidant Activity

2.3.1 DPPH radical assay

DPPH free radical-scavenging activity of saponins-rich extracts was assessed using a stable radical DPPH: 2,2-diphenyl-1-picrylhydrazyl [13,14]. Briefly, fifty microliters of saponins extracts at different concentrations ranging from 10 to 1000 µg/ml were mixed with 2 ml of DPPH methanol solution (60 µM). After 20 min of incubation in darkness, at room temperature, the absorbance was measured at 517 nm. A blank sample containing the same amount of methanol and DPPH solution was used as negative control. Synthetic antioxidant reagent Butylated hydroxytoluene (BHT) and quercetin were used as positive controls. All tests were carried out in triplicate and the results were expressed as mean±SD. The percentage of inhibition of the DPPH radical was calculated according to the formula:

DPPH scavenging effect (%) = $[(A_0 - A_1)*100]/A_0$

Where: A_0 is the absorbance of the control at 20 min, and A_1 is the absorbance of the sample at 20 min. IC_{50} is the concentration of antioxidant required for 50% scavenging of DPPH radicals and was calculated by plotting inhibition percentages against concentrations of the sample.

2.3.2 ß-Carotene/linoleic acid bleaching assay

The β-carotene–linoleic acid bleaching assay was assessed as described by Miraliakbari and Shahidi (2008) with slight modifications [15]. A solution of β-carotene–linoleic acid mixture was prepared as following: 0.5 mg of β-carotene was

dissolved in 1 ml of chloroform (HPLC grade), 25 µl of linoleic acid and 200 mg of Tween 40 was added. The chloroform was evaporated under vacuum using a rotary evaporator at 40°C. Then, 100 ml of distilled water was added and the mixture was shaking vigorously to form a clear yellowish emulsion (A). 2500 µl of this emulsion was dispersed in test tubes and 350 µl of various concentrations ranging from 10 to 1000 µg/ml of saponins extracts prepared previously in water was added. The test tubes were incubated for 2 h in a water bath at 50°C. The same procedure was repeated with positive control BHT and quercetine and with negative control (blank). A second emulsion (B) consisting of 25 µl of linoleic acid, 200 mg of Tween 40, 1 ml of chloroform and 100 ml of distilled water was prepared to adjust the zero of spectrophotometer. The absorbance values were measured at 470 nm immediately at the beginning of the experiment (t=0) and after 2h of incubation. Antioxidant activities (percentage inhibition I%) of the samples was calculated using the following equation:

I% = (A β-carotene after 2 h assay /A initial β-carotene) ×100

Where A β-carotene after 2 h assay is the absorbance values of β-carotene after 2 h assay remaining in the samples and A initial β-carotene is the absorbance value of β-carotene at the beginning of the experiment.

The antioxidant activity was expressed as 50% inhibition concentration (IC_{50}). The IC_{50} was calculated by plotting inhibition percentage against the extract concentration. All tests were carried out in triplicate and IC_{50} values were reported as means ±SD of triplicates.

2.3.3 Reducing power determination

The determination of reducing power was evaluated as described by Oyaizu (1986) [16]. Different concentrations ranging from 10 to 1000 µg/ml of saponins extracts were mixed with phosphate buffer (2.5 ml, 0.2 mol/L, pH 6.6) and potassium ferricyanide (K Fe $(CN)_6$) (2.5 mL, 1%). The mixture was incubated at 50°C for 20 min. Then, 2.5 mL of trichloroacetic acid (10%, w/v) was added to the mixture to stop the reaction, and the mixture was centrifuged at 650 × g for 10 min. At last, 2.5 mL of the supernatant was mixed with distilled water (2.5 mL) and ferric chloride $FeCl_3$ (0.5 mL, 1%) and the absorbance was measured at 700 nm against a blank. BHT and quercetin were used as reference compound. The extract concentration providing 0.5 of absorbance (IC_{50}) was calculated by plotting absorbance at 700 nm against the corresponding extract concentration. The test was carried out in triplicate and IC_{50} values were reported as means±SD.

2.4 Antimicrobial Activity

The crude saponins were screened against two Gram-negative bacteria: *Escherichia coli* (ATCC 25922), and a clinically isolated strain *Klebsiella pneumoniae*, three Gram-positive bacteria: *Micrococcus luteus* (ATCC 10240), *Staphylococcus aureus* (CCMM B3) and *Bacillus cereus* (ATCC 14579) and four candida: *Candida albicans* (CCMM L4), *Candida glabrata* (CCMM L7), *Candida krusei* (CCMM L10) and *Candida parapsilosis* (CCMM L18).

2.4.1 Disc diffusion method

The disc diffusion method is carried out to evaluate the antimicrobial activity of saponins extracted from *P. argentea* and *S. marginata* [17]. Suspensions prepared from overnight cultures of each microorganism were uniformly spread on a Mueller Hinton Agar (MHA) for bacteria and Sabouraud Dextrose Agar (DSA) for yeasts. Sterile paper discs (6mm in diameter) impregnated with 20 µl of saponins-rich extracts corresponding to 6 mg/disc of saponins extracts, were placed on the surface of each inoculated agar plates. Plates were placed at 4°C for 4 h and incubated for 24 h at 37°C for bacteria strains and 28°C for *Candida* strains. After incubation, the diameters of inhibition zones were measured in millimeter. Disc impregnated with sterile distilled water served as negative control and disc impregnated with antibiotics (Ciprofloxacin 5 µg/disc, Kanamycin 30 µg/disc, and Cefixime 10 µg/disc and Fluconazole 40 µg/disc) served as positive control. Each assay was performed in triplicates.

2.4.2 Determination of the minimum inhibitory concentration

MIC assay of saponins-rich extracts were assessed using micro-well dilution method [18]. Two-fold serial dilutions of saponins-rich extracts ranging from 1 mg/mL to 128 mg/mL were prepared in sterile distilled water. Then, three to four colonies of overnight cultures of each microorganism was inoculated into 5 ml of sterile nutrient broth and incubated for 3 to 5 h. 50 µl of this suspension was diluted in twice concentrated Mueller-Hinton Broth (MHB) for bacteria and Sabouraud dextrose broth (SDB) for yeasts to adjusted the culture to 10^6 CFU/mL for bacteria and $1-2 \times 10^3$ cells/mL for candida. Microwells containing 100 µl of saponin dilution were, separately, inoculated with 100 µl of bacterial or yeasts suspensions initially prepared. The inoculated microplates were incubated at 37°C for 18–24 h. The minimum inhibitory concentration (MIC) was defined as the lowest concentration of saponins-rich extracts inhibiting visible growth of the tested strains. The Minimum bactericidal concentration (MBC) and minimum fungicidal concentration (MFC) were determined by sub-culturing 10 µl of the MIC test solutions on nutrient agar plate for bacteria or PDA for yeasts and the plates were incubated in the same conditions. The MBC and MFC were defined as the lowest bactericidal and fungicidal concentration. Ciprofloxacin, cefixime, kanamycin and fluconazole were served as conventional antibiotics. All tests were performed in duplicate and repeated three times at least and the results were averaged.

2.4.3 Synergetic interaction

The synergistic interactions between conventional antibiotics (ciprofloxacin, kanamycin, and cefixime), and a classical antifungal (fluconazole), and saponin extracts from *P. argentea* and *S. marginata* were tested using the checkerboard essay method [19]. Synergy between antibiotics and saponins-rich extracts at low concentration (fraction of the MIC: MIC/4) was studied using microdilution assay. 50 µl of the saponins-rich extracts at MIC/4 were added to microwells containing, separately, 50 µl of antibiotics or antifungal dilutions, and inoculated with 100 µl of cell suspension of approximately 10^6 CFU/ml for bacteria and $1-2 \times 10^3$ cells/ml for yeasts. Then, the microwells were incubated in the same condition. All assays were performed in duplicate and repeated thrice.

-The gain was determined as MIC of antibiotic alone/MIC of antibiotic in combination with saponins extracts.

-Fraction inhibitory concentration index (FICI) was calculated by the method reported by Didry et al. [20], according to the following formula:

$$FICI = MIC_{A/B} /MIC_A + MIC_{B/A}/ MIC_B$$

where MIC_A = MIC of the compound A alone and $MIC_{A/B}$ is the MIC of compound A in combination with compound B. MIC_B and $MIC_{B/A}$ are defined in the same way as for compound A.

Total synergism (FICI ≤ 0.5), partial synergism (0.5<FICI ≤0.75), no effect (0.75 < FICI ≤ 2) or antagonism (FICI > 2) were evaluated.

3. RESULTS AND DISCUSSION

3.1 Detection of Saponins in Crude Extracts

As shown in Table 1, the yield of saponins crude extract of *P. argentea* was higher than that of *S. marginata*. However, the presence of persistent foam in aqueous extracts of both plants, calculated using the foaming index which was higher than 100%, indicated the presence of saponins.

The first indication of the presence of saponins in crude saponin extracts can be obtained by spraying Godin reagent on the TLC chromatogram. As can be seen from the TLC chromatogram (Fig. 1), crude saponins of *P. argentea* and *S. marginata* showed different spots with different Rf and colors (Table 2). Blue and purple blue spots indicated the presence of triterpenoids saponins [5]. This is in accordance with the result obtained with foaming index assay, which showed the presence of foam in aqueous extracts of the studied plants (foaming index higher than 100).

3.2 Antioxidant Activity

The antioxidant activity of saponins extracted from *P. argentea* and *S. marginata* was evaluated by three complementary tests: DPPH free radical scavenging, β-carotene-linoleic acid and reducing power activities [21]. DPPH was used to test the Free radical scavenging ability of tested saponins. As shown in Table 3, both saponins-rich extracts had a potent antioxidant activity, exhibiting ability to reduce the stable radical DPPH. Saponin-rich extract of *P. argentea* (IC_{50}=19.08 μg/ml±0.62) have a higher antioxidant activity than that from *S. marginata* (IC_{50}=29.65 μg/ml±0.40). Comparing IC_{50} values of saponins with those of synthetic antioxidant, the tested extracts were less potent than BHT and quercetin (4.21 μg/ml±0.08 and 1.07 μg/ml±0.01 respectively).

However, the results for β-carotene/linoleic acid bleaching test showed that saponin extract from *P. argentea* exhibited ability to inhibit conjugated dienehydroperoxides formation than that obtained from *S. marginata* with IC_{50} values of 98.24±0.48 μg/ml and 614±0.17 μg/ml respectively. Saponins-rich extracts were found to possess less antioxidant activity in comparison with BHT and quercetin (7.09 μg/ml±0.10 and 2.29 μg/ml±0.10 respectively).

Besides, the ability of saponins-rich extracts to donate an electron or hydrogen to Fe^{3+} to reduce Fe^{2+} was investigated. It can be seen from Table 3 that saponins extracted from *P. argentea* (27.22 μg/ml±0.57) and those from *S. marginata* (61.44 μg/ml±0.19) exhibited a potent capacity to reduce Fe^{3+}. Although, these saponins was less effective than BHT and quercetin (7.09 μg/ml± 0.10 and 2.29 μg/ml±0.10 respectively).

To our knowledge, no results from experiments with antioxidant activity of saponins extracted from *P. argentea* and *S. marginata* have been reported. While previous studies were conducted only on the antioxidant activity of *P. argentea* and *S. rubia* (same genus as *S. marginata*) methanolic and water extracts and demonstrated great activity for these extracts [3-22].

Many saponins are known by their antioxidant activity which can be related to the structure of their aglycones and the number of attached sugar residue [23]. As discussed above, saponins extracts of *P. argentea* and *S. marginata* exhibited high antioxidant activity, this is could be due to their structure and their surface-active. Huong et al. [24] have investigated the antioxidant activity of saponins from Vietnamese ginseng; and found that saponins exerted protective action against free radical-induced tissue injury. Another study reported that Triterpene saponins from *Butyrospermum parkii* of Cameroon showed an antioxidant activity using DPPH method [25].

3.3 Antimicrobial Activity

The antimicrobial and synergistic interactions with antibiotics were assayed *in vitro*. The crude saponins were screened against Gram-negative bacteria (*Escherichia coli*, and *Klebsiella pneumoniae*), Gram-positive bacteria (*Micrococcus luteus*, *Staphylococcus aureus* and *Bacillus cereus*) and candida (*Candida albicans*, *Candida glabrata*, *Candida krusei* and *Candida parapsilosis*). The results of disc diffusion method (Table 4) demonstrated that Gram-positive bacteria were the most sensitive being inhibited by the tested saponins extracts. *M. luteus* was the most sensitive with inhibition zones of 11.10±0.35 mm and 14.50±0.76 mm respectively for saponin extract of *P. argentea* and *S. marginata*. The studied saponin extracts had a weak effect on *E. coli* and no effect on *K. pneumoniae*. The inhibition zones of *Candida* strains showed an inhibition zone ranging from 10.37 to 15.73 mm and from 9.40 to 13.07 mm for extracts from *S. marginata* and *P. argentea* respectively.

Moreover, the results obtained for micro-well dilution method (Table 5), showed that both saponins-rich extracts were found to be active against all *Candida* strains except *C. krusei*. In fact, saponins-rich extract from *P. argentea* exhibited higher activity against *Candida* strains than those from *S. marginata*. The highest MIC value (4 mg/mL) was observed for extract from *S. marginata* against *C. albicans*, followed by *C. glabrata* and *C. parapsilosis*.

Table 1. Percentage yield and foaming index of crude saponins

	Yield of crude extract (%)	Foaming index (%)
P. argentea	3.2±0,41	275
S. marginata	2.5±0,15	200

Table 2. Rf values for crude saponin extracts on TLC silica gel

P. argentea crude saponins		*S. marginata* crude saponins	
Rf values	Spot color	Rf values	Spot color
0.13	Blue	0.11	Blue
0.30	Blue	0.34	Blue
0.44	Yellow	0.68	Blue
0.58	Blue	0.69	Blue
0.69	Blue	0.75	Blue
0.77	Yellow	0.85	Blue
0.90	Purple blue	0.90	Blue

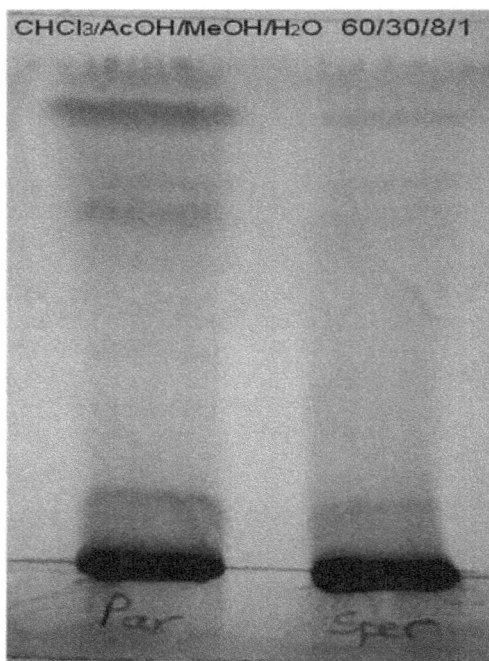

Fig. 1. TLC chromatogram of crude saponins extract on silica gel sprayed with the godin reagent. Chloroform / ethyl acetate / methanol / water (60: 30: 8: 1) used as solvent. par: crude saponin extract of *P. argentea*; Sper: saponin extract of *S. marginata*

Both saponins-rich extracts showed antimicrobial activity against tested Gram-positive bacteria. The MIC values for *P. argentea* were 8 and 16 mg/mL respectively for *M. luteus*, *B. cereus* and *S. aureus*. While the MIC values for those of *S. marginata* were 8 mg/mL for all Gram-positive bacteria. Furthermore, the crude saponins extracts had no effect on gram-negative bacteria

The MIC was equivalent to the MBC and MFC for *S. marginata* extract principally against *M. luteus*, *C. albicans* and *C. parapsilosis*, indicating a bactericidal action.

Synergistic interaction between antibiotics and saponins-rich extracts from *P. argentea* and *S. marginata* was also evaluated in this study. The results were presented in Table 6. For bacteria strains, 30 combinations were studied, 17 (56.66%) combinations had total synergism, 7 (23.33%) had partial synergism, 4 (13.33%) had no effect and 2 (6.66%) had antagonism effect. For Gram-positive bacteria, the best synergistic antibacterial action were obtained with the combination saponins-cefixime with total synergistic effect (FICi ranging from 0.38 to 0.49), followed by the combination saponins-kanamycin.

For *E. coli*, the best combination was saponins-ciprofloxacin with partial synergism (FICi=0.5). However, the three combinations of the both saponins-rich extracts and antibiotics had no effect on *K. pneumoniae*. For *Candida* strains, 8 combinations of saponins extracts and fluconazole are tested. All of these combinations (100%) exhibited a total synergism with FICi ranging from 0.31 to 0.50 (Table 7).

The obtained results showed that saponins extracted from *P. argentea* and *S. marginata* had an inhibitory effect on the growth of Gram-positive bacteria and no effect on Gram-negative bacteria. While, the tested extracts exhibited an anticandidal activity against *Candida* strains used in the study except *C. krusei*.

Several studies reported that saponins have antibacterial, antifungal and antiviral activities [10-26]. Our finding is in agreement with other study conducted on the crude saponins and saponins-rich fraction from *Guar meal*, which showed that crude saponins from this plant were active only against Gram-positive bacteria and not on Gram-negative ones. In contrast, saponin-rich fractions of Guar meal were active against both Gram-positive bacteria and Gram-negative bacteria [11]. Another study proved that saponins of *Sorghum bicolor* have an inhibitory effect on gram-positive bacteria but not on gram-negative one and fungi [10]. Whereas, saponins from *Anabasis articulate* exhibited a potent antimicrobial activity against Gram-negative and Gram-positive bacteria and *Candida albicans* [27].

The differences on ineffectiveness may be due to the degradation of saponins by some glucosidase enzymes produced by Gram-negative bacteria or may be saponins extracts could not be able to penetrate the cell membranes of the microorganisms [28]. In fact, Gram-negative bacteria are known by their resistance for commercial antibiotics. This could be explained by the structure of cell envelope; Gram-negative bacteria possess an additional membrane, termed outer membrane, delineating the periplasmic space with the cytoplasmic membrane that restricts diffusion of hydrophobic compounds [29].

Combined antibiotic therapy has been shown to delay the emergency of bacteria resistance and may also produce favorable synergistic effects in the treatment of bacterial infection. Drug synergism between known antibiotics and bioactive plant extracts is one of the novel ways to overcome the resistance mechanisms of bacteria. In this study, synergistic effect resulting from the combination of antibiotics and the crude saponins was studied. Our results showed that saponins extracts combined with antibiotics exhibited a high synergistic effect against most microbial strains and the MICs of antibiotic were reduced. Several studies on the interaction between plant extracts and antibiotics indicated a synergistic interaction [19,30,31]. Synergism effect between antimicrobial agent and water extracts of some plants was occurred in both sensitive and resistant strains but the magnitude of minimum fold inhibition in resistant strains was higher than the sensitive strains [32]. In fact, plant extracts combined with antibiotics showed a decrease in MIC and this can be explained by the presence of different phytochemicals product [33], which might inhibit bacteria by different mechanisms. The double attack of both agents on different target sites of the bacteria could theoretically lead either an additive or synergistic effect [34].

Table 3. Antioxidant activity of saponin extracts, BHT and quercetin

Tests	IC$_{50}$ µg/ml			
	Saponin extract of *P. argentea*	Saponin extract of *S. marginata*	BHT	Quercetin
DPPH	19.08±0.62	29.65±0.4	4.21±0.08	1.07±0.01
β-carotene-linoleic acid	98.24±0.48	614±0.17	4.30±0.33	0.95±0.02
Reducing power	27.22±0.57	61.44±0.19	7.09±0.1	2.29±0.10

Values represent means ± standard deviations for triplicate experiments

Table 4. Antimicrobial activity of saponin extracts and reference antibiotics against bacteria and *Candida* strains using disc diffusion method

Test bacteria	Saponin extracts		Inhibition zone diameter (mm)			
			Antibiotics			
	P. argentea (6 mg/disc)	*S. marginata* (6 mg/disc)	Cefixime (10 µg/disc)	Ciprofloxacin (5 µg/disc)	Kanamycin (30 µg/disc)	Fluconazole (40 µg/disc)
E. coli ATCC25922	7.00±0.10	8.17±0.17	19.33±0.80	30±0.58	22.00±1.15	
K. pneumoniae	NI	NI	10.33±0.30	7.83±0.93	NI	
M. luteus ATCC10240	11.10±0.35	14.50±0.76	20.17±0.44	29.67±0.88	25.00±1.15	NT
S. aureus CCMM B3	9.83±0.20	10.17±0.60	15.17±0.10	27.67±0.67	23.33±1.66	
B. cereus ATCC14579	7.90±0.46	9.33±0.33	26.33±0.30	35.67±0.88	37.00±2.19	
C. albicans CCMM L4	13.07±0.12	15.73±0.43				23.33±1.76
C. glabrata CCMM L7	11.17±0.17	13.25±0.20	NT			19.00±0.58
C. krusei CCMM L10	7.73±0.15	10.73±0.15				28.00±0.76
C. parapsilosis CCMM L18	9.40±0.10	12.20±0.12				32.17±0.73

-Values represent averages ±standard deviations for triplicate, -Inhibition zone including disc diameter (6 mm), - NI: No inhibition, NT: not tested

Table 5. Antimicrobial activity of antibiotics and saponins extracted from *P. argentea* and *S. marginata* using micro-well dilution method

	Saponin extracts				Antibiotics							
	P. argentea mg/ml		*S. marginata* mg/ml		Ciprofloxacin mg/ml		Cefixime mg/ml		Kanamycin mg/ml		Fluconazole mg/ml	
	MIC	MBC	MIC	MBC	MIC	MBC	MIC	MBC	MIC	MBC	MIC	MFC
E. coli ATCC25922	32	64	32	64	0.008	0.015	0.015	0.062	0.015	0.031		
K. pneumonia	64	>64	64	>64	0.250	>0.250	1	>1	0.500	>0.500		
S. aureus CCMM B3	16	32	8	16	0.031	0.125	0.062	0.125	0.125	>0.125	NT	
M. luteus ATCC10240	8	16	8	8	0.015	0.062	0.031	0.062	0.062	0.125		
B. cereus ATCC14579	16	32	8	32	0.015	0.031	0.015	0.062	0.062	0.125		
C. albicans CCMM L4	8	8	4	4							0.031	0.031
C. glabrata CCMM L7	8	32	8	16							0.500	>0.500
C. parapsilosis CCMM L18	16	32	8	8							0.062	0.125
C. krusei CCMM L10	>64	>64	>64	>64							0.250	0.500

NT: not tested. MIC: Minimum Inhibitory Concentration, MBC: Minimum Bactericidal Concentration, MFC: Minimum Fungicidal Concentration

Table 6. Synergistic interaction between *Paronychia argentea* and *Spergularia marginata* saponin extracts and antimicrobial agents against selected bacteria

strains	PA+ C		PA+CP		PA+K		SM+C		SM+CP		SM+K	
	FICi	Gain	FICi	Gain	FICi	Gain	FICi	Gain	FICi	Gain	FICi	Gain
E. coli	0.52b	4	0.50a	4	0.78b	2	0.78b	2	0.50 a	4	0.78b	2
K. pneumoniae	1.25c	1	2.30d	1	1.25c	1	1.25c	1	2.30 d	1	1.25c	1
S. aureus	0.49a	4	0.50a	4	0.75b	2	0.38 a	8	0.50 a	4	0.75b	2
M. luteus	0.38a	8	0.50a	4	0.38a	8	0.38 a	8	0.40 a	8	0.38a	8
B. cereus	0.38a	8	0.40a	8	0.49a	4	0.52b	4	0.50 a	4	0.49a	4

PA: saponins of P. argentea; SM: saponins of S. marginata; C: Cefixime ; CP: Ciprofloxacin; K: Kanamycin; FICi: Fractional inhibitory concentration. [a]Total synergism / [b]Partial synergism/ [c]No effect/. [d]Antagonism index, NT: not tested

Table 7. Synergistic interaction between *Paronychia argentea* and *Spergularia marginata* saponin extracts with fluconazole antimicrobial agent against selected yeasts

fungi	PA+F		SM+F	
	FICi	Gain	FICi	Gain
C. albicans	0.50a	4	0.38a	8
C. glabrata	0.31a	16	0.31a	16
C. parapsilosis	0.50a	4	0.38a	8
C. krusei	0.49a	4	0.50a	4

PA: saponins of *P. argentea*; SM: saponins of *S. marginata*; ; F: Fluconazole. FICi: Fractional inhibitory concentration. [a] Total synergism / [b] Partial synergism/ [c] No effect/. [d] Antagonism index, NT: not tested

The moderate activity of crude saponins extracted from *P. argentea* and *S. marginata* against some strains used in this study can be explained by the fact that the crude saponin extract is a mixture of several fractions each one could be as effective as antibiotics or even more effective than the popular antibiotics. In our laboratory fractionation of crude extracts is being undertaken in order to separate fractions more active than the crude extracts. Subsequently, fractionation may lead to pure saponins with a strong activity.

4. CONCLUSION

The results obtained in this study demonstrated that both crude saponins extracts had a remarkable antioxidant and antimicrobial activities. Saponins-rich extract from *Paronychia argentea* were more effective than that from *Spergularia marginata* as antioxidant. Furthermore, both saponin extracts was found to be active against the majority of *Candida* strains and Gram-positive bacteria. However, crude saponin extracted from *S. marginata* was more active on microorganisms than that of *P. argentea*.

In addition, the combinations between saponins-rich extract and classical antibiotics exhibited synergistic interactions against resistant bacteria and candida. The results founded suggested that further work should be performed on the isolation and identification of the antioxidative and antimicrobial components of these saponins extracts.

ACKNOWLEDGEMENTS

The authors are grateful to Centre National de la Recherche Scientifique et Technique (CNRST) in Morocco (URAC35) for financial support.

CONSENT

It is not applicable.

ETHICAL APPROVAL

It is not applicable.

COMPETING INTERESTS

Authors have declared that no competing interests exist.

REFERENCES

1. Bellakhdar J. La pharmacopée marocaine traditionnelle. Médecine arabe ancienne et savoirs populaires - Saint –Etienne, Edit. Ibis Press. 1997;249.
2. Bouanani S, Henchiri C, Migianu-Griffoni E, Aouf N, Lecouvey M. Pharmacological and toxicological effects of *Paronychia argentea* in experimental calcium oxalate nephrolithiasis in rats. J Ethnopharmacol. 2010;129(1):38-45.
3. Ferreira A, Proenca C, Serralheiro MLM, Ara´ujo MEM. The *In vitro* screening for acetylcholinesterase inhibition and antioxidant activity of medicinal plants from Portugal. J Ethnopharmacol. 2006;108(1):31-7.
4. Afifi FU, Al-Khalidi B, Khalil E. Studies on the in vivo hypoglycemic activities of two medicinal plants used in the treatment of diabetes in Jordanian traditional medicine following intranasal administration. J Ethnopharmacol. 2005;100(3):314-8.
5. Hostettman KA, Marston A. Chemistry and pharmacology of natural products, Saponins. Cambridge University Press, Cambridge; 1995.
6. Sparg SG, Light ME, van Staden J. Biological activities and distribution of plant saponins. J Ethnopharmacol. 2004;94(2):219–243.
7. Chapagain BP, Wiesman Z. Phyto-saponins as a natural adjuvant for delivery of agromaterials through plant cuticle

membranes. J Agric Food Chem. 2006; 54(17):6277-85.

8. Man S, Zhang WGY, Huang L, Liu C. Chemical study and medical application of saponins as anti-cancer agents and antiproliferative. Fitoterapia. 2010;81(7): 703-14.

9. Yannai EB, Ben-Shabat S, Goldschmidt N, Chapagain BP, Liu RH, Wiesman Z. Antiproliferative activity of steroidal saponins from *Balanites aegyptiaca*—An in vitro study. Phytochem. Lett. 2011;4(1): 43–47.

10. Soetan k, Oyekunle MA, Aiyelaagbe OO, Fafunso MA. Evaluation of the antimicrobial activity of saponins extract of *Sorghum bicolor* L. Moench. Afr. J. Biotechnol. 2006;5(23):2405-2407.

11. Hassan SM, Haq AU, Byrd JA, Berhow MA, Cartwright AL, Bailey CA. Haemolytic and antimicrobial activities of saponin-rich extracts from *Guar meal*. Food Chem. 2010;119(2):600–605.

12. Shah KK, Shiradkar MR, Bindu H V. Transdermal delivery of Aceclofenac: Effect of *Gymnema sylvestre* and *Caralluma adscendens* With Its Mechanism of Action. RJPBCS. 2011;2 (3):762-772.

13. Burits M, Bucar F. Antioxidant activity of *Nigella sativa* essential oil. Phytother Res. 2000;14(5):323-8.

14. Sahin F, Güllüce M, Daferera D, Sökmen A, Sökmen M, Polissiou M. Biological activities of the essential oils and methanol extract of *Origanum vulgare* ssp. vulgare in the Eastern Anatolia region of Turkey. Food Control. 2004;15(7):549–557.

15. Miraliakbari H, Shahidi F. Antioxidant activity of minor components of tree nut oils. Food Chem. 2008;111(2):421-427.

16. Oyaizu M. Studies on product of browning reaction prepared from glucose amine. Jpn J Nutr. 1986;44(6):307-315.

17. NCCLS– National Committee for Clinical Laboratory Standards. Performance Standards for Antimicrobial Disk Susceptibility Test, 6th ed. Approved Standard M2-A6, Wayne, PA; 1997.

18. Fadli M, Chevalier J, Saad A, Mezrioui NE, Hassani L, Pages JM. Essential oils from Moroccan plants as potential chemosensitisers restoring antibiotic activity in resistant Gram-negative bacteria. Int J Antimicrob Agents. 2011; 38(4):325-330.

19. Fadli M, Chevalier J, Saad A, Mezrioui NE, Hassani L, Pages JM. Antibacterial activity of *Thymus maroccanus* and *Thymus broussonetii* essential oils against nosocomial infection – bacteria and their synergistic potential with antibiotics. J Phymed. 2012;19(5):464-471.

20. Didry N, Dubreuil L, Pinkas M. Antibacterial activity of thymol, carvacrol and cinnamaldehyde alone or in combination. Pharmazie. 1993;48(4):301-304.

21. Aruoma OI. Methodological considerations for characterizing potential antioxidant actions of bioactive components in plant food. Mutat Res-Fund Mol M. 2003; 523(524):9-20.

22. Vinholes J, Grosso C, Andrade PB, Gil-Izquierdo A, Valentao P, Guedes de Pinho P, Ferreres F. *In vitro* studies to assess the antidiabetic, anti-cholinesterase and antioxidant potential of *Spergularia rubra*. Food Chem. 2011;129(2):454-462,

23. Ryu CS, Kim CH, Lee SY, Lee KS, Choung KJ, Song GY, Kim BH, Ryu SY, Lee HS, Kim SK. Evaluation of the total oxidant scavenging capacity of saponins isolated from *Platycodon grandiflorum*. Food Chem. 2012;132(1):333-337.

24. Huong NT, Matsumoto K, Kasai R, Yamasaki K, Watanabe H. *In-vitro* anti-oxidant activity of Vietnamese Ginseng saponin and its components. Biol Pharm Bull. 1998;21(9):978-81.

25. Tapondjou LA, Nyaa LB, Tane P, Ricciutelli M, Quassinti L, Bramucci M, Lupidi G, Ponou BK, Barboni L. Cytotoxic and antioxidant triterpene saponins from *Butyrospermum parkii* (Sapotaceae). Carbohydr Res. 2011;346(17):2699-2704.

26. Killeen G, Madigan C, Connolly C, Walsh G, Clark C, Hynes M, Timmins B, James P, Headon D, Power R. Antimicrobial saponins of *Yucca schidigera* and the implications of their in vitro properties for their in- vivo impact. J Agric Food Chem. 1998;46(8):3178–3186.

27. Maatalah M, Bouzidi NK, Bellahouel S, Merah B, Fortas Z, Soulimani R, Saidi S, Derdour A. Antimicrobial activity of the alkaloids and saponin extracts of *Anabasis articulate*. J Biotech and Pharm Res. 2012; 3(3):54-57.

28. Soetan KO. Evaluation of some pharmaceutical and haematological activities of saponins in guinea corn (*Sorghum bicolor* L Moench) M.Sc

Dissertation, Department of Biochemistry, College of Medicine, University of Ibadan; 2003.

29.   Tian F, Li B, Ji B, Yang J, Zhang G, Chen Y, Luo Y. Antioxidant and antimicrobial activities of consecutive extracts from *Galla chinensis*: the polarity affects the bioactivities. Food Chem. 2009;113,(1): 173–179.

30.   Nazer AI, Kobilinsky A, Tholozan JL, Dubois-Brissonnet F. Combinations of food antimicrobials at low levels to inhibit the growth of *Salmonella* sv. *Typhimurium*: a synergistic effect. Food Microbiol. 2005; 22(5):391–398.

31.   Rosato A, Vitali C, De Laurentis N, Armenise D, Milillo MA. Antibacterial effect of some essential oils administered alone or in combination with norfloxacin. Phytomed. 2007;14(11):727-732.

32.   Adwan G, Mhanna M. Synergistic Effects of Plant Extracts and Antibiotics on *Staphylococcus aureus* Strains Isolated from Clinical Specimens. Middle East J Sci Res. 2008;3(3):134-139.

33.   Duke JA, JoBogenschutz-Godwin M, DuCellier J, Duke PAK. CRC Handbook of Medical Plant. CRC press, Boca Raton, FL. 2003;348.

34.   Esimone CO, Iroha IR, CO Ude IG, Adikwu MU. In vitro interaction of ampicillin with ciprofloxacin or spiramycin as determined by the Decimal assay for additivity technique. Niger J Health biomed Sci. 2006;5(1):12–16.

10

Composition of Fatty Acids and Tocopherols Content in Oilseeds of Six Wild Selected Plants from Kahuzi-Biega National Park/DR. Congo

Kazadi Minzangi[1], Pius T. Mpiana[2], Bashwira Samvura[3], Archileo N. Kaaya[4], Matthäus Bertrand[5] and Justin N. Kadima[6*]

[1]*Department of Biology, Research Centre in Natural Substances CRSN/Lwiro, Official University of Bukavu, RD Congo.*
[2]*Faculty of Sciences, University of Kinshasa, P.O.BOX 190, Kinshasa XI, RD Congo.*
[3]*Department of Chemistry, Institute of Pedagogy Bukavu, RD Congo.*
[4]*Department of Food Technology and Nutrition, Makerere University, Kampala, Uganda.*
[5]*MRI - Max Rubner-Institut, Bundesforschungsinstitut für Ernährung und Lebensmittel, Food Department Working Group for Lipid Research, Schützenberg 12, 32756 Detmold, Germany.*
[6]*Department of Pharmacy, School of Medicine and Pharmacy, University of Rwanda, Rwanda.*

Authors' contributions

This work was carried out in collaboration between all authors. Authors KM, BS, JNK and PTM conceived experiment and designed the experiments. Authors KM, BS and MB performed experiments. Authors KM, JNK, MB, ANK and PTM analyzed the data. Authors KM, JNK, MB and PTM wrote the paper. All authors read and approved the final manuscript.

Editor(s):
(1) Marcello Iriti, Faculty of Plant Biology and Pathology, Department of Agricultural and Environmental Sciences, Milan State University, Italy.
Reviewers:
(1) Anonymous, Brazil.
(2) Anonymous, India.
(3) Zoue Lessoy Yves Thierry, University Felix Houphouet Boigny, Cote D'ivoire.

ABSTRACT

Objective: Kahuzi-Biega National Park (KBNP) in Democratic Republic of the Congo is packed with fantastic oilseed plants that need to be analysed in order to promote a sustainable exploitation for both commercial and food supply purposes. The study aimed to determine the content of Fatty acids (FAs) and Tocopherols in the oilseeds from *Eckebergia capensis* Sparrman (Meliaceae), *Entada abyssinica* Steud. ex A. Rich (Leguminosae), *Macaranga kilimandscharica* Pax

Corresponding author: E-mail: kntokamunda48@yahoo.com, kntokamunda@ur.ac.rw

(Euphorbiaceae), *Prunus africana* (Rosaceae), *Sesbania sesban* L. (Fabaceae) and *Telfairia pedata* (Cucurbitaceae) using gas liquid chromatography and HPLC.

Results: The respective oil yields for the six studied plants ranged from a minimum of 7.2% for *S. sesban* seeds to a maximum of 42.2% for *P. africana* seeds. Eighteen FAs were detected, of which, five saturated (SFAs), six monounsaturated (MUFAs) and seven polyunsaturated (PUFAs). The SFAs fraction was dominated by stearic acid varying from 5.95 % in *M. kilimandscharica* oil to 76.19% in *P. africana* oil. The content in PUFAs fraction represented by linoleic acid an omega-6 fatty acid varied from 3.19% in *P. africana* oil to 58.82% in *S. sesban* oil while alpha-linolenic acid an omega-3 accounted for 0.32% in *P. africana* oil to 5.88% in *S. sesban* oil. The MUFAs fraction represented by oleic acid an omega-9 fatty acid varied from 3.4% in *P. africana* oil to 41.77% in *T. pedata* oil. The highest content of tocopherols was 10.9 mg/100 g in *S. sesban* oil, followed by *E. abyssinica* (7.9 mg/100 g) and *M. kilimandscharica* oil (4.9 mg/100 g).

Conclusion: The findings will help select the appropriate plant for specific desired FAs and tocopherols.

Keywords: Oilseed plants; Kahuzi-Biega National Park; fatty acids; tocopherols.

1. INTRODUCTION

Many studies have reported about the nutritional, medical and industrial benefits of oilseed plants [1-5]. The profiles of FAs give good information on both the nutritional quality and the performance of raw materials used for industrial applications [6]. At the public health level, it has been claimed that about one-third of the world's population –mostly children and women – are deficient in at least one essential nutriment that can be provided by consuming oilseeds [7]. Oilseeds contain energy, nutrients including vitamins and minerals, and other health beneficial components such as antioxidants.

Edible vegetable oils mainly consist of triglycerides with various fatty acids (FAs) which are responsible for their nutritional and physicochemical properties. Besides the major FAs present, several phytochemical detectable in oils may include phenolic and polyphenolic compounds, tocopherols and carotenoids as active molecules [8]. There is direct relationship between total phenolic content and antioxidant capacity of food. Carotenoids and tocopherols are essential vitamins that have particular nutritional and protective properties from their antioxidant activity. Tocopherols are kind of fat-soluble vitamin-E isomers. They possess potent antioxidant properties that make them anti-inflammatory, antimutagenic and antitumor potentials [9,10].

Nowadays, as the global human population continues growing, there is steadily more need to find alternative sources of FAs and tocopherols

that could be used as food supplement without increasing final product costs.

Kahuzi-Biega National Park (KBNP) in the Democratic Republic of the Congo (DRC) is packed with fantastic oilseed plants that need to be analysed in order to promote a sustainable exploitation for both commercial and food supply purposes. KBNP is a very vast expanse of dense primary tropical forest situated within the species-rich Albertine Rift. The Park is home of Grauer's Gorilla endemic to the region. KBNP has an exceptional high floral diversity with over 1,100 recorded species, of which 145 are endemic to the Albertine Rift [11]. Situated in one of the most densely populated regions of DRC, the threats for KBNP are settlements and land clearing for agriculture, poaching and hunting for bush meat, logging and mineral extraction [12]. Thus some important plant species in KBNP and surrounding areas are threatened with extinction [13].

A series of endeavours and studies have been undertaken to scientifically highlight the value of oilseed plants growing in KBNP by documenting their nutriment composition in order to validate and valorise their uses [6]. In the present study we have selected six wild plants surrounding KBNP, used by the local populations mainly for nutrition and medical purposes, to evaluate the oil yield and determine the composition of FAs and tocopherols in those species. These plants are: *Eckebergia capensis* Sparrman (Meliaceae); *Entada abyssinica* Steud Ex.A.Rich (Leguminosae); *Macaranga kilimandscharica* Pax (Euphorbiaceae); *Prunus africana* (Rosaceae); *Sesbania sesban* L. (Fabaceae);

and *Telfairia pedata* (Cucurbitaceae). Their photos in Fig.1 could help recognize them. They are all evergreen trees found in Afromontane forests that are growing in different parts of Africa and some are commercialized [14-19]. They are resorted in folk medicines to be aperient, diuretic, emetic, emmenagogue, febrifuge, laxative, tonic, antiviral, etc. *Prunus africana* is used to treat benign prostate hyperplasia. *Telfairia* seeds are eaten raw or cooked and nuts are especially mentioned as source of food for women during the lactating period. After oil extraction the residue makes a valuable cake for livestock feeding [20]. Some studies have been undertaken on species from other countries to identify the bioactive chemicals from bark extracts and FAs from oilseeds, but not yet on the species from KBNP.

2. MATERIALS AND METHODS

2.1 Oil Extraction and Quantification

Around 500 g of oilseeds were handily harvested from wild plants in the park and brought to the phytochemistry laboratory of CRSN/L "Centre de Recherche en Sciences Naturelles de Lwiro" where they were before sun dried during 5-8

days and then completed at 105°C in oven for 1-3 hours (model Boekel, Arthur H. Thomas Co. Philadelphia, USA). After drying, the seeds were shelled by hand to expel the kernels and then crushed with a coffee-mill (model Corona 01 Landers & CIA.SA) to produce fine seed flours. The respective fine flours were extracted by repeated washing with petroleum ether (boiling point 40⁻60°C) using the Soxhlet's procedure [20] for 8 hours. The oil dissolved in petroleum ether was filtered through filter paper and the solvent evaporated under vacuum in a rotary evaporator model Eyala of Tokyo Rikakikai Co. Ltd. The remaining solvent traces were removed by heating the flask containing the oil in water bath (50°C). The oil content was weighted and the yield expressed as percent of the fine flour mass.

2.2 Determination of Fatty Acids Content by GC

The fatty acid composition was determined following the ISO standard ISO 5509:2000 [21]. In brief, one drop of the oil was dissolved in 1 mL of n-heptane; 50 µg of sodium methylate was added, and the closed tube was agitated vigorously for 1 min at room temperature.

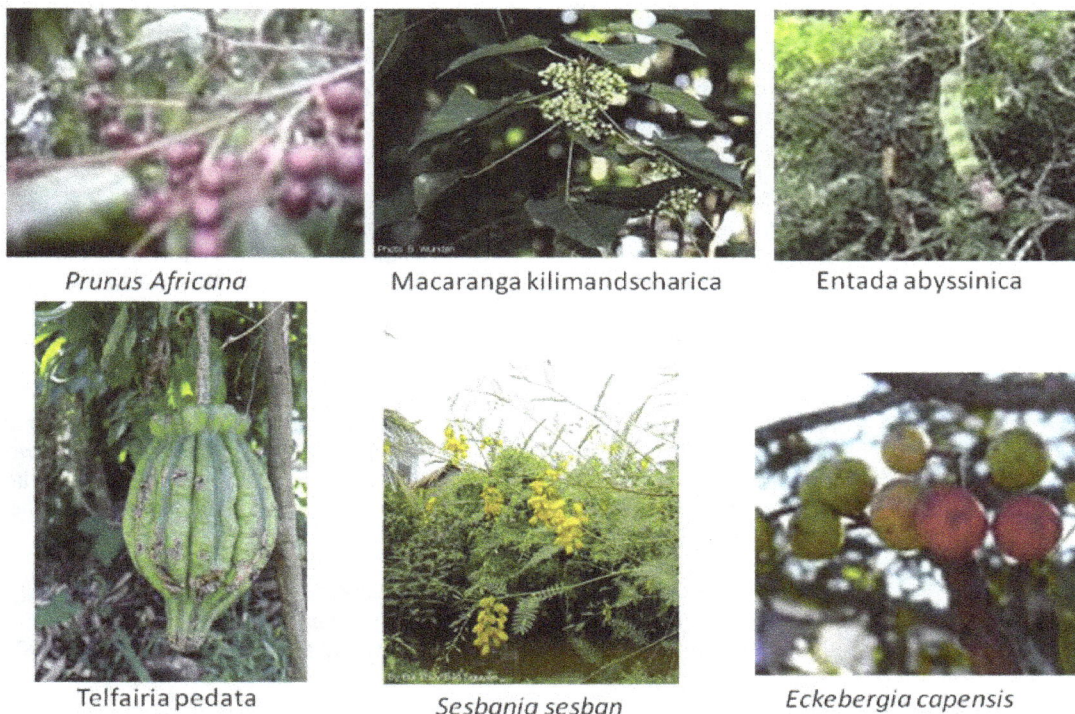

Prunus Africana   Macaranga kilimandscharica   Entada abyssinica

Telfairia pedata   *Sesbania sesban*   *Eckebergia capensis*

Fig. 1. Photography of the six studied plants

After addition of 100 µL of water, the tube was centrifuged at 4500 g for 10 min and the lower aqueous phase was removed. Then 50 µL of HCl (1 mol with methyl orange) was added, the solution was shortly mixed, and the lower aqueous phase was rejected. About 20 mg of sodium hydrogen sulphate (monohydrate, extra pure; Merck, Darmstadt, Germany) was added, and after centrifugation at 4500 g for 10 min, the top n-heptane phase was transferred to a vial and injected in a Varian 5890 gas chromotograph with a capillary column, CP-Sil 88 (100 m long, 0.25 mm ID, film thickness 0.2 µm). The temperature program was as follows: from 155°C; heated to 220°C (1.5°C/min), 10 min isotherm; injector 250°C, detector-FID 250°C; carrier gas 36 cm/s hydrogen; split ratio 1:50; detector gas 30 mL/min hydrogen; 300 mL/min air and 30 mL/min nitrogen; manual injection volume less than 1 µL. The peak areas were computed by the integration software, and percentages of fatty acid methyl esters (FAMEs) were obtained as weight percent by direct internal normalization (methyl tricosanoate C23:0 internal standard). The peaks were recognized, based on their retention times (RT) using standard FAMEs.

2.3 Determination of Tocopherols Content

For determination of tocopherols, the DGF F-II 4a method was used [22,23]. In brief, a solution of 250 mg of oil in 25 mL of n-heptane was directly used for the HPLC. The HPLC analysis was conducted using a Merck-Hitachi low-pressure gradient system, fitted with a L-6000 pump (Merck-Hitachi, Darmstadt, Germany), a Merck-Hitachi F-1000 fluorescence spectrophotometer (Darmstadt, Germany, detector wavelengths for excitation 295 nm, for emission 330 nm), and a ChemStation integration system (Agilent Technologies Deutschland GmbH, Böblingen, Germany). The samples in the amount of 20 µL were injected by a Merck 655-A40 autosampler (Merck-Hitachi, Darmstadt, Germany) onto a Diol phase HPLC column 25 cm × 4.6 mm ID (Merck, Darmstadt, Germany) used with a flow rate of 1.3 mL/min. The mobile phase used was n-heptane/tert-butyl methyl ether (99 + 1, v/v). The mobile phase used was 99 mL n-heptane + 1 mL tert-butyl methyl ether. The mean values were given in the tables, without the standard deviation, because this

value would represent only the deviation of the method and not the variation of the appropriate sample.

3. RESULTS

The respective oil yields for the six plants studied are shown in the Table 1. These values ranged from a minimum of 7.2% for S. sesban seeds to a maximum of 42.2% for P. africana seeds.

Fig. 2 shows that P. africana and E. capensis seed oils are rich in saturated FAs (SFAs), while mono-unsaturated (MUFAs) were in T. pedata and M. kilimandscharica oils and polyunsaturated (PUFAs) in S. sesban oil.

Table 2 shows the distribution of the eighteen FAs detected, of which, five were SFAs including Palmitic (16:0), Stearic (18:0), Arachidic (20:0), Behenic (22:0), and Lignoceric (24:0); six were MUFAs including Palmitoleic (16:1D9), Elaidic (18:1), Oleic(18:1D9), Vaccenic (18:1D11, Eicosenoic (20:01), 11-Eicosenoic (20:1 11); and seven were PUFAs consisting of Linoelaidicic (18:2trans1), Linoleic (18:2), α-Linolenic (18:3), Eicosadienoic (20:2 11,14), Eicosatrienoic (20:3 5,11,14), Eicosatetraenoic (20:4 5,11,14,17) and Eicosatetraenoic (20:4).

The SFAs fraction was dominated by stearic acid (C18:0) varying from 5.95 % in M. kilimandscharica to 76.19% in P. africana oils. The fraction of MUFAs is represented by linoleic acid (LA 18:1 D9) an omega-6 from 3.19% in P. africana oil to 58.82% in S. sesban oil. The PUFAs fraction is represented by linoleic acid (C18:2) an omega-9 fatty acid from 3.4% for P. africana oil to 41.77% for T. pedata oil. Alpha-linolenic acid (ALA 18:3) an omega-3 accounted from 0.32% for P. africana to 5.88% for S. sesban oil.

In addition to the common FAs, very long-chain FAs (VLCFAs) with 20 carbons or more were detected in the investigated samples particularly in M. kilimandscharica and P. africana, and less in S. sesban oil.

Table 3 indicates that the high content of tocopherols was in S. sebsban oil (10.9mg/100g), E. abyssinica oil (7.9 mg/100 g) and M. kilimandscharica oil (4.9 mg/100 g).

Table 1. Scientific name, local name and seed oil content of wild oilseed plants from Kahuzi-Biega National Park, kivu, DR. Congo

Plant scientific name		Family	Local name	Oil yield (%W/W)
EC	Eckebergia capensis Sparrman	Meliaceae	Kaobeobe	22.3%
EA	Entada abyssinica Steud. ex A. Rich	Leguminosae	Cishangishangi	36.1%
MK	Macaranga kilimandscharica Pax	Euphorbiaceae	Mushesha (Shi)	9.2%
PA	Prunus africana	Rosaceae	Muhumbahumba	42.2%
SS	Sesbania sesba L.	Fabaceae	Munyegenyege	7.2%
TP	Telfairia pedata	Cucurbitaceae	Muhirehire	29.3%

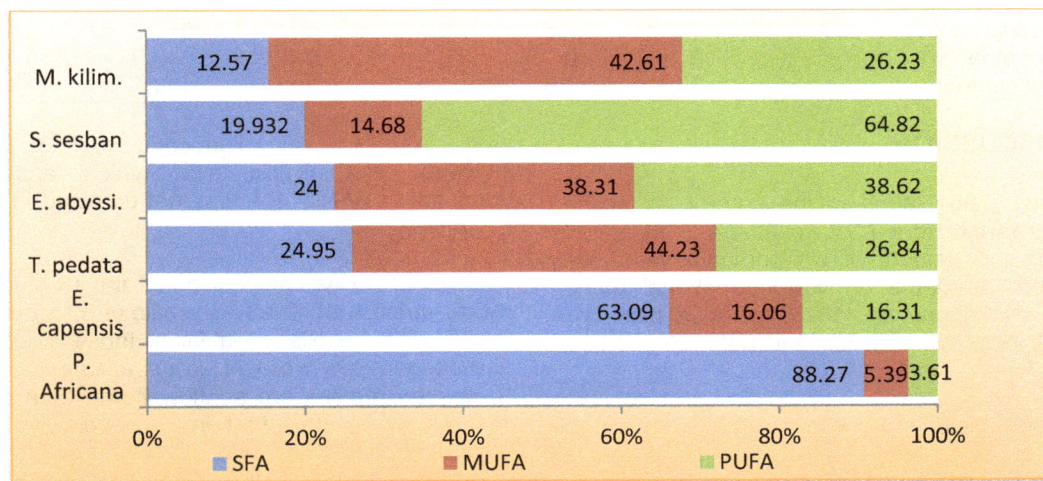

Fig. 2. Variation of saturated (SFAs), monounsaturated (MUFAs) and polyunsaturated (PUFAs) Fatty acid fractions in oils of six wild oilseed plants from KBNP/ DR. Congo

Table 2. Fatty acids composition (%w/w) in oils of six wild oilseed plants from KBNP/DR. Congo

Fatty acids	Plant abbreviation and content in % (w/w)					
	EC.	EA.	MK.	PA.	SS.	TP.
Palmitic (16:0)	6.83	11.00	4.22	3.78	13.32	14.06
Palmitoleic (16:1D9)	0.14	-	-	0.85	-	0.6
Stearic (18:0)	51.12	8.36	5.95	76.19	5.98	9.13
Elaidic (18:1)	-	-	8.23	-	-	-
Oleic (18:1 D9)	14.46	37.09	32.00	3.40	13.73	41.77
Vaccenic (18:1 D11)	0.32	0.52	0.23	0.12	0.63	0.68
Linoelaidicic (18:2 trans1)	-	-	2.66	-	-	-
Linoleic (18:2)	14.66	36.77	12.63	3.19	58.82	22.03
α-Linolenic (18:3)	1.17	0.42	1.07	0.32	5.88	0.74
Arachidic (20:0)	5.03	2.34	0.82	8.18	0.53	0.88
Eicosenoic (20:01)	0.57	-	-	-	-	-
11-Eicosenoic (20:1 11)	0.57	0.7	2.15	1.02	0.32	1.18
Eicosadienoic (20:2 11,14)	0.19		3.25		0.12	1.17
5,11,14-Eicosatrienoic (20:3 5,11,14)	-	-	2.34	-	-	-
5,11,14,17-Eicosatetraenoic (20:4 5,11,14,17)	0.29	-	3.64	-	-	2.22
Behenic (22:0)	0.11	-	1.05	0.12	0.39	0.88
Eicosatetraenoic (20:4)	-	1.43	0.64	0.1	-	0.68
Legnoceric (24:0)	-	2.3	0.53	-	-	-

EC (eckebergia capensis sparrman) , EA (entada abyssinica steud. ex A. Rich) , MK (macaranga kilimandscharica pax), PA (prunus africana), SS (sesbania sesba L.) TP (telfairia pedata)

Table 3. Tocopherols content in oils of six wild oilseed plants from KBNP/ DR. Congo

Tocopherols type	Plants and tocopherols content (mg/100g oil)					
	EC	EA	MK	PA	SS	TP
α-Tocopherol	0	0.1	0.1	0	3.8	0.3
α-Tocotrienol	0.1	0.1	0.1	0.1	0.2	0.1
β-Tocopherol	2.2	2.3	3.2	1.8	1.7	1.4
γ-Tocopherol	0.1	3.9	0	0	4.4	0.1
β-Tocotrienol	0	0	0	0	0	0
Plastochromanol-8	0	0.1	0.1	0	0	0
γ-Tocotrienol	0.8	0.8	1.5	0.6	0.7	0.5
δ-Tocopherol	0	0.6	0	0	0	0
δ-Tocotrienol	0	0	0	0	0	0
Total content	3.2	7.9	5.0	2.5	10.8	2.4

4. DISCUSSION

The oil yields found in the current six studied plants range from 7.2% to 42.2%. This yield is satisfactory enough if we compare with many oilseeds available on the international market such as cottonseed (18-25%), soya bean (15-20%), peanut (45-55%), and palm oil (30-60%) [24-27].

The oil yield may vary with the extractive methods used. For example, Malimo sylvia [28] compared the yield of extraction of oyster nut (*Telfairia pedata* Sims Hook) and found that Soxhlet process was the best of the three methods used. It gave an oil yield of 63.9% while the biotechnical rotar evaporation gave 28.0% and with centrifugation, it gave 30.3% oil yield. The oil yield by soxhlet method combined with rotar evaporation in our *T. pedata* species averaged 30%.

The content of FAs in oilseeds may vary with the origin of the plants. For instance *T. pedata* seed oil has been reported by Okoli [29] as containing linoleic acid (32.5%), palmitic acid (24.5%), stearic acid (18%), oleic acid (11.5%) and 5% of Alpha-linoleic acid. In the current species, we have found linoleic acid (22%), palmitic acid (14%), stearic acid (9%) and oleic acid (42%) not mentioning polyunsaturated derivatives.

Abyssinian oil (Lotioncrafter LLC) was promoted as new natural seed *oil* with an ultra light, non-greasy skin feel as it contains a high percentage of unsaturated C22 fatty acids [15]. The fatty acid profile of the marketed FANCOR® Abyssinian Oil is typically presented as containing palmitic (1-4%), palmitoleic (0.1-0.5%), stearic (0.5-2%), oleic (10-25%), linoleic (7-15%), linolenic (2-5%), arachidic (0.5-2%), eicosenoic (2-6%), eicosadienoic (0-0.5%), behenic (1-3%), erucic

acid (50-65%), and lignoceric (0-1%) [15]. However, the Erucic acid which appears dominant in FANCOR® was not detected in our *E. abyssinica* oil.

The profile of FAs composition of the six studied plants varied a lot. The FAs profile of *E. capensis* and *P. africana* oils is similar to those of butter and coconut oils while *M. kilimandscharica* and *S. sesban* profiles are sunflower and corn oils-like. Fig. 1 showed that in *T. pedata* and *E. abyssinica* oils there was equilibrium between SFAs, MUFAs and PUFAs fractions while SFAs dominate in *E. capensis* and *P. africana*, MUFAs in *M. kilimandscharica* and PUFAs in *S. sesban*.

Thus, *T. pedata*, *S. sesban* and *E. abyssinica* oils could have great economic value as oleic acid sources in comparison to 59-75% found in the pecan oil, 61% in canola oil, or 20-85% reported for peanut oil and sunflower oil [30].

Stearic acid is the highest molecular weight SFA occurring abundantly in fats and oils. It occurs in small quantities in seed and marine oils. Besides its major food sources for adults that are meat/poultry/fish, grain products, and milk/milk products, stearic acid is also found in Cocoa butter (55%), Mutton tallow(41%), Beef tallow(38%), Lard(34%), Butter(19%), Soybean oil(26%), Coconut oil(3%), Olive oil(14%) and Corn oil(14.%) [30]. In the current studied plant oils, *P. africana* and *E. capensis* oils are rich in stearic acid (76.2% and 51.1% respectively), making them worth sources for this FA.

Unlike other predominant long-chain SFAs – palmitic (C16:0), myristic (C14:0), and lauric (C12:0) acids - which increase blood cholesterol levels - stearic acid has been shown to have a neutral effect on blood total and low density lipoprotein (LDL) cholesterol levels [31,32].

Stearic acid's neutral effect on blood total and LDL cholesterol levels implies that this long-chain SFA may not increase the risk for cardiovascular disease. For this reason, it has been suggested that stearic acid not be grouped with other long-chain SFAs, although to date this recommendation has not been implemented in dietary guidance or nutrition labeling [31,32].

The study of Dambatt and Ogah in Kenya [33] found that the oil content of the *S. sesban* seed extracted with 40/60 petroleum ether in a Soxhlet apparatus yielded 4.6% and FAs detectable by GLC were oleic (87.4%), palmitic (10.8%), caprylic (0.4%), and caproic (0.8%). For this study, *S. sesban* oil yielded 7.2% and the major FA is lineloic acid (55%); palmitic and oleic acid accounted instead for only 13% each. Furthermore, the oil of *S. sesban* species contains enough amount of omega-3 ALA (5.88%) compared to soybean which is commercial source of ALA or to other commercial oils such as peanut oil (0.4%), sesame oil (0.4%) and sunflower oil (0.5%).

However the ratio of omega-6 to omega-3 FAs is 12:1 for *M. kilimandscharica*, 10:1 for *P. Africana*, 10:1 for *S.sesban*, 20:1 for *T. pedata*, 13:1 for *E. capensis*, and 88:1 for *E. abyssinica*. The current recommended dietary ratio of omega-6:omega-3 FAs is about 10:1 according to FAO guideline while Modern Western diets exhibit omega-6: omega-3 ratios ranging between 15:1 and 17:1[34,35]. Thus only *T. pedata*, and *E. abyssinica* have bad ratios. It has been said that excessive amount of LA and a very high LA/ALA ratio could trigger or enhance the pathogenesis of many diseases, including coronary heart disease (CHD), cancer, inflammation and autoimmune diseases [35]. Due to the opposing effects of omega-3 and omega-6 fatty acids, a healthy diet should contain a balanced omega-6: omega-3 ratio. Epidemiology and dietary intervention studies have demonstrated that while an exceptionally high omega-6: omega-3 ratio promotes the development of many chronic diseases, a reduced omega-6: omega-3 ratio can prevent or reverse these diseases [35].

Groundnut oil which has arachidic acid (AA) content ranging from 2 to 4% is known as the vegetable source of this FA. In the studied plants, *E. abyssinica*, *E. capensis* and *P. africana* oils had 2.34%, 5.03% and 8.18% of AA respectively.

There is surprisingly very high amount of *trans*-FAs in *S. sesban* seed oil containing 8.23% of *trans*-oleic (Elaidic acid) and 2.66% of *trans*-LA (Linoelaidicic acid). High amounts of *trans* fats correlate with circulatory diseases such as atherosclerosis and chronic heart disease more than the same amounts of non-*trans* fats [33-37]. The maximum content recommended for *trans*-acids in food products is 1.0% [36]. Dietary *trans*-acids come mainly from oil partial hydrogenation, in dairy fats where they are formed by bio-hydrogenation in the rumen, and through exposure to high temperatures [38-40]. Thus, the presence of trans-FAs in *S. sesban* oil could be attributed to erroneous exposition to high temperature during the processing method precisely during oil extraction.

In addition to the common FAs, very long-chain FAs (VLCFAs) with aliphatic tails longer than 22 carbons were detected in the investigated samples particularly in *M. kilimandscharica* seed oil and *P. africana* seed oil. *M. kilimandscharica* seed oil and *P. africana* seed oil as new sources of VLCFAs oils for industry.

VLCFAs are important in the oleo-chemical industry where they cover about 6% of the industry requirements in FAs [41,42]. They are used specifically in the manufacturing of some products such as high-grade candles. There are comparatively few common vegetal fats that contain appreciable amounts of VLCFAs. They are currently produced by transgenetic modification of some plant species [41]. However, for nutrition, unlike most fatty acids, VLCFAs are too long to be metabolized in the mitochondria, and must be metabolized in peroxisomes. Certain peroxisomal disorders, such as adrenoleukodystrophy, can be associated with an accumulation of VLCFAs [43].

Tocopherols and Tocotrienols are natural form of vitamin E. The main recognized biochemical function of tocopherols is the protection of polyunsaturated FAs against peroxidation. They display antioxidant activity which protects the body tissues against the damaging effects, caused by the free radicals resulting from many normal metabolic functions [44-46]. Most food plants contain low to moderate levels of vitamin E activity. Soybean oil is the most consumed vegetable oil in the world, representing 30% of the consumption in the worldwide market. Soybean deodorizer distillate (SODD), a deodorized byproduct is an alternative to marine animals as natural source of squalene and as a good raw material for the production of fatty acid steryl esters (FASEs), free phytosterols, and tocopherol [47].

In the investigated plants, *S. sesban* seed oil is rich in tocopherols content (10.7 mg/100 g) followed by *E. abyssinica* seed oil (7.9 mg/100 g) and *M. kilimandscharica* seed oil (4.9 mg/100 g). Plastochromanol-8 which is among the major vitamin E components in olive oil is only in traces in *E. abyssinica* and *M. kilimandscharica* (0.1 mg /100 g). Moreover, *E. abyssinica* is rich in beta (2.3 mg/100 g) and gamma (3.9 mg/kg) tocopherols, while *S. sesban* oil has mixed alpha (3.8 mg/kg), and gamma (4.4 mg/100 g) tocopherols. *S. sesban* and *E. abyssinica* oils are the most appropriate as sources of tocopherols.

Alpha-tocopherol is the form of vitamin E that is the most active tocopherol against peroxyl radicals (LOO·); delta-tocopherol is the least active (alpha>beta=gamma>delta) [48,49]. Beta-tocopherol is a natural tocopherol with less antioxidant activity than alpha-tocopherol. Gamma-tocopherol is the major form of vitamin E in many plant seeds and in the US diet, but has drawn little attention compared with alpha-tocopherol [48]. Despite the fact that studies are controversial, recent studies indicate that gamma-tocopherol may be important to human health and that it possesses unique features that distinguish it from alpha-tocopherol. Unlike alpha tocopherol, gamma tocopherol is a potent defender against reactive nitrogen oxides. Furthermore, gamma tocopherol has been found to reduce inflammation, regulate factors that guard against certain cancers and activate genes involved in protecting against Alzheimer's disease [48]. Mixed tocopherols help prevent cardiovascular disease.

5. CONCLUSION

The findings could help select the appropriate plant for specific desired FAs. *Eckebergia capensis and Entada abyssinica* have arachidic acid content similar and even above that of groundnut oil and can serve as alternative sources of that fatty acid. *Telfairia pedata, Sesbania sesban* and *Entada abyssinica* oils could be considered as new sources of oleic acid while *Prunus africana* and *Eckebergia capensis* oils rich in stearic acid can be replacer of commercial oil sources of this last fatty acid. *Sesbania sesban* and *Entada abyssinica* seed oils may be suitable oil seed crop for the various industries due to their very low content of

linolenic and high content of linoleic acid. The fatty acid profiles of *Eckebergia capensis* and *Prunus Africana* seed oils are similar to those of Butter and coconut oil while those of *Macaranga kilimandscharica* and *Sesbania sesban* are similar to those of Sunflower and Corn oils. Thus they can be substitutes to these expensive fats and oils.

CONSENT

It is not applicable.

ETHICAL APPROVAL

It is not applicable.

COMPETING INTERESTS

Authors have declared that no competing interests exist.

REFERENCES

1. Riediger ND, Othman RA, Suh M, Moghadasian MH. A systemic review of the roles of n-3 fatty acids in health and disease. J Am Diet Assoc. 2008;109(4): 668-79.
2. Bazinet RP, Layé S. Polyunsaturated fatty acids and their metabolites in brain function and disease. Nature Reviews Neuroscience. 2014;15:771–785.
3. Chen Z, Zhang Y, Jia C, Wang Y, Lai P, Zhou X, Wang Y, Song Q, Jun Lin, Ren Z, Gao Q, Zhao Z, Zheng H, Wan Z, Gao T, Zhao A, Dai Y, Bai X. mTORC1/2 targeted by n-3 polyunsaturated fatty acids in the prevention of mammary tumorigenesis and tumor progression. Oncogene. 2014;33: 4548–4557.
4. Akoh CC, Min DB, et al. Food Lipids: Chemistry, Nutrition, and Biotechnology, 2nd ed., Marcel Dekker, Inc., New York; 2002.
5. Scrimgeour C. Chemistry of Fatty Acids Scottish Crop Research Institute Dundee, Scotland.
   Available:www.media.johnwiley.com.au/pr oduct_data/excerpt/22/.../0471385522.pdf; accessed March 3rd 2015.
6. Bavhure B, Kasali FM, Mahano AO, Kazadi M, Matabaro A, Mwanga I, Kadima, NJ. Fatty Acid Composition of *Lebrunia bushiae* Staner and *Tephrosia vogelii* Hook.f. Seed Oils. European Journal of Medicinal Plants. 2014;4(7):844-853.

7.   Tulchinsky. Micronutrient deficiency conditions: global health issues. Public Health Reviews. 2010;32:243-255.

8.   Onyeike EN, Acheru GN. Chemical composition of selected Nigerian oil seeds and physicochemical properties of the oil extracts. Food Chemistry. 2002;77(4):431–437.

9.   Tangkanakul P, Trakoontivakorn G, Saengprakai J, Auttaviboonkul P, Niyomwitoon N, Nakahara K. Antioxidant capacity and anti-mutagenicity of Thermal processed Thai foods. JIRCAS J. 2011; 45(2):211-218.

10.   Dauqan E, Abdullah HS, Abdullah A, Muhamad H, Top GM. Vitamin E and Beta Carotene Composition in four Different Vegetable Oils. Am. J. Appl. Sci. 2011;8(5):407-412.

11.   Basabose AK. Diet composition of chimpanzees inhabiting the montane forest of Kahuzi, DR Congo. Am. J. Primatol. 2002;58(1):1–21.

12.   UNESCO. World Heritage in the Congo Basin, UNESCO World Heritage Centre, Paris; 2010. Consulted on February 26; 2015.
Available:http://whc.unesco.org/en/list/137

13.   Plumptre AJ, Eilu G, Ewango C, Ssegawa P, Nkuutu D, Gereau R, Beentje H, Poulsen AD, Fischer E, Goyder D, Pearce TR, Hafashimana D. The biodiversity of the Albertine Rift. Section 7: Plants. Albertine Rift Technical Reports Series. 2003;3:68-77.

14.   Kadu CA, Parich A, Schuele, S, Konrad H, Muluvi GM, Eyog-Matig O, Muchugi A, Williams VL, Ramamonjisoa L, Kapinga C, Foahom B, Katsvanga C, Hafashimana D, Obama C, Vinceti B, Schumacher R, Geburek T. Bioactive constituents in *Prunus africana*: geographical variation throughout Africa and associations with environmental and genetic parameters. Phytochemistry. 2012;83:70-8.

15.   Research and Development Report FANCOR ABYSSINIAN OIL Crambe Abyssinica Seed Oil.
Available:www.essentialingredients.com/pdf/AbyssinianOilResearchReport.pdf
3/3/2015

16.   Vadivel V, Ami Patel, Biesalski HK. Effect of traditional processing methods on the antioxidant, α-amylase and α-glucosidase enzyme inhibition properties of *Sesbania sesban* Merrill seeds. CyTA - Journal of Food. 2012;10(2):128-136.

17.   Orwa C, Mutua A, Kindt R, Jamnadass R, Simons A. Agroforestree Database: A tree reference and selection guide version 4.0; 2009.
Available:http://www.worldagroforestry.org/af/tree accessed February 20, 2015.

18.   Available:http://www.theseedybusiness.com/the-seed-book/rrsatkzp458h2upnrg4q0mor6y2lf9 February 16, 2015.

19.   Cos P, Hermans N, De Bruyne T, Apers S, Sindambiwe JB, Vanden Berghe B, Pieters L, Vlietinck AJ. Further evaluation of Rwandan medicinal plant extracts for their antimicrobial and antiviral activities. Journal of Ethnopharmacology. 2002; 79(2):155 –163.

20.   Barthet VJ, Chornick T, Daun JK. Comparison of methods to measure the oil contents in oilseeds. J. Oleo Sci. 2002;51: 589-597.

21.   International Standard ISO 659: - Oilseeds – Determination of hexane extract (or light petroleum extract), called "oil content", ISO, Geneva; 1998.

22.   Balz M, Schulte E, Their H-P Trennung von Tocopherolen und Tocotrienolen durch HPLC. Fat Sci. Technol. 1992;94:209-213.

23.   Matthäus B, Özcan MM. Determination of fatty acid, tocopherol, sterol contents and 1,2- and 1,3-diacylglycerols in four different virgin olive oil. J. Food Process Technol. 2011; 2:117.

24.   Abraham G, Hron RJ. Oil seeds and their oils In: Encyclopedia of Food Science and Technology. Hui YJ. (Ed.), John Wiley and Sons Inc. 1992;1904–1907.

25.   Dubois V, Breton S, Linder M, Fanni J, Parmentier M. Fatty acid profiles of 80 vegetable oils with regard to their nutritional potential. Eur. J. Lipid Sci. Technol. 2007;109:710–732.

26.   Sekhar SC, Rao BVK. Cottonseed oil as health oil. Pertanika J. Trop. Agric. Sci. 2011;34(1):17-24.

27.   Top-Notch Technology In Production.
Available:http://www.chempro.in/fattyacid.htm accessed February 16, 2015.

28.   Malimo Sylvia. Extraction and analysis of oyster nut (telfairia pedata) oil.
Available:http://chemistry.uonbi.ac.ke/sites/default/files/cbps/sps/chemistry/Fourth%20Year%20Project-2006-2595.pdf accessed February 20, 2015.

29.   Okoli BE. Protabase Record display for Telfairia pedata. Protabase. prota.org. Retrieved November 2; 2012.

30. AUS Fat. Stearic Acid–A. Available:www.beefnutrition.org./StearicAcid.pdf

31. Pearson TA. (Ed). Stearic acid: a unique saturated fatty acid. Am. J. Clin. Nutr. 1994;60(suppl):983s-1072s.

32. Mensink RP. Effects of stearic acid on plasma lipid and lipoproteins in humans. Lipids. 2005;40:1201-1205.

33. Dambatt BB, Ogah SU. Extraction and characterization of oil from the seed of *Sesbania sesban* Linn shrubs. Discovery and Innovation. 2000;12(3/4):153-157.

34. Wijendran V, Hayes KC. Dietary n-6 and n-3 FA balance and cardiovascular health. Annu. Rev. Nutr. 2004;24:597–615.

35. Available:http://www.gbhealthwatch.com/Science-Omega3-Omega6.php Accessed Mars 2, 2015.

36. Chardigny JM, Destaillats F, Malpuech-Brugère C, Moulin J, Bauman DE. Lock AL, et al. Do trans fatty acids from industrially produced sources and from natural sources have the same effect on cardiovascular disease risk factors in healthy subjects? Am. J. Clin. Nutr. 2008;87:558–566.

37. Sebedio JL, Christie WW. Trans Fatty acids in Human Nutrition, The Oily Press, Dundee. D. Firestone and A. Sheppard, Advances in Lipid Methodology — One (ed. W.W. Christie). The Oily Press; 1998.

38. Tang TS. Fatty acid composition of edible oils in the Malaysian market, with special reference to trans-fatty acids. J. Oil Palm Res. 2002;14(1):1-8.

39. C̆molík J, Pokorny´ J. Physical refining of edible oils. Eur. J. Lipid Sci. Technol. 2000;102:472–486.

40. De Greyt W, Kellens M. Refining practice. In: Edible Oil Processing. Hamm W., Hamilton R. J. ed. Danvers: Blackwell. 2000;281.

41. Hirsinger F. Oleochemical raw materials and new oilseed crops. *Oléagineux.* 1986; 641(7):345-352.

42. Taylor DC, Guo YV. Katavic V, Mietkiewska E, Francis T, Bettger W. New seed oils for improved human and animal health and as industrial feedstocks: Genetic manipulation of the Brassicaceae to produce oils enriched in nervonic acid, in Modification of Seed Composition to Promote Health and Nutrition, edited by A.B. Krishnan, ASA-CSSA-SSSA Publishing, Madison, Wisconsin, USA. 2009;219-233.

43. Very long-chain acyl-CoA dehydrogenase deficiency. Genetics Home Reference, National Institutes of Health. Retrieved 28 March; 2013.

44. Emmanuel AO, Mudiakeoghene O. The use of antioxidants in vegetable oils. Afr. J. Biotech. 2008;7(25):4836-4842.

45. Matthäus B, Özcan MM. Fatty acid, tocopherol and squalene contents of Rosaceae seed oils. Botanical Studies. 2014;55(48):1-6.

46. Vitamine-E. Available :http://fr.wikipedia.org/w/index.php?title=Vitamine_E&oldid=108789880. Accessed 6th November 2014.

47. Soybean. Available:https://www.novapublishers.com/catalog/product_info.php?products_id=25983 accessed March 2, 2015.

48. Jiang Q, Christen S, Shigenaga MK, Ames BN. gamma-tocopherol, the major form of vitamin E in the US diet, deserves more attention. Am J Clin Nutr. 2001;74(6):714-22.

49. Lyle MacWilliam. What Makes Gamma Tocopherol Superior to Alpha Tocopherol Life Extension Magazine. Available:http://www.lef.org/magazine/2006/4/report_gamma/Page-01

11

Chemical Composition and Antioxidant Property of Two Species of Monkey Kola (*Cola rostrata* and *Cola lepidota* K. Schum) Extracts

Emmanuel E. Essien[1*], **Nimmong-uwem S. Peter**[1] **and Stella M. Akpan**[1]

[1]*Department of Chemistry, University of Uyo, Akwa Ibom State, Nigeria.*

Authors' contributions

This work was carried out in collaboration among all authors. Author EEE designed the study, wrote the protocol, and the first draft of the manuscript. Authors NSP and Author SMA conducted experimental work, managed the analyses of the study and literature searches. All authors read and approved the final manuscript.

Editor(s):
(1) Marcello Iriti, Department of Agricultural and Environmental Sciences, Milan State University, Italy.
Reviewers:
(1) Anonymous, Egypt.
(2) Anonymous, Nigeria.

ABSTRACT

Aims: To determine the total phenols content and antioxidant activity of *Cola rostrata* and *C. lepidota* seeds and fruit pulp methanol extracts.

Study Design: *In vitro* evaluation of antioxidant assays; phytochemical screening, quantitative determination of total phenolics and flavonoids content of seeds and fruit pulp extracts.

Place and Duration of Study: Department of Chemistry, University of Uyo, Nigeria (July – October, 2014).

Methodology: Standard methods were employed in the phytochemical screening, quantitative phenols and flavonoid determination and antioxidant assays (DPPH radical, ferric reducing and metal chelating activity).

Results: Alkaloids, saponins, terpenoids, carbohydrates and flavonoids were detected in the seeds and fruit pulp extracts of the studied plants. Fruit pulp of *C. rostrata* and seeds of *C. lepidota* contained the highest amount of flavonoids (60.5 µgQE/g) and phenolics (72.9 µgGAE/g) respectively. The extracts exhibited significant DPPH radical and ferric reducing activity with IC_{50} values 50-66.5 µg/mL and 60.0-63.0 µg/mL respectively. The *Cola* extracts also demonstrated

Corresponding author: E-mail: emmaflowus1@yahoo.co.uk

metal chelating activity (11.49-34.83%) at 100 µg/mL.

Conclusion: The results of this study substantiates a probable role of the seeds and edible fruit pulp of *C. rostrata* and *C. lepidota* as natural sources of antioxidants which could be further exploited for their potential biological activity.

Keywords: Sterculiaceae; Cola rostrata; Cola lepidota; antioxidant activity.

1. INTRODUCTION

The genus *Cola* of the family Sterculiaceae is indigenous to tropical Africa and has its centre of greatest diversity in West Africa [1]. About 40 *Cola* species have been described in West Africa. In Nigeria about twenty three (23) species are known and some are used in traditional medicine as stimulant, to prevent dysentery [2], headache [3] and to suppress sleep [4]. *Cola rostrata* and *C. lepidota* (CL) K. Schum are perennial trees popularly known as monkey cola and cockroach kola [5]. Monkey kola is a common name given to a number of minor relatives of the *Cola* spp. that produce edible tasty fruits. Native people of southern Nigeria and the Cameron relish the fruits, as well as some wild primate animals especially monkeys, baboons and other species. Seeds of the monkey kola species are obliquely ovoid with two flattered surfaces, rough and reddish brown or green; but not edible unlike the seeds of kola nut (*C. nitida*). The aril (waxy mesocarp) form the edible portion of the follicle, and varied in colour, with the *C. rostrata* having whitish aril, while *C. lepidota* is characterized by yellowish aril. *Cola lepidota* is reported to be employed in Nigerian folk medicine as febrifuges, for pulmonary problems and cancer related ailments [6,7].

Free radicals contribute to more than one hundred disorders in humans including atherosclerosis, arthritis, ischemia and reperfusion injury of many tissues, central nervous system injury, gastritis and cancer [8,9]. Antioxidant activity [7], anticancer [6,10] and acute toxicity [11] of the leaf and stem bark extracts of *C. lepidota* have been studied. Phytochemical screening and acute toxicity of *C. rostrata* root bark have also been reported by Odion et al. [4]. Literature search reveals that there is paucity of information as regards the antioxidant potential of *C. rostrata* and *C. lepidota* seeds and fruit aril coupled with the increase in demand for herbs and the urgent need to evaluate nature's repository of chemicals in plants for their potential value in health care. This present study was designed to evaluate the phytochemicals, phenolics, flavonoids content and antioxidant activity of the seeds and fruit pulp of *C. rostrata* and *C. lepidota*.

2. MATERIALS AND METHODS

2.1 Samples Collection and Extraction

The fruits of *C. rostrata* and *C. lepidota* were purchased from local markets in Uyo and Essien Udim Local Government Area of Akwa Ibom State in July, 2014. The plants were identified and authenticated by Dr. (Mrs.) M. E. Bassey, a taxonomist in the Department of Botany and Ecological Studies, University of Uyo, Nigeria where voucher specimens were deposited. The fruit pulp and seeds were separated, chopped into small pieces and oven dried at 40°C. The samples were pulverized and extracted with methanol using a Soxhlet apparatus. The extract was concentrated under vacuum using a rotator evaporator. All chemicals and solvents used in this study were of analytical reagent grade and were purchased from Merck (Darmstadt, Germany) and Sigma Aldrich (St. Louis, MO). Standard antioxidant compounds were obtained from laboratory stock, acquired from commercial sources. All solutions were made in distilled water.

2.2 Phytochemical Screening

Standard methods for phytochemical screening (alkaloids, flavonoids, saponins, tannins, carbohydrates, phlobatannins, sterols and triterpenes) were employed. Alkaloids determination was done using Mayer's and Dragendoff's reagents following the methods of Kapoor et al. [12] and Odebiyi and Sofowora [13]; tannins and phlobatannins [13]. The methods described by Kapoor et al. [12] were used for determining flavonoids. The persistent frothing test as described by Kapoor et al. [12] and Odebiyi and Sofowora [13] were used for saponins. Carbohydrates determination was done using Fehling's reagent following the method described by Harbone [14]. Sterols and triterpenes were determined following the

Eiebemann-Burchard test as described by Odebiyi and Sofowora [13] and Harbone [14].

2.3 Determination of Total Phenolics

The concentration of phenolics was expressed as µg gallic acid equivalent per gram of the extract. The method of Singleton and Rossil was used [15]. Solution (1 mg) containing extract (1 mg) in methanol was added to distilled water (46 ml) and FCR (1 ml) then mixed thoroughly. After 3 mins, sodium carbonate (2%, 3 ml) was added to the mixture and shaken intermittently for 2 hrs at room temperature. The absorbance was read at 760 nm. Gallic acid was used as a standard and a calibration curve was plotted.

2.4 Determination of Total Flavonoids

Measurement of flavonoid concentration of extracts was based on the method of Park et al. [16] expressed as quercetin equivalent. An aliquot of the solution (1 ml) containing the extract (1 mg) in methanol was added to test tubes containing aluminium nitrate (10%, 0.1 ml), potassium acetate (1 M, 0.1 ml) and ethanol (3.8 ml). After 40 mins at room temperature, the absorbance was determined at 415 nm. Quercetin was used as a standard and a calibration curve was plotted.

2.5 DPPH Radical Scavenging Activity

DPPH radical scavenging activity of each extract was determined according to the method of Blois [17]. DPPH (0.1 mM) in methanol was prepared and the solution (1 mL) was mixed with crude extracts (1.0 mL) prepared in methanol at different concentrations (20, 40, 60, 80, and 100 µg/ mL). The mixture was shaken and kept for 30 mins at room temperature. The decrease of solution absorbance due to proton donating activity of components of each extract was determined at 517 nm. Ascorbic acid and Butylated hydroxyanisole were used as the positive control. The DPPH radical scavenging activity was calculated using the following formula:

$$\% \text{ inhibition} = \frac{A_{control} - A_{sample}}{A_{control}} X \ 100$$

2.6 Ferric Reducing Capacity

The reducing power of each sample was determined according to the method of Oyaizu [18]. Sample solutions of different concentrations were mixed with phosphate buffer (0.2 M, 2.5 mL, pH 6.6) and potassium ferric cyanide (1%, 2.5 mL). After the mixture was incubated at 50°C for 20 mins, trichloroacetic acid (TCA) (10%, 2.5 mL) was added and the mixture was centrifuged for 10 mins. The upper layer (2.5 ml) was mixed with distilled water (2.5 ml) and ferric chloride (0.1%, 2.5 mL), and the absorbance was measured at 700 nm against. Higher absorbance of the reaction mixture indicated greater reducing power. BHA was used as positive control.

2.7 Metal Chelating Activity

The method of Dinis et al. [19] was used. Crude extract (0.5 g) was mixed with $FeCl_2$ (2 mM, 0.05 ml) and Ferrozine (5 mM, 0.2 mL). The total volume was diluted with methanol (2 mL). The mixture was shaken vigorously and left standing at room temperature for 10 mins. After the mixture had reached equilibrium, the absorbance of the solution was measured at 562 nm in a spectrophotometer. The percentage inhibition of ferrozine Fe^{2+} complex was calculated using the formula:

$$\% \text{ inhibition of ferrozine} - Fe2+ = \frac{A_{control} - A_{sample}}{A_{control}} X \ 100$$

3. RESULTS AND DISCUSSION

The phytochemical profile of *C. rostrata* and *C. lepidota* extracts are presented in Table 1. The four extracts contained high amount of alkloids, saponins, terpenoids, carbohydrates and flavonoids, while anthraquinones were detected exclusively in *C. rostrata* seed extract. Tannins were also not detected in the edible fruit pulp of both samples whereas the seeds contained appreciable quantity of tannins. Similar phytochemical data for *C. lepidota* seeds and root bark of *C. rostrata* have been reported by Burkill [20] and Odion [4] respectively; *C. nitida* nut varieties [21]. The relative high amount of carbohydrates in *C. lepidota* fruit may be due to the natural sugary taste of the succulent white pulp as compared with the pale yellow fruit pulp of *C. rostrata*. Therefore, the varying degree of phytochemical constituents may confer different levels of antioxidant activity on the studied plant extracts especially, polyphenolic components which have been implicated in recent studies as antioxidants via other mechanisms to prevent disease processes [22]. They are capable of removing free radicals, chelating metal catalysts, activating antioxidant enzymes, reducing α-tocopherols and inhibiting oxidases [23].

The Folin-Ciocalteu method is a rapid and widely-used assay in investigating the total phenolic content, but it is known that different phenolic compounds gave different responses with this method [24]. Table 2 indicates the total phenols and flavonoids content of *C. rostrata* and *C. lepidota* methanol extracts. In this study, total phenolics content ranged from 33.1-72.9 µg/GAE/g while flavonoids content was 18.9-51.4 µgQE/g. Fruit pulp of *C. rostrata* and seeds of *C. lepidota* constituted the highest amount of flavonoids (60.5 µgQE/g) and phenolics (72.9 µgGAE/g) respectively. The antioxidant activity of plant extracts containing polyphenol components is due to their capacity to be donors of hydrogen atoms or electrons and to capture the free radicals [25].

DPPH radical was used as a stable free radical to determine antioxidant activity. Fig. 1 illustrates the concentration of DPPH radical due to the scavenging ability of seed and fruit pulp extracts of *C. rostrata* and *C. lepidota*. Standards BHA and vit C were used as references. Ascorbic acid is a known and potent antioxidant agent used in medicines [26]. The percentage inhibition of the free radical was dose dependent. Increase in concentration gave corresponding increased % inhibition. The DPPH radical scavenging capacity (IC_{50}) of the extracts was found to range from 50.0 – 66.5 µg/ml (Table 3) which is the concentration that decreases the initial DPPH radical concentration by 50% in each extract. On the other hand the (IC_{50}) of vit C and BHT was 22.0 and 16.0 µg/ml respectively. The effectiveness of antioxidant properties is inversely correlated with IC_{50} values. Thus, BHA exhibited higher DPPH scavenging effect than ascorbic acid and extracts in the study.

Table 1. Phytochemical analysis of *C. rostrata* and *C. lepidota* methanol extracts

Test	*C. rostrata* extracts		*C. lepidota* extracts	
	Seeds	Fruit Pulp	Seeds	Fruit Pulp
Alkaloids	++	+++	+++	+++
Flavanoids	+++	++	++	+
Saponins	+++	+++	+	+++
Terpenes/steroids	+++	+++	+	+++
Cardiac glycosides	++	+	++	++
Tannins	++	-	+	-
Phlobatannins	+	-	++	-
Anthraquinones	+++	-	-	-
Carbohydrate	++	++	++	+++
Deoxy sugars	+++	++	++	+++

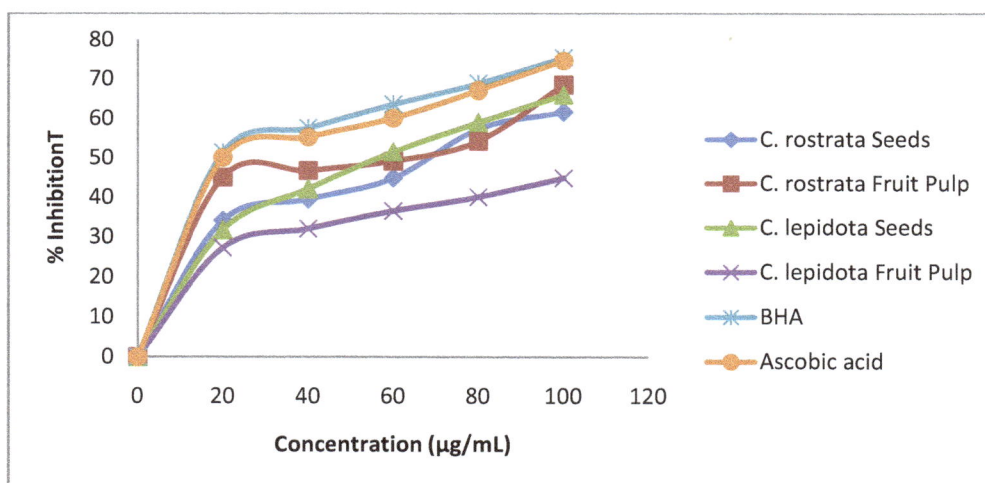

Fig. 1. Percentage DPPH scavenging activity of *Cola rostrata* and *C. lepidota* extracts/standards

The antioxidant power has also been reported by some investigators to be concomitant with the development of reducing power [27]. Reductones, which have strong reducing power, are generally believed not only to react directly with peroxides but also to prevent peroxide formation by reacting with certain precursors [28]. Furthermore, these *Cola* extracts are suggested to act as electron donors, reacting with free radicals and converting them to more stable products, which can terminate radical chain reaction. As shown in Fig. 2, in a concentration of 100 µg/mL of seeds, fruit pulp extracts and standard BHA, the descending order of reducing power is as follows: BHA (6.921) > *C. rostrata* seed (4.955) > *C. lepidota* seed (4.327) > *C. rostrata* fruit (4.174) > *C. lepidota* fruit (3.394). This study also reveals that the *Cola* extracts demonstrated strong metal chelating activity (Fig. 3) compared with standard EDTA at 100 µg/mL. The metal chelating activity of both fruit pulp extracts were similar and about 3-fold that observed for the seed extracts.

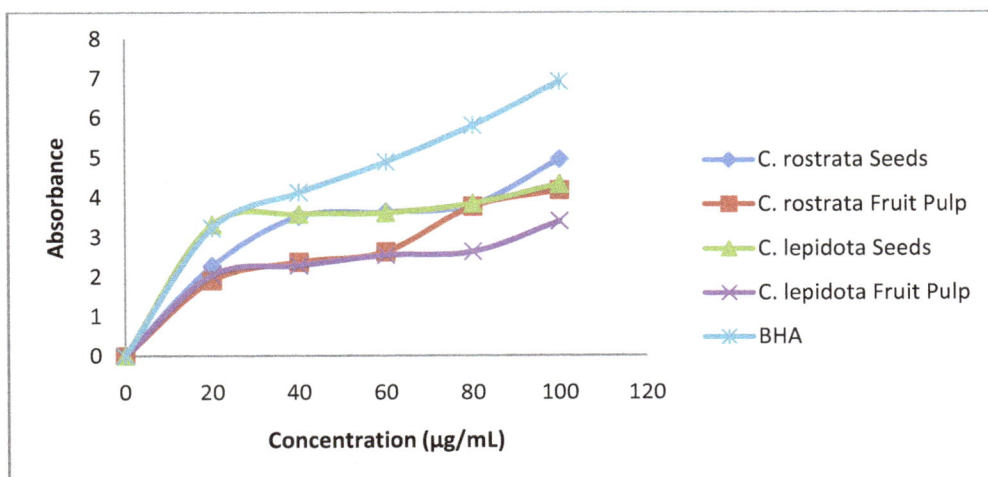

Fig. 2. Ferric reducing activity of *Cola rostrata* and *C. lepidota* extracts/standards

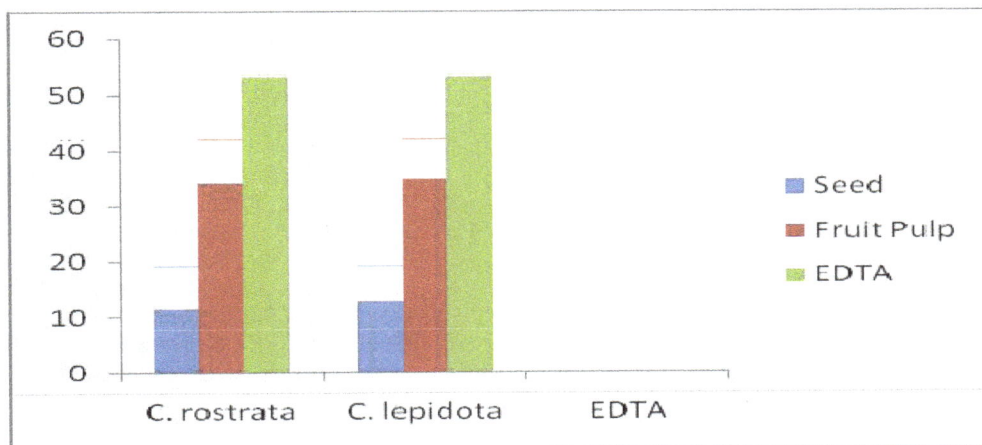

Fig. 3. Metal chelating activity of *C. rostrata* and *C. lepidota* extract/standard (100 µg/mL)

Table 2. Total phenolics and flavonoid content of *C. rostrata* and *C. lepidota* extracts

Methanol extracts	*C. rostrata*		*C. lepidota*	
	Total phenolics (µg/GAE/g)	Total flavonoids (µgQE/g)	Total phenolics (µg/GAE/g)	Total flavonoids (µgQE/g)
Seed	55.00	25.75	72.90	51.40
Fruit pulp	60.50	48.60	30.10	18.90

Table 3. IC_{50} (μg/ mL) of *C. rostrata* and *C. lepidota* extracts

Activity	C. rostrata extracts		C. lepidota extracts		Standards	
	C. rostrata Seeds	C. rostrata Fruit Pulp	C. lepidota Seeds	C. lepidota Fruit Pulp	BHA	Ascobic acid
DPPH	66.5	50.0	60.0	58.0	16.0	22.0
Ferric Reducing	60.0	62.0	60.0	63.0	50.0	-

4. CONCLUSION

The reducing power of the studied *Cola* extracts correlated well with the DPPH radical scavenging activity. It indicated that the marked antioxidant activity of these extracts may be as a result of their reducing power. It is interesting to note that *C. lepidota* seed and *C. rostrata* fruit pulp extracts with significant amount of polyphenols displayed relative corresponding antioxidant activity, moderately comparable with the pure standard compounds. The results of this study substantiates a probable role of the seeds and edible fruit pulp of *C. rostrata* and *C. lepidota* as natural sources of antioxidants which could be further exploited for their potential biological activity.

CONSENT

It is not applicable.

ETHICAL APPROVAL

It is not applicable.

COMPETING INTERESTS

Authors have declared that no competing interests exist.

REFERENCES

1. Rusell TA. The *cola* of Nigeria and Cameroon.Trop Agric. 1955;32:210-240.
2. Morton JF. Widespread tannin intake via stimulants and masticatories, especially guarana, kola nut, betel vine and accessories. Basic Life Sci. 1992;739-765.
3. Seitz R, Gehrmann B, Krauss L. Cola. In: Hänsel R, Rimpler H, Keller K, Schneider G, editors. Hager's handbook of pharmaceutical practice. Drugs A-D. Springer-Verlag, Berlin – Heidelberg. 1992;4:940-946.
4. Odion EE, Poh CF, Falodun A, Adelusi SA. *Cola rostrata*: Phytochemical and toxicity studies. J Appl Sci Environ Manage. 2013;17(4):603-607.
5. Keay RWJ. Trees of Nigeria. Oxford: Claredon Press. 1989;131-135.
6. Engel N, Opermann C, Falodun A. Udo K. Proliferative effects of five traditional Nigerian medicinal plant extracts on human breast and bone cancer cell lines. J Ethnopharmacol. 2011;137:1003-1010.
7. Oghenerobo VI, Falodun A. Antioxidant activities of the leaf extract and fractions of *Cola lepidota* K. Schum (Sterculiaceae). Nig J Biotech. 2013;25:31-36.
8. Kumpulainen JT, Salonen JT. Natural antioxidants and anticarcinogens in nutrition health and disease. The Royal Society of Chemistry UK. 1999;178-187.
9. Cook NC, Samman S. Flavonoids-chemistry, metabolism, cardioprotective effects, and dietary sources. Nutri Biochem. 1996;7:66-76.
10. Imieje V, Erharuyi O, Engel N, Falodun A. Antiproliferative and apoptotic activities of *Cola lepidota* against estrogen receptor positive breast cancer cells. Scientia Africana. 2014;13(1):1-8.
11. Imieje V, Igbe I, Falodun A. Phytochemical screening, proximate analysis and acute toxicity studies of leaves of *Cola lepidota* K. schum (Sterculiaceae). J Pharma and Allied Sci. 2013;10(1):1684-1689.
12. Kapoor DI, Singh AL, Kapoor IS, Svivaslava NS. Survey of Indian plants for saponins, alkaloids and flavonoids. Lioydia. 1969;32:297-304.
13. Odebiyi OO, Sofowora EE. Phytochemical screening of Nigerian medicinal plants. Lioydia. 1978;41:234-246.
14. Harbone JB. Phytochemical Methods. 2nd edition. Chapman and Hall. Hong Kong; 1991.
15. Singleton VL, Rossi JA. Colorimetry of total phenolics with phosphomolybdic phosphotungstic acid reagents. Am J Enology and Viticulture. 1965;16:144-158.
16. Park YK, Koo MH, Ikegaki M, Contado JL. Comparison of the flavonoid aglycone contents of *Apismellifera propolis* from

various regions of Brazil. Brazilian Arch Biol Technol. 1997;40:97-106.

17. Blois MS. Antioxidants determination by the use of a stable free radical. Nature. 1958;46:1199-1200.

18. Oyaizu M. Studies on product of browning reaction prepared from glucose amine. Japanese J Nutr. 1986;44:307-315.

19. Dinis TCP, Madeira VMC, Almeida LM. Action of phenolics derivates (acetoaminophen, salicylate and 5-aminosalicylate) as inhibitors of membrane lipid peroxidation and as peroxyl radical scavengers. Arch Biochem Biophy. 1994;315:161-169.

20. Burkill HM. The useful plants of west tropical Africa. Royal Botanic Gardens: Kew. 1985;5.

21. Nyamien Y, Adje F, Niamké F, Chatigre O, Adima A, Biego GH. Caffeine and phenolic compounds in *Cola nitida* (Vent.) Schott and Endl and *Garcinia kola* Heckel grown in Côte d'Ivoire. Brit J Appl Sci Tech. 2014;4(35):4846-4859.

22. Oboh G, Rocha JB. Polyphenols in red pepper [*Capsicum annuum* var. aviculare (Tepin)] and their protective effect on some prooxidants induced lipid peroxidation in brain and liver. Eur Food Res Technol. 2007;225:239-247.

23. Cheplick S, Kwon YI, Bhowmik P, Shetty K. Phenolic-linked variation in strawberry cultivars for potential dietary management of hyperglycemia and related complications of hypertension. Bioresource Technol. 2010;101:404-413.

24. Upadhyay M, Ahmad kanie S, Agnihotri RK, Sharma R. Studies on antioxidant activity and total phenolic content of *Tinospora cordifolia* (Miers.). Am J Phytomed Clin Therap. 2013;1(8):617-627.

25. Ozcelik D, Ozara SR, GurelZ, Uzun H and Aydin S. Copper mediated oxidative stress in rat liver. Biol Trace Elements Res. 2003;96:209-15.

26. Jain A, Soni M, Deb L, Rout S, Gupta V, Krishna K. Antioxidant and hepatoprotective activity of ethanolic and aqueous extracts of *Momordica dioica* leaves. J Ethnopharmacol. 2008;115:61-66.

27. Sultana B, Anwar F, Ashraf M. Effect of extraction solvent/technique on the antioxidant activity of selected medicinal plant extracts. Molecules. 2009;14:2167-2180.

28. Oh PS, Lim KT. Antioxidant activity of *Dioscorea batatas* decne glycoprotein. Eur Food Res Technol. 2008;226:507–515.

12

Comparative Study on the Phytochemical Compositions and Antihyperglycemic Potentials of the Leaves Extracts of *Combretum paniculatum* and *Morinda morindoides*

Akintayo L. Ogundajo[1], Mutiu I. Kazeem[2], Jude E. Evroh[1], Mayowa M. Avoseh[1] and Isiaka A. Ogunwande[1*]

[1]Department of Chemistry, Natural Products Research Unit, Faculty of Science, Lagos State University, Badagry Expressway, P.M.B. 0001 LASU Post Office, Ojo, Lagos, Nigeria.
[2]Department of Biochemistry, Antidiabetic Drug Discovery Group, Faculty of Science, Lagos State University, Badagry Expressway, P.M.B. 0001 LASU Post Office, Ojo, Lagos, Nigeria.

Authors' contributions

This work was carried out in collaboration with all authors. Authors ALO and IAO designed the study and supervised the whole research. Authors MMA and JEE performed the extraction and participated in all the experimental works. Author MIK carried out the hypoglycemic analysis, performed the statistical analysis and wrote initial draft of the manuscript. Author IAO managed the literature searches and wrote the final draft of the manuscript. All authors read and approved the final manuscript.

Editor(s):
(1) Marcello Iriti, Department of Agricultural and Environmental Sciences, Milan State University, Italy.
Reviewers:
(1) Indra Prasad Tripathi, Faculty of Science & Environment, Mahatma Gandhi Chitrakoot Gramoday Vishwavidyalaya, Chitrakoot, India.
(2) Victor Y. A. Barku, Department of Chemistry, University of Cape Coast, Ghana.

ABSTRACT

The phytocheimcal components and antihyperglycemic potential of methanol and ethanol leaves extracts of *Combretum paniculatum* Vent (*Combretaceae*) and *Morinda morindoides* (Baker) Milne-Redh (*Rubiaceae*) grown in Nigeria have been studied. The phytochemical composition was determined by established methods while the *in vitro* hypoglycemic effect was performed by determining the inhibitory potentials of the extracts on α-amylase and α-glucosidase. Results

Corresponding author: E-mail: isiaka.ogunwande@lasu.edu.ng

showed that the ethanol extract of *C. paniculatum* displayed the most potent inhibition of both α-amylase (IC_{50}: 5.06 mg/mL) and α-glucosidase (IC_{50}: 1.96 mg/mL). The ethanol extract of *C. paniculatum* inhibited α-amylase and α-glucosidase in a non-competitive and mixed non-competitive manner. The presence of phytochemicals such as phenols, steroids, flavonoids and athraquinones were confirmed in the extracts.

Aims: To determine the phytochemical compositions and hypoglycemic potentials of the methanol and ethanol leaves extracts of *Combretum paniculatum* and *Morinda morindoides*.

Study Design: Extraction of the air-dried and pulverized leaves of *C. paniculatum* and *M. morindoides* with both methanol and ethanol, and testing the various extracts for the phytochemical composition and hypoglycemic potentials.

Place and Duration of Study: The leaves of *C. paniculatum* were collected from Ibefun, Oyo State, in May 2013 while those of *M. morindoides* were collected from Etegbin Area, Shibiri, Lagos, State, Nigeria, in June 2013.

Methodology: The pulverized leaves were extracted separately with ethanol and methanol for 24 h. The resulting infusions were decanted, filtered and evaporated in a rotary evaporator. The dried extracts were weighed and dissolved in dimethylsulphoxide (DMSO) to yield a stock solution from which lower concentrations were prepared. Phytochemical compositions of the extracts were determined using the methods described previously. Moreover, the hypoglycemic potentials were evaluated as described previously.

Results: The ethanol extract of *C. paniculatum* possessed mild inhibition of α-amylase and strong inhibition of α-glucosidase compared to other extracts.

Conclusion: The present results justify the use of *C. paniculatum* in the treatment of sugar related disorders in Nigeria.

Keywords: Combretum paniculatum; Morinda morindoides; hyperglycemia; phytochemical composition; hypoglycemic activity.

1. INTRODUCTION

Type 2 diabetes mellitus is a disorder of the endocrine system, majorly characterized by glycemic imbalance, which stimulates several metabolic errors and finally results into oxidative stress and chronic complications [1]. Current statistics suggests that about 382 million people are living with diabetes around the globe and this number is projected to increase to 471 million in 2035. South Africa tops the list of diabetics in Africa with prevalence of 8.27% followed by Nigeria with 4.99% of the population [2]. In fact, this disease is associated with a reduced quality of life and increased risk factors for mortality and morbidity among its sufferers, who are mostly poor and socially disadvantaged [2].

Glycemic control is the most important goal in diabetes care as its impairment leads to several complications such as nephropathy, neuropathy and cardiovascular disease in diabetic patients [3]. Different classes of drugs such as biguanides, insulin secretagogues, thiazolidinediones and α-glucosidase inhibitors have been used widely to manage this condition. However, these antidiabetic drugs produced undesirable side effects such as hypoglycaemia, weight gain and gastro-intestinal disturbances

[4]. Due to these, the use of herbal agents in the management of diabetes mellitus has gained prominence in all parts of the world, and some of the plants used include *Combretum paniculatum* and *Morinda morindoides*.

Combretum paniculatum is a shrub with vivid scarlet flowers attaining 15 m length and is widespread in tropical Africa. A high degree of antiviral activity against HIV-2 was achieved with the acetone extract of *C. paniculatum* [5]. The aqueous extract of inflorescences of the plant has anti-tumor activity against carcinoma of the lung [6]. The antimicrobial, anti-inflammatory, antishistosomal, anti-HIV and central nervous system stimulation activities of *C. paniculatum* have been documented [7]. The cytotoxic activity of pheophorbide-a and pheophorbide a-methyl ester isolated from the leaves of *C. paniculatum* have been reported [8]. Other compounds such as cyanidin 3,5-O-β-D-diglu-copyranoside and pelargonidin 3,5-O-β-D-diglucopyranoside [9], as well as cholest-5-en-3-ol, 2-phyten-1-ol, isoquercitrin, p-coumaric acid, 2, 3, 8-tri-O-methylellagic acid, beta-sitosterol, gallocatechin, apigenin and apigenin-7-glucoside [10] were characterised from the plant. Till moment, the authors are unaware of any analysis on the hypoglycemic activity of this plant.

Extracts and compounds of *M. morindoides* are known to possess antimicrobial [11-13], antidiarrheal [14], anticomplimentary [15], xanthine oxidase inhibiting and superoxide scavenging activity [16], antimalarial [17-20], antispermatogenic [21,22], cytotoxic effects [23] and possesses biochemical effects on lipid profile, bilirubin and some marker enzymes level in the plasma of male albino rats [24]. The plant contains antimalarial iridoids [19], quercetin, quercetin-7,4'-dimethylether, luteolin-7-glucoside, apigenin-7-glucoside, quercetin-3-rhamnoside, kaempferol-3-rhamnoside, quercetin-3-rutinoside, kaempferol-3-rutinoside, chrysoeriol-7-neohesperidoside and kaempferol-7-rhamnosylsophoroside [25,26]. Though studies have been performed on the antidiabetic efficacy of the root [27] and leaf extracts [28] of this plant confirming the claim of the traditional healers, no work could be found on the mechanism by which the extract elicit this potential.

Despite the usage of these plants in the management of sugar-related disorders in Nigeria, there is dearth of information on their efficacy and possible mechanism of antidiabetic action. Therefore, this study aimed to determine the phytochemical and hypoglycemic potential of *C. paniculatum* and *M. morindoides* leaf extracts and the mechanism by which they elicit this action. This is in continuation of our previous studies on the hypoglycaemic potentials of some Nigerian medicinal plants [29,30].

2. MATERIALS AND METHODS

2.1 Chemicals and Reagents

Porcine pancreatic α-amylase, rat intestinal α-glucosidase and paranitrophenyl-glucopyranoside were products of Sigma-Adrich Co., St Louis, USA while starch soluble (extra pure) was obtained from J. T. Baker Inc., Phillipsburg, USA. Other chemicals and reagents were of analytical grade and the water used was glass-distilled.

2.2. Plants Collection

The leaves of *C. paniculatum* were collected in Ibefun, Oluyole Local Government, Oyo State, Nigeria. The plant was identified and authenticated by Dr. S. O. Shosanya, a taxonomist at the Forestry Research Institute of Nigeria (FRIN), Ibadan, Nigeria where a voucher specimen FHI 109950 was deposited in the

Institute's herbarium. The leaves of *M. morindoides* were obtained from Etegbin area, Shibiri, Ojo Local Government area, Lagos State. Botanical authentication was achieved at the Herbarium, Department of Botany, University of Lagos, Nigeria, where a voucher specimen LUH 5618, was also deposited. The leaves were air-dried, pulverized and kept in airtight plastic bags till moment of analysis.

2.3 Preparation of Plant Extracts

The pulverized leaves were divided into two portions of 10 g each and extracted separately with ethanol and methanol for 24 h. The flasks were shaken and kept still to allow the plant material settle at the bottom of the flask. The resulting infusions were decanted, filtered and evaporated in a rotary evaporator (Cole Parmer SB 1100, Shangai, China). The dried extracts were weighed and dissolved in dimethylsulphoxide (DMSO) to yield a stock solution from which lower concentrations were prepared.

2.4 Phytochemical Screening

Phytochemical compositions of the leaf extracts were determined using the methods described previously [31,32].

2.5 Hypoglycemic Potentials of the Extracts

2.5.1 α-Amylase inhibitory assay

This assay was carried out using a modified procedure of McCue and Shetty [33]. A total of 250 µL of extract was placed in a test tube and 250 µL of 0.02 M sodium phosphate buffer (pH 6.9) containing α-amylase solution (0.5 mg/mL) was added. This solution was pre-incubated at 25°C for 10 min, after which 250 µL of 1% starch solution in 0.02 M sodium phosphate buffer (pH 6.9) was added at timed intervals and then incubated at 25°C for 10 min. The reaction was terminated by adding 500 µL of dinitrosalicylic acid (DNS) reagent. The tubes were then incubated in boiling water for 5 min and cooled to room temperature. The reaction mixture was diluted with 5 mL distilled water and the absorbance was measured at 540 nm using a spectrophotometer (Spectrumlab S23A, Globe Medical England). The control and blank were prepared using the same procedure replacing the extract with DMSO and distilled water respectively. The α-amylase inhibitory activity was calculated as percentage inhibition, thus;

% Inhibition = $[(\Delta A_{control}-\Delta A_{extract})/A\Delta_{control}]$ x 100 where $\Delta A_{control} = A_{control} - A_{blank}$ and $\Delta A_{extract} = A_{extract} - A_{blank}$

Concentrations of extracts resulting in 50% inhibition of enzyme activity (IC_{50}) were determined graphically.

2.5.1.1 Mode of α-amylase inhibition

The mode of inhibition of α-amylase by the leaf extract was conducted using the most potent extract according to the modified procedure previously described [34]. Briefly, 250 µL of the (5 mg/mL) extract was pre-incubated with 250 µL of α-amylase solution (0.5 mg/mL) for 10 min at 25°C in one set of tubes. In another set of tubes α-amylase was pre-incubated with 250 µL of phosphate buffer (pH 6.9). 250 µL of starch solution at increasing concentrations (0.3–5.0 mg/mL) was added to both sets of reaction mixtures to start the reaction. The mixture was then incubated for 10 min at 25°C, and then boiled for 5 min after addition of 500 µL of DNS to stop the reaction. The amount of reducing sugars released was determined spectrophotometrically using a maltose standard curve and converted to reaction velocities. A double reciprocal (Lineweaver-Burk) plot (1/v versus 1/[S]) where v is reaction velocity and [S] is substrate concentration was plotted to determine the mode of inhibition.

2.5.2. α-Glucosidase inhibitory assay

The effect of the plant extracts on α-glucosidase activity was determined according to an established procedure [35]. The substrate solution, p-nitropheynyl glucopyranoside (pNPG) was prepared in 20 mM phosphate buffer, pH 6.9. 100 µL of α-glucosidase (E.C. 3.2.1.20) (0.5 mg/mL) was pre-incubated with 50 µL of the different concentrations of the extracts for 10 min. Then 50 µL of 3.0 mM pNPG dissolved in 20 mM phosphate buffer (pH 6.9) was added to start the reaction. The reaction mixture was incubated at 37°C for 20 min and stopped by adding 2 mL of 0.1 M Na_2CO_3. The α-glucosidase activity was determined by measuring the yellow coloured para-nitrophenol released from pNPG at 405 nm. The control and blank were prepared using the same procedure by replacing the extract with DMSO and distilled

water respectively. Percentage inhibition was calculated thus;

% Inhibition = $[(\Delta A_{control}-\Delta A_{extract})/A\Delta_{control}]$ x 100 where $\Delta A_{control} = A_{control} - A_{blank}$ and $\Delta A_{extract} = A_{extract} - A_{blank}$

Concentrations of extracts resulting in 50% inhibition of enzyme activity (IC_{50}) were determined graphically.

2.5.2.1 Mode of α-glucosidase inhibition

The mode of inhibition of α-glucosidase by the extracts was determined using the extract with the lowest IC_{50} according to the modified method described above [34]. Briefly, 50 µL of the (5 mg/mL) extract was pre-incubated with 100 µL of α-glucosidase solution (0.5 mg/mL) ofor 10 min at 25°C in one set of tubes. In another set of tubes, α-glucosidase was pre-incubated with 50 µL of phosphate buffer (pH 6.9). 50 µL of pNPG at increasing concentrations (0.63 - 2.0 mg/mL) was added to both sets of reaction mixtures to start the reaction. The mixture was then incubated for 10 min at 25°C and 500 µL of Na_2CO_3 was added to stop the reaction. The amount of reducing sugars released was determined spectrophotometrically using a para-nitrophenol standard curve and converted to reaction velocities. A double reciprocal (Lineweaver-Burk) plot (1/v versus 1/[S]) where v is reaction velocity and [S] is substrate concentration was plotted to determine the mode of inhibition.

2.6 Statistical Analysis

Statistical analysis was performed using GraphPad Prism 5 statistical package (GraphPad Software, USA). The data were analysed by one way analysis of variance (ANOVA) followed by Bonferroni test. All the results were expressed as mean ± SEM for triplicate determinations.

3. RESULTS AND DISCUSSION

The management of hyperglycemia is the hallmark of treatment in diabetes and one of the therapeutic approaches for decreasing postprandial hyperglycemia is to retard the digestion and absorption of carbohydrates by the inhibition of carbohydrate hydrolyzing enzymes, α-amylase and α-glucosidase, in the digestive tract [36]. Though, synthetic α-glucosidase inhibitors such as acarbose and voglibose are presently in use but are bedeviled by undesirable side effects such as nausea, diarrhoea and liver failure [37], which necessitated this study.

Table 1 showed the phytochemical composition of different extracts of *C. paniculatum* and *M. morindoides*. Steroid was detected in all the tested extracts while flavonoid was conspicuously absent in all the extracts. Phenolic compounds and tannins were detected in both the methanol and ethanol extracts of *C. paniculatum* while saponins and anthraquinones were detected in all the extracts except ethanol extract of *C. paniculatum*.

The result of percentage inhibition of α-amylase by methanol and ethanol extracts of *C. paniculatum* and *M. morindoides* leaves is shown in Figs. 1(a) and 1(b). With the exception of 0.32 mg/mL, methanol extract of *C. paniculatum* possessed significantly higher percentage inhibition ($P = .05$) of the enzyme than ethanol extract. However, for *M. morindoides*, at all concentrations tested, there was no significant difference between the two extracts. Table 2

showed the IC_{50} values for the inhibition of α-amylase and α-glucosidase by *C. paniculatum* and *M. morindoides*. Among the extracts tested, methanol extract of *C. paniculatum* had the lowest IC_{50} for α-amylase inhibition and this is lower than the standard, acarbose.

Figs. 2(a) and 2(b) shows the percentage inhibition of α-glucosidase by the extracts of *C. paniculatum* and *M. morindoides* leaves. At lower concentrations (0.32 - 0.63 mg/mL), there was no significant difference between the percentage inhibition of the ethanol and methanol extracts of *C. paniculatum*. At higher concentrations, there was significant difference ($P= .05$) between the inhibitions of the enzyme by ethanol and methanol extracts. With regards to *M. morindoides* extracts, there was no significant difference between the ethanol and methanol extracts at all concentrations tested. Ethanol extract possessed the lowest IC_{50} for α-glucosidase inhibition but it is higher than that of acarbose (Table 2).

Table 1. Phytochemical composition of *C. paniculatum* and *M. morindoides* leaves

Phytochemicals	C. paniculatum		M. morindoides	
	Methanol	**Ethanol**	**Methanol**	**Ethanol**
Tannins	+	+	-	-
Steroids	+	+	+	+
Phenolics	+	+	+	-
Saponins	+	-	+	+
Anthraquinones	+	-	+	+
Flavonoids	-	-	-	-

*+ **High concentration**; + Low concentration; - Absent*

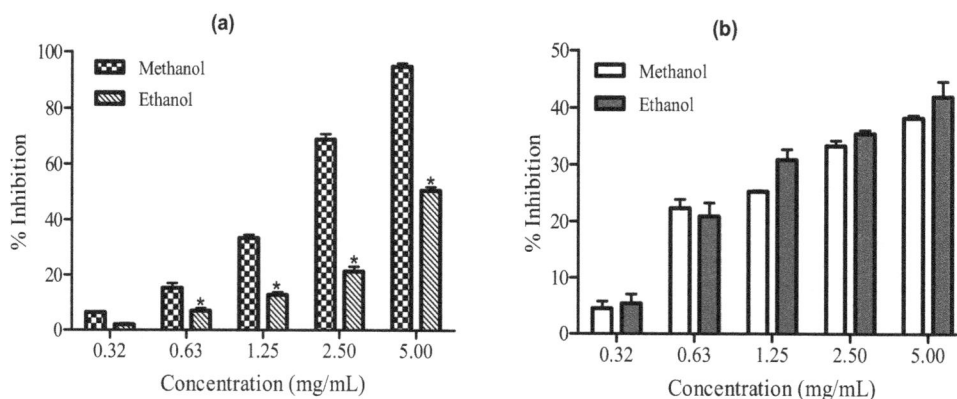

Fig. 1. Inhibitory potency of (a) *C. paniculatum* and (b) *M. morindoides* leaves extracts against α-amylase activity. The values are expressed as means ± SEM of triplicate determinations
Significantly different at the same concentration (P= .05)

Table 2. IC$_{50}$ values of α-amylase and α-glucosidase inhibition by *C. paniculatum M. morindoides* leaf extracts

Extracts	IC50 (mg/mL)	
	α-Amylase	α-Glucosidase
C. paniculatum methanol	2.27±0.02[a]	2.50±0.02[a]
C. paniculatum ethanol	5.06±0.03[b]	1.96±0.01[b]
M. morindoides methanol	6.43±0.01[c]	2.05±0.01[b]
M. morindoides ethanol	5.63±0.02[b]	2.68±0.02[a]
Acarbose	2.60±0.01[a]	0.63±0.00[c]

We found that methanol extract of *C. paniculatum* displayed the highest inhibition of α-amylase while both extracts of *M. morindoides* possessed less than 50% inhibition of the enzyme. The result culminated in the low IC$_{50}$ (2.27 mg/mL) obtained for the methanol extract of *C. paniculatum*. The possession of a lower IC$_{50}$ similar to the standard, acarbose suggests that the extract provides similar physiological as well as side effects, arising from the excessive inhibition of α-amylase [38]. Therefore, ethanol extract of *C. paniculatum* was selected for further study because a good antidiabetic agent should necessarily be a mild inhibitor of this enzyme so as to prevent the side effect of synthetic agents like acarbose [39]. Ethanol extract of *C. paniculatum* also displayed the best inhibition of α-glucosidase and this resulted in its lowest IC$_{50}$. This is because it is desirable of a potent antidiabetic drug to be a strong inhibitor of α-glucosidase.

Figs. 3(a) and 3(b) showed the mode(s) of inhibition of both α-amylase and α-glucosidase by the ethanol extract of *C. paniculatum*. These show that ethanol extract of *C. paniculatum* inhibited α-amylase non-competitively while α-glucosidase was inhibited in a mixed non-competitive manner.

The pure non-competitive inhibition of α-amylase by the ethanol extract of *C. paniculatum* indicated that the active components in the extract also binds to a site other than the active site of the enzyme and combines with either free enzyme or the enzyme-substrate complex, possibly interfering with the action of both [40]. However, the inhibitor had equal affinity for both the free enzyme and enzyme-substrate complex. Similarly, the mixed non-competitive inhibition of α-glucosidase by the ethanol extract also suggests that the inhibitory components in the extract also bind to a site other than the active site of the enzyme but has different affinities for the free enzyme and enzyme-substrate complex [41].

The effect of oral administration of ethanol extract of *C. paniculatum* on starch-loaded postprandial hyperglycemia is shown in Fig. 4. At all durations tested, the extract-treated group had significantly lower (*P*= .05) blood glucose level compared to the control animals.

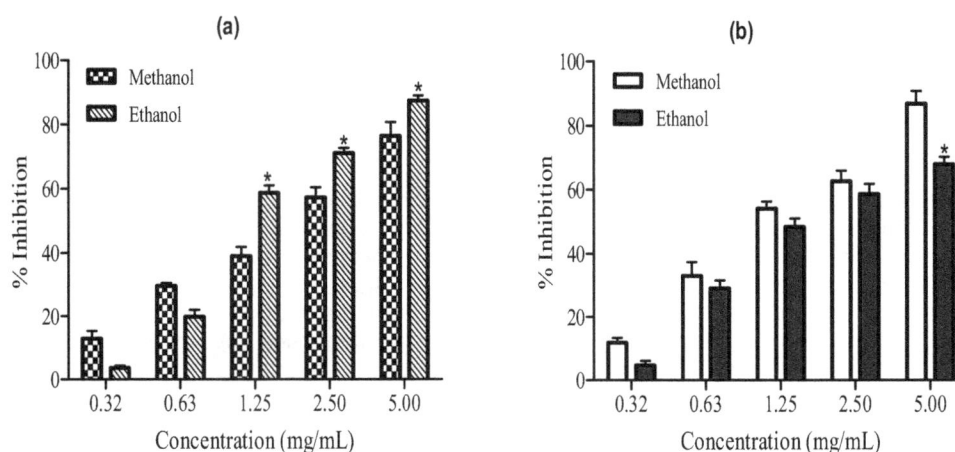

Fig. 2. Inhibitory potency of (a) *C. paniculatum* and (b) *M. morindoides* leaves extracts against α-glucosidase activity. The values are expressed as means ± SEM of triplicate determinations
Significantly different at the same concentration (P= .05)

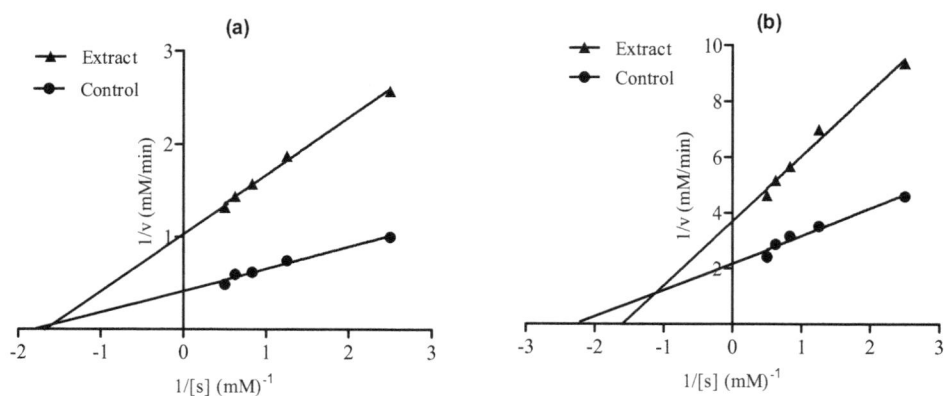

Fig. 3. Mode of inhibition of (a) α-amylase and (b) α-glucosidase by ethanol extract of *C. paniculatum* leaves

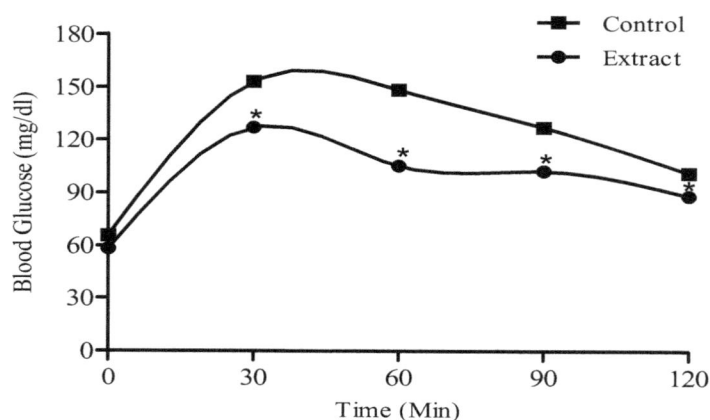

Fig. 4. Effect of administration of ethanol extract of *C. paniculatum* on blood glucose level of starch - loaded rats
* Values are significantly different from the control

In order to ascertain the antihyperglycemic effect of *C. paniculatum*, ethanol extract of the plant was orally administered to starch-loaded rats. The significant reduction in the postprandial blood glucose level of the extract-treated rats compared to the control suggests the plant possesses antihyperglycemic potential [38]. Therefore, we inferred that the antihyperglycaemic effect of the extract may be due to the inhibition of the pancreatic α-amylase and intestinal α-glucosidase in the rats, thereby lowering their blood glucose levels.

The α-amylase and α-glucosidase inihibitory effect as well as the antihyperglycemic potential of the ethanol extract of *C. paniculatum* may be due to the presence of phytochemicals such as tannins, phenolics and steroids in the plant. Tannins have been found to induce phosphorylation of insulin receptors and translocation of glucose transporter, thereby helping in the reduction of blood glucose level [42] while phenolics have been found to possess antioxidant, hypoglycemic and antiglycation potentials [43]. Steroids on the other hand, are involved in the stimulation of pancreatic β-cells and subsequent secretion of insulin [44]. It can therefore be concluded that the antihyperglycemic potential of the ethanol extract of *C. paniculatum* may be due to the presence of these phytochemicals present in it.

4. CONCLUSION

This study revealed that out of all the extracts of plants tested, ethanol extract of *C. paniculatum* displayed mild and strong inhibition of α-amylase and glucosidase respectively. *M. morindoides* extracts did not exhibited potent inhibition of both enzymes. Ethanol extract of *C. paniculatum* also inhibited both enzymes in a non-competitive manner and reduces postprandial blood glucose level of starch-loaded rats. It can be concluded that ethanol extract of *C. paniculatum* possesses hypoglycemic potential and its mode of antidiabetic action may be due to inhibition of pancreatic α-amylase and intestinal glucosidase.

CONSENT

It is not applicable

ETHICAL APPROVAL

All authors hereby declare that "Principles of laboratory animal care" (NIH publication No. 85-23, revised 1985) were followed.

COMPETING INTERESTS

Authors have declared that no competing interests exist.

REFERENCES

1. American Diabetes Association, Diagnosis and classification of diabetes mellitus, Diabetes Care. 2011;34(1):s62-s69.
2. International Diabetes Federation, IDF Diabetes Atlas, 6th Edition, Brussels, Belgium; 2013.
3. Turchin A, Matheny ME, Shubina M, Scanlon JV, Greenwood B, Pendergrass ML. Hypoglycemia and clinical outcomes in patients with diabetes hospitalized in the general ward. Diabetes Care. 2009;32(7):1153-1157.
4. Adisakwattana S, Roengsamran S, Hsu WH, Yibchok-anun S. Mechanisms of antihyperglycemic effect of p-methoxycinnamic acid in normal and streptozotocin-induced diabetic rats. Life Sci. 2005;78(4):406-412.
5. Asres K, Bucar F, Kartnig T, Witvrouw M, Pannecoupe C, De Clercq E. Antiviral activity against human immunodeficiency virus type 1 (HIV-1) and type 2 (HIV-2) of ethnobotanically selected Ethiopian medicinal plants. Phytother Res. 2001;15(1):62-69.
6. Abbot BJ, Leiter J, Hartwel L, Caldwell ME, Beal JL, Perdue RE, et al. Screening data from the cancer chemotherapy national service center screening laboratories. XXXIV. Plant extracts. Cancer Res. 1966;26(3):207-366.
7. De Morais Lima GR, de Sales IRP, Caldas-Filho MRD, de Jesus NZT, de Sousa- Falcão H, Barbosa-Filho JM, et al. Bioactivities of the Genus *Combretum* (*Combretaceae*): A Review. Molecules. 2012;17(8):9142-9206
8. Sowemimo A, Van de Venter M, Baatjies L, Koekemoer T, Adesanya S, Lin W. Cytotoxic compounds from the leaves of *Combretum paniculatum* Vent. Afr J Biotech. 2012;11(20):4631-4635.
9. Hema A, Palé E, Duez P, Luhmer M, Nacro M. Two diglucosylated anthocyanins from *Combretum paniculatum* flowers. Nat Sci. 2012;4(3):166-169.
10. Samdumu FB. Characterization of antimicrobial compounds from *Combretum paniculatum*, a plant with anti-HIV replication activity. Ph.D Thesis, University of Pretoria, South Africa; 2007.
11. Moroh JL, Bahi C, Dje K, Loukou YG, Guede-Guina F. Study of the antibacterial activity of *Morinda morindoides* (Baker) Milne-Readhead (*Rubiaceae*) acetatique extract (ACE) on *in vitro* growth of *Escherichia coli* strains. Bull Soc Roy Sci Liege. 2008;77(1):44-61.
12. Koffi AE, Yapi HF, Bahi C, Guessend KN, Djaman JA, Guede-Guina F. Antimicrobial activity of *Morinda morindoides* on *in vitro* growth of vibrio cholerae in Côte d'Ivoire]. Med Trop (Mars). 2010;70(1):53-56. French.
13. Bagre I, Bahi C, Gnahoue, Djaman AJ, Guede-Guina F. Phytochemical composition and evaluation of in vitro antifungal activity of leaves of *Morinda morindoides* (Baker) Milne-redh (*Rubiaceae*) against *Aspergillus fumigatus* and *Candida albicans*. J Sci Pharm Biol. 2007; 8(1):15-23.
14. Meite S, N'guessan JD, Bahi C, Yapi HF, Djaman AJ, Guede-Guina F. Antidiarrheoal activity of the ethyl acetate extract of *Morinda morindoides* in rats. Trop J Pharm Res. 2009;8(3):201-207
15. Cimanga K, De Bruyne T , Lasure A, Poel BV, Pieters L, van den Berghe D, et al. *In vitro* anticomplementary activity of

constituents from *Morinda morindoides*. J Nat Prod. 1995;58(3):372-378.

16. Cimanga K, de Bruyne T, Hu JP, Cos P, Apers S, Pieters L. et al. Constituents from *Morinda morindoides* leaves as inhibitors of xanthine oxidase and scavengers of superoxide anions. Pharm Pharmacol Comm. 1999;5(6):419-424.

17. Zirihi GN, Mambu L, Guede-Guede F, Bodo B, Grellier P. *In vitro* antiplasmodial activity and cytotoxicity of 33 West African plants used for the treatment of malaria. J Ethnopharmacol. 2005;98(3):281-285.

18. Cimanga RK, Tona GL, Kambu OK, Mesia GK, Muyembe JJT, Apers S. et al. Antimalarial activity of some extracts and isolated constituents from *Morinda morindoides* leaves. J Nat Med. 2008;8(2):191-202.

19. Satoru T, Bruno KK, Sawako I, Toshihiro H, Muzele KT, Nobutoshi M. New anti-malarial phenylpropanoid conjugated iridoids fromMorinda morindoides. Bioorg Med Chem Lett. 2010;20(5):1520-1523.

20. Dawet A, Yakubu P. Antiplasmodial efficacy of stem bark extracts of *Pseudocedrela kotschyi* in mice infected with *Plasmodium berghei berghei*. British J Pharm Res. 2014;4(5):594-607.

21. Adenubi OT, Olukunle JO, Abatan MO, Ajayi OL, Adeleye OE, Kehinde OO. Antispermatogenic activity of *Morinda morindoides* root bark extract in male wistar rats. J Nat Sci Engr Tech. 2010;9(1):99-105.

22. Cimanga KR, Mukenyi PNK, Kambu KO, Tona LG, Apers S, Totte J. et al. The spasmolytic activity of extracts and some isolated compounds from the leaves of *Morinda morindoides* (Baker) Milne-Redh. (Rubiaceae). J. Ethnopharmacol. 2010; 127(2):215-220.

23. Marie-Genevieve OA, Ongoka PR, Gatouillat G, Attibayeba, Lavaud C, Madoulet C. Cytotoxic effect induced by *Morinda morindoides* leaf extracts in human and murine leukemia cells. Afr J Biotech. 2010;9(39):6560-6565.

24. Balogun EA, Akinloye DI. Biochemical effects of methanolic extract of *Morinda Morindoides* and *Morinda lucida* leaves on lipid profile, bilirubin and some marker enzymes. Asian J Med Res. 2012;1(1):12-16.

25. Harisolo R, Chardin SS, Philomène AY, Timothé O, Vincent AA, Léon AD, Antoin AC. A ketosteroid isolated from *Morinda morindoides*. Europ J Sci Res. 2009;28(4):622-627.

26. Cimanga K, De Bruyne T, Lasure A, Li Q, Pieters L, Claeys M, Vanden BD, Kambu K, Tona L, Vlietinck AJ. Flavonoid o-glycosides from the leaves of *Morinda morindoides*. Phytochem. 1995;38(5): 1301-1303.

27. Koffi KJ, Doumbia I, Méité S, Yapi HF, Djaman AJ, N'guessan JD. Phytopharmacological evaluation of *Morinda morindoides* for anti-hyperglycemic activity in normal rabbits. Int Res J Biochem Bioinform. 2012;2(1):16-21.

28. Olukunle JO, Abatan MO, Adenubi OT, Amusan TA. Hypoglycaemic and hypolipidaemic effects of crude extracts and chromatographic fractions of *Morinda morindoides* root bark in diabetic rats. Acta Vet Brno. 2012;81:259-274. DOI:10.2754/avb201281030269.

29. Kazeem MI, Adamson JO, Ogunwande IA. Modes of inhibition of α-amylase and α-gluscosidase by aqueous extracts of *Morinda lucida* Benth. leaf. Biomed Res Int; 2013. Article ID 527570:6. Available:http://dx.doi.org/10.1155/2013/52 7570

30. Ogunwande IA, Matsui T, Fujise T, Matsumoto K. α-Glucosidase inhibitory profile of Nigerian medicinal plants in immobilized assay system. Food Sci Technol Res. 2007;13(2):169-172.

31. Trease GE, Evans WC. Pharmacognosy, WB Saunders: Philadelphia, USA; 1996.

32. Sofowora A. Medical Plants and Traditional Medicine in Africa. Spectrum Books: Ibadan, Nigeria; 1996.

33. Mccue PP, Shetty K. Inhibitory effects of rosmarinic acid extracts on porcine pancreatic α-amylase *in vitro*. Asia Pac J Clin Nutr. 2004;13(1):101-106.

34. Ali H, Houghton PJ, Soumyanath A. Alpha-amylase inhibitory activity of some Malaysian plants used to treat diabetes with particular reference to *Phyllanthus amarus*. J Ethnopharmacol. 2006;107(3): 449-55.

35. Kim YM, Jeong YK, Wang MH, Lee WY, Rhee HI. Inhibitory effects of pine bark extract on alpha-glucosidase activity and postprandial hyperglycemia. Nutr. 2005; 21(6):756-61.

36. Matsui T, Ogunwande IA, Abesundara KJM, Matsumoto K. Anti-hyperglycemic

potential of natural products. Mini Rev Medic Chem. 2006;6(3):349-356.

37. Auwal IA, Islam MS. Butanol fraction of *Khaya senegalensis* root modulates β-cell function and ameliorates diabetes-related biochemical parameters in a type 2 diabetes rat model. J Ethnopharmacol. 2014;154(3):832-838.

38. Adisakwattana S, Yibchok-Anun S, Charoenlertkul P, Wongsasiripat N. Cyanidin-3-rutinoside alleviates postprandial hyperglycemia and its synergism with acarbose by inhibition of intestinal α-glucosidase. J Clin Biochem Nutr. 2011;49(1):36-41.

39. Kwon YI, Vattem DA, Shetty K. Evaluation of clonal herbs of Lamiaceae species for management of diabetes and hypertension. Asia Pac J Clin Nutr. 2005;15(1):107-108.

40. Shai LJ, Masoko P, Mokgotho MP, Magano SR, Mogale AM, Boaduo N, et al. Yeast alpha glucosidase inhibitory and antioxidant activities of six medicinal plants collected in Phalaborwa, South Africa. South Afr J Bot. 2010;76(3):465-70.

41. Dixon M, Webb EC. Enzyme inhibition and activation, In *Enzymes*, 3rd edition. New York: Academic Press Inc. 1999;332-380.

42. Liu X, Kim JK, Li Y, Li J, Liu F, Chen X. Tannic acid stimulates glucose transport and inhibits adipocyte differentiation in 3T3-Li cells. J Nutr. 2005;135(2):165-171.

43. Han X, Shen T, Lou H. Dietary polyphenols and their biological significance. Int J Molec Sci. 2007;8(9):950-988.

44. Daisy P, Jasmine R, Ignacimuthu S, Murugan E. A novel steroid from *Elephantopus scaber* L. an ethnomedicinal plant with antidiabetic activity. Phytomed. 2009;16(2-3):252-257.

13

Antibacterial Activity and Phytochemical Screening of *Goniothalamus sesquipedalis* (Wall.) Hook. f. & Thomson Extracts from Manipur, North East India

Sanjita Chanu Konsam[1], Sanjoy Singh Ningthoujam[2*] and Kumar Singh Potsangbam[1]

[1]*Department of Life Sciences, Manipur University, Canchipur, Imphal, India.*
[2]*Department of Botany, Ghanapriya Women's College, Imphal, India.*

Authors' contributions

This work was carried out in collaboration between all authors. Authors SSN and KSP designed the experiment and managed the analysis of the study. Author SCK wrote the protocol, performed the experiment and wrote the first draft of the manuscript. Author SSN performed the statistical analysis. All authors read and approved the final manuscript.

Editor(s):
(1) Marcello Iriti, Faculty of Plant Biology and Pathology, Department of Agricultural and Environmental Sciences, Milan State University, Italy.
Reviewers:
(1) Armando Zarrelli, Department of Chemical Science, University of Naples, Italy.
(2) Anonymous, Sao Paulo State University, Brazil.

ABSTRACT

Aims: To screen the phytochemical constituents and study the antibacterial properties of the *Goniothalamus sesquipedalis* (Wall.) Hook.f. & Thomson used in the traditional medicine in the North East India.
Place and Duration of Study: Plant samples were collected from different parts of Manipur during May 2013 to February 2014. Experiments were performed at Department of Life Sciences, Manipur University, Canchipur, Imphal.
Methodology: Antibacterial activities were analyzed by well diffusion method against the pathogen *Bacillus subtilis* and *Escherichia coli* by using different concentrations of methanolic extracts. Phytochemical screening was performed on the extracts of different solvents viz. chloroform, ethanol, methanol, petroleum ether and water.
Results: Methanolic extract exhibited higher inhibition zones in *Escherichia coli* with 10.03, 12.01,

Corresponding author: E-mail: ningthouja@hotmail.com

13.04, 14.04, 15.03 and 16.04 mm as compared to *Bacillus subtilis* which showed 3.00, 4.04, 6.03, 7.04, 8.03 and 10.01 mm against extract concentrations of 20, 40, 60, 80, 100 and 120 µl respectively. Alkaloids, flavonoids and terpenoids were detected in all the solvents used. Glycosides were not detected in chloroform extracts while phenols and tannins were absent in water extract. Phytosterol and saponins were detected in ethanol, water and petroleum ether extracts.

Conclusion: The present study showed that the *Goniothalamus sesquipedalis* is potential source of antibacterial agents and reaffirms its importance in traditional medicine.

Keywords: Goniothalamus sesquipedalis; antibacterial activity; phytochemical screening; North East India; traditional medicine.

1. INTRODUCTION

Medicinal plants are important component in the traditional medicine which have been practiced in many developed and developing countries [1]. Plants associated with ethnomedicinal practices are the potential target for drug discovery programmes with the anticipation that these plants might possess bioactive compounds or potential lead compounds. However, intense studies of these ethnomedicinal plants are required to determine whether these usage are actually related to their medicinal properties or placebo effects associated with their folklore. For validating the traditional uses as well as providing insights in drug discovery programmes, biochemical screening of ethnomedicinal plants used by different communities remain significant.

The genus *Goniothalamus* Hk. f. et Thoms. (family: Annonaceae) consists of about 130 shrubs and tree species growing in the rainforest of tropical Asia [2]. This genus has wide distribution covering Eastern India, Myanmar, Bangladesh and Malayan archipelago [3-5]. Many species of the genus are used in fiber, timber source, ornamental and medicinal purposes in different countries. Species of this genus are known for wide ranging biological activities such as immunosuppressive and anti-inflammatory, anti-malarial, anticancer and larvicidal activity [6]. Root of *G. cheliensis* from the Yunnan province of China were used for treatment of cancer, malaria, edema, rheumatism and as pesticide [7,8]. Seeds of *G. amuyon* [9] from Taiwan was used in the treatment of edema and rheumatism. Stem bark decoction of *G. laoticus* in Thailand were used as febrifuge. In Malaysia, *G. scortechinii* was used in abortion, post-natal treatment and insect repellents [10] while *G. macrophyllus* was used in colds, fever, malaria, cholera and post-partum treatments [11,12]. Roots of *G. giganteus* were also used for treatment of colds, swellings and as abortifacient

[2]. In Indonesia, an infusion of the roots of *G. tapis* was used to treat typhoid fever [13]. Out of 130-140 species of the genus, about thirty seven species of the genus have been studied for phytochemical and pharmacological properties [14]. Because of the presence of cytotoxic acetogenins and styryl-lactones in the genus, the various species are considered to be potential source of anticancer and antibacterial drugs [2].

In the North East India, various species of the *Goniothalamus* are available. Out of these species, *Goniothalamus sesquipedalis* (Wall.) Hook.f. & Thomson is one important species that is used for various utilities. This glabrous shrub is sparingly branched and extends up to 50 to 120 cm [5,15]. Leaves are oblong, acuminate, coriaceous and minutely pellucid punctuate [3,5,15]. The flowers are solitary and axillary, often greenish yellow in colour [3-5,15] with pedicels 0.2-0.4 cm long [5]. Flower buds are triquetrous and valvate. Calyx consists of three sepals, each with 0.4 cm length [3,5] and shining interior [15]. The corolla consists of two series of three petals which are glabrous [3]. The androecium comprises of many stamens [3] and the gynoecium consists of carpels which are ovoid, glabrous, very short stalked orange red with 5 in number varying from 3-4 or 8-10 [3,4,15]. Fruit orange red with short stalked, 3-4 or 8-10 cm, mucronate, granulate [3,5]. Ovaries are golden strigose, narrow, and cylindrically recurved [4]. Flowering and fruiting occur between May and September [5].

G. sesquipedalis has wide ranging applications in traditional medicine in the North East Indian region. Traditional applications ranged from cough and urinary problems [16], insecticide and blood purifier [17], sleep inducer and asthma [18], post-natal treatments [19] to leucorrhoea [20]. Moreover, *G. sesquipedalis* along with another species of Lamiaceae, *Isodon ternifolius* were used in Manipur, one of the states of the

North East India, in pre and post-natal care as well as in traditional fumigation (Fig. 1). Traditional people believed that both of these species have properties that act against pathogens and possess other disease causing materials. Considering the phytochemical and pharmacological properties of other species of the genus and the traditional uses associated with this plant, it is highly probable that *G. sesquipedalis* might have possess antibacterial properties. With this perspective, an attempt has been made to study the antibacterial properties of the *G. sesquipedalis* and characterize the phytochemical constituents.

2. MATERIALS AND METHODS

2.1 Plant Collection and Storage

G. sesquipedalis plants were collected from different parts of Manipur, India from May 2013 to February 2014. Plants were identified and deposited (Voucher No. SCK-012) in the Department of Life Sciences, Manipur University, Canchipur, India. The plant materials were washed properly and grind to powder after drying. Then, the materials were stored in closed containers at room temperature until used.

2.2 Preparation of Extracts

The extracts were prepared by soaking 5 g of the powdered materials in 50 ml each of different solvents, viz. chloroform, ethanol, methanol, petroleum ether and water for 24 hr. The extracts were then filtered using Whatman Filter Paper which was concentrated to half of the volume. Filtrates were centrifuged at 1000 rpm for 30 min. It is again filtered, concentrated to dried residue and then stored in airtight containers separately till use [21].

2.3 Phytochemical Analysis

Extracts of different solvents were analyzed for the detection of various constituents. Test for alkaloid was done by using Dragendroff and Wagner Reagent method [21], Glycosides Salkowski's Test was also performed to determine the presence of phytosterol and terpenoids [22]. Froth Test and Foam Test were conducted for the presence of saponin with slight modification [21]. Estimation were also done for the presence of glycosides [1,23,24], flavonoids, phenol and tannins [25]. Estimations were done in triplicates.

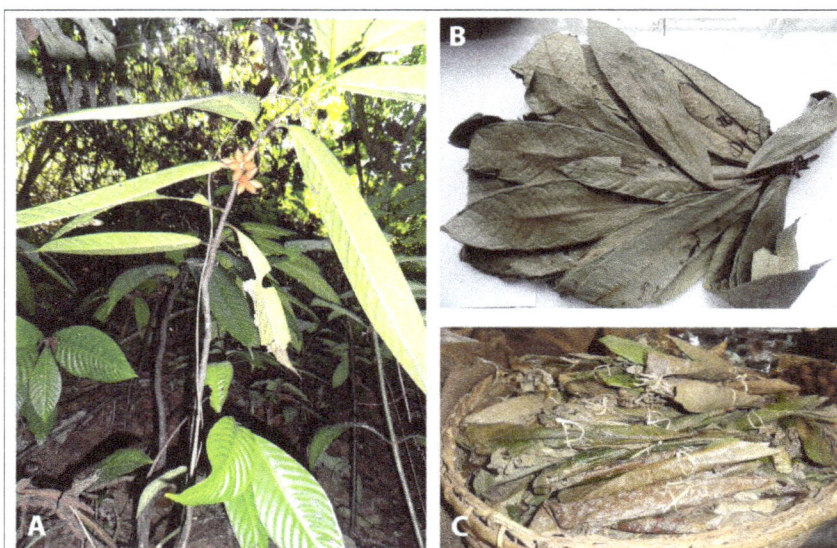

Fig. 1. (a) *Goniothalamus sesquipedalis* growing in the wild, (b) Dry leaves of *G. sesquipedalis* and (c) dry leaves of *G. sesquipedalis* and *Isodon ternifolius* selling in the market of Manipur, North East India

2.4 Bacterial Strains

The antibacterial activity of *G. sesquipedalis* leaf extract was tested against gram positive *Bacillus subtilis* (MUBS052) and gram negative *Escherichia coli* (MUEC045). The strains were provided by the Plant Pathology Laboratory, Life Sciences Department, Manipur University and were maintained in the Mueller Hinton agar medium at 4°C. Inoculums were prepared by growing cells in Mueller Hinton broth (MHB) for 24 hours at 37°C.

2.5 Determination of Antibacterial Activity

The antibacterial activity was evaluated in the methanolic extracts by the agar well diffusion method using Muller-Hinton agar plates [26]. The agar plates were swabbed with *B. subtilis* and *E. coli* by using sterile cotton swab and wells of 6 mm diameter were punched in each plate using a sterile cork borer. Then, 0.3 g of dried methanolic extract was dissolved in 1.5 ml of DMSO (dimethyl sufoxide) which served as the stock solution. The extracts were then transferred into the wells with different concentrations of 20, 40, 60, 80, 100 and 120 µl and incubated at $37^\circ C$ for 24 h. After incubation, the diameter of the zone of growth of inhibition of the plant extracts were compared with that of DMSO as negative control [26,27].

2.6 Statistical Analysis

Experiments were carried out in triplicates and results are expressed as the mean ± SD (standard deviation). ANOVA tests were performed to test the significance difference between the different means at $p=0.05$. Statistical analyses were done in SPSS Version 19.0.

3. RESULTS AND DISCUSSION

Methanolic extract of the leaves of *G. sesquipedalis* have been tested against the *B. subtilis* and *E. coli*. The results from the present study showed that the extracts have antibacterial activities against both tested organisms. However, the activities differed according to the tested organisms and the concentrations of extracts. Methanolic extract showed less activities in gram positive *B. subtilis* as compared to gram negative *E. coli* (Table 1).

Methanolic extract of the *G. sesquipedalis* inhibited the growth of two tested organisms in dose-dependent manner (Fig. 2). It was observed that zone of inhibition at different well increased markedly corresponding to drug concentration. These inhibitions were observed to significantly different at $p = 0.05$ in both the organisms.

Table 1. Antibacterial activity of methanolic extract of *G. sesquipedalis* leaves against *E. coli* and *B. subtilis*

Organisms	Zone of Inhibition (in mm)
Escherichia coli	10.03 ± 0.05
Bacillus subtilis	3.00 ± 0.01

The results of phytochemical screening of *G. sesquipedalis* showed the presence of alkaloids, flavonoids and terpenoids in all the extracts used (Table 2). Glycosides were detected in all extracts except in chloroform. Phenols and tannins were not detected in water extract. Phytosterols and saponins were found to be present in ethanol, water and petroleum ether extracts.

In the present study, methanolic extract had been used for testing the antibacterial properties of the species. This organic solvent has been selected because of its capability of solubilizing the various active components belonging to alkaloids, flavonoids, glycosides, phenols, tannins and terpenoids [28]. The *G. sesquipedalis* methanolic extract has shown to exhibit antibacterial activities against two test organisms. These bioactivities can be compared to similar activities reported in other species [2,29]. Methanolic extracts of *G. scortechinii* exhibited mean zone of inhibition 20 mm and 13 mm against *Bacillus sp.* and *Escherichia coli* in Disc diffusion method [2], while *G. umbrosus* exhibited mean zone of inhibition 15 mm in dichloromethane extract [6] while using 20 mg/ml of the extracts.

Application of plant extract with known antimicrobial properties are significant for further therapeutic treatments. Antimicrobial activities of the *G. sesquipedalis* could be ascribed to the presence of different compound such as goniopedaline, aristololactam A-II, taliscanine, aurantiamide acetate, beta sitosterol [30]. Among the phytochemicals present, alkaloids were known for antibacterial properties in many plants. Presence of alkaloids were also characterized from other species of the genus such as *G. griffithii* [31] and *G. laoticus* [32] which also exhibited antimicrobial properties.

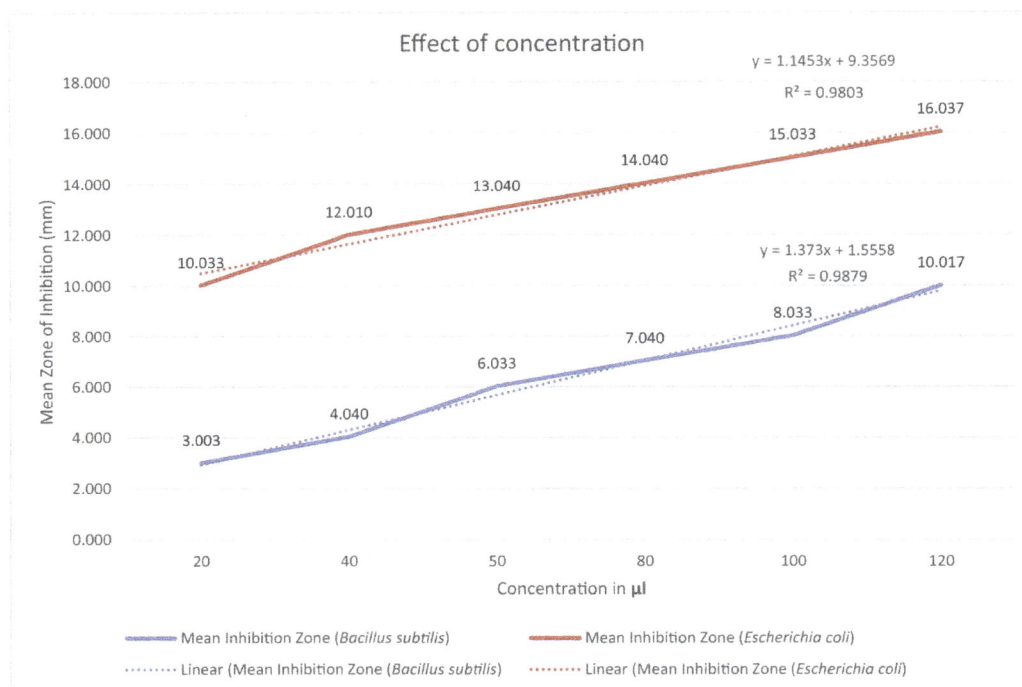

Fig. 2. Effect of concentration of crude extract on inhibition zone

Table 2. Phytochemical groups present in different extracts of *G. sesquipedalis*

Solvents	Alkaloids	Flavonoids	Glycosides	Phenols	Phytosterols	Saponins	Tannins	Terpenoids
Ethanol	+	+	+	+	+	+	+	+
Water	+	+	+	-	+	+	-	+
Methanol	+	+	+	+	-	-	+	+
Petroleum ether	+	+	+	+	+	+	+	+
Chloroform	+	+	-	+	-	-	+	+

Presence of flavonoids in the methanolic extract might be another result as these compounds are known to possess anti-allergic, anti-inflammatory, anti-microbial and anti-cancer properties [33]. Flavonoids can act as bacteriostatic compounds by restricting the number of viable colonies and can also act as energy metabolism inhibitor. Terpenoids present in the methanolic extract might have also contributed to the antibacterial properties as these compounds are active against bacteria and fungi [2].

With regard to antibacterial property, one compound altholactone, a styryl-lactone isolated from *G. mayalayanus* was observed to be effective against both Gram positive and Gram negative bacteria [34]. This compound is yet to be isolated from *G. sesquipedalis*, though many species of this genus are believed to possess different compounds belonging to stylryl-lactone

[35,36]. Exact mechanism of the antibacterial activity in this species are yet to be confirmed as there are chances of synergistic relationship between different compounds [29].

4. CONCLUSION

The present study affirmed the antibacterial activity of *G. sesquipedalis* species growing in North East India. These antibacterial activities which might be the reason for preference of this species as fumigants in traditional post-partum management. The study also highlighted the possible utilization of this species in future drug discovery processes from the natural resources from Manipur. Future direction calls for isolation and characterization of the individual components present in this species for drug discovery processes.

ETHICAL APPROVAL

No human and animal subjects were used in the experiment. Authors have followed National and International ethical standard while performing the experiment and writing the manuscript.

COMPETING INTERESTS

Authors have declared that no competing interests exist.

REFERENCES

1. WHO. National policy on traditional medicine and regulation of herbal medicines: Report of a WHO global survey. Geneva: World Health Organization; 2005.
2. Wiart C. Goniothalamus species: A source of drugs for the treatment of cancers and bacterial infections? Evid Based Complement Alternat Med. 2007;4(3):299-311.
3. Oinam KS. Floristic study of Tamnenglong district, Manipur with ethnobotanical notes. Department of Life Sciences, Manipur University, (Ph.D. Thesis Unpublished); 1990.
4. Hooker JD. The Flora of British India. London: L. Reeve & Co. 1875;1.
5. Singh NP, Chauhan AS, Mondal MS. Flora of Manipur. Calcutta: Botanical Survey of India. 2000;1.
6. Wahab SIA, Abdul AB, Fong HK, Mohan S, Elhassan MM, Zubairi ASA, et al. Antimicrobial and free radical scavenging activities of the dichloromethane extract of Goniothalamus umbrosus. Int J Trop Med. 2009;41:32-6.
7. Jiang MM, Feng YF, Gao H, Zhang X, Tang JS, Yao XS. Three new bis-styryllactones from Goniothalamus cheliensis. Fitoterapia. 2011;82(4):524-7.
8. Jiang MM, Feng YF, Zhang X, Zhao LL, Yao XS. Furanofurone-type styryllactones from Goniothalamus cheliensis. Biochem Syst Ecol. 2011;39(4-6):846-8.
9. Li X, Chang CJ. Antitumor cytotoxicity and stereochemistry of polyketides from Goniothalamus amuyon. Nat Prod Lett. 1996;8(3):207-15.
10. Burkill IH. A dictionary of the economic products of the Malay Peninsula. A Dictionary of the Economic Products of the Malay Peninsula. 2nd edition; 1966.
11. Izaddin SA, Ee GCL, Rahmani M. Bioactive compound from Goniothalamus andersonii. Proceedings of the International Seminar on Chemistry. Jatinangor; 2008.
12. Abdullah N, Sahibul-Anwar H, Ideris S, Hasuda T, Hitotsuyanagi Y, Takeya K, et al. Goniolandrene A and B from Goniothalamus macrophyllus. Fitoterapia. 2013;88:1-6.
13. Efdi M, Fujita S, Inuzuka T, Koketsu M. Chemical studies on Goniothalamus tapis Miq. Nat Prod Res. 2010;24(7):657-62.
14. Choo CY, Abdullah N, Diederich M. Cytotoxic activity and mechanism of action of metabolites from the Goniothalamus genus. Phytochem Rev. 2014;13(4):835-51.
15. Kanjilal UN, Kanjilal PC, Das A. Flora of Assam I. Delhi: Taj Offset Press; 1982.
16. Imotomba RK, Devi LS. Creation of geo-spatial data base of medicinal plants of Senapati district, Manipur. Nat J Chem Biosis. 2011;2(2):17-36.
17. Sanglakpam P, Mathur RR, Pandey AK. Ethnobotany of chothe tribe of Bishnupur district (Manipur). Indian J Nat Prod Resour. 2012;3(3):414-25.
18. Rai PK, Lalramnghinglova H. Ethnomedicinal plants of india with special reference to an Indo-Burma hotspot region: An overview. Ethnobot Res Appl. 2011;9:379-420.
19. Meetei SY, Singh PK. Survey for medicinal plants of Thoubal district, Manipur. Flora Fauna. 2007;13(2):355-8.
20. Shil S, Choudhury MD. Indigenous knowledge on healthcare practices by the Reang Tribe of Dhalai district of Tripura, North East India. Ethnobot Leaflets. 2009;13:775-90.
21. Latha B, Rumaisa Y, Soumya CK, Shafeena S, Sadhiya N. Phytochemical studies on Leucas aspera. J Chem Pharma Res. 2013;5(4):222-8.
22. Singh D, Singh P, Gupta A, Solanki S, sharma E, Nema R. Qualitative estimation of the presence of bioactive compound in Centella asiatica: An important medicinal plant. Int J Life Sci Med Sci. 2012;2(1):5-7.
23. Kinnings SL, Liu N, Buchmeier N, Tonge PJ, Xie L, Bourne PE. Drug discovery using chemical systems biology: Repositioning the safe medicine comtan to treat multi-drug and extensively drug resistant tuberculosis. PLoS Comput Biol. 2009;5(7):e1000423.

24. Manalisha D, Chandra KJ. Preliminary phytochemical analysis and acute oral toxicity study of *Clitoria ternatea* Linn. root in albino mice. Int Res J Pharm. 2011;2(12):139-40.

25. Menon AV, Vijayalakshmi S, Ranjitha J. Preliminary phytochemical screening and heavy metal analysis of leaf extracts of *Hippophae rhamnoides* Linn. Int J Pharm Sci Rev Res. 2014;25(2):76-9.

26. Karthikeyan A, Shanthi V, Nagasathaya A. Preliminary phytochemical and antibacterial screening of crude extract of the leaf of *Adhatoda vasica* L. Int J Green Pharm. 2013;3(1):78-80.

27. Mandal S, Patra A, Samanta A, Roy S, Mandal A, Mahapatra TD, et al. Analysis of phytochemical profile of *Terminalia arjuna* bark extract with antioxidative and antimicrobial properties. Asian Pac J Trop Biomed. 2013;3(12):960-6.

28. Bauer AW, Kirby WM, Sherris JC, Turck M. Antibiotic susceptibility testing by a standardized single disk method. Am J Clin Pathol. 1966;45(4):493-6.

29. Humeirah AS, Azah MN, Mastura M, Mailina J, Saiful J, Muhajir H, et al. Chemical constituents and antimicrobial activity of *Goniothalamus macrophyllus* (Annonaceae) from Pasoh Forest Reserve, Malaysia. Afr J Biotechnol. 2010;9(34): 5511-5.

30. Talapatra SK, Basu D, Chattopadhyay P, Talapatra B. Aristololactams of *Goniothalamus sesquipedalis* wall. Revised structures of the 2-oxygenated aristololactams. Phytochemistry. 1988; 27(3):903-6.

31. Zhang Y-J, Kong M, Chen R-Y, Yu D-Q. Alkaloids from the roots of *Goniothalamus griffithii*. J Nat Prod. 1999;62(7):1050-2.

32. Lekphrom R, Kanokmedhakul S, Kanokmedhakul K. Bioactive styryllactones and alkaloid from flowers of *Goniothalamus laoticus*. J Ethnopharmacol. 2009;125(1): 47-50.

33. Joselin J, Brintha TSS, Florence AR, Jeeva S. Screening of select ornamental flowers of the family Apocynaceae for phytochemical constituents. Asian Pac J Trop Dis. 2012;2:S260-S4.

34. Al Momani F, Alkofahi AS, Mhaidat NM. Altholactone displays promising antimicrobial activity. Molecules. 2011; 16(6):4560-6.

35. Cao SG, Wu XH, Sim KY, Tan B, Pereira J, Goh SH. Styryl-lactone derivatives and alkaloids from *Goniothalamus borneensis* (Annonaceae). Tetrahedron. 1998;54(10): 2143-8.

36. Hisham A, Toubi M, Shuaily W, Bai MA, Fujimoto Y. Cardiobutanolide, a styryllactone from *Goniothalamus cardiopetalus*. Phytochemistry. 2003;62(4): 597-600.

Chemical Composition of Essential Oils of *Plumeria rubra* L. Grown in Nigeria

Oladipupo A. Lawal[1*], Isiaka A. Ogunwande[1] and Andy R. Opoku[2]

[1]*Department of Chemistry, Natural Products Research Unit, Faculty of Science, Lagos State University, Badagry Expressway, PMB 0001 LASU Post office, Ojo, Lagos, Nigeria.*
[2]*Department of Biochemistry and Microbiology, University of Zululand, KwaDlangezwa 3886, South Africa.*

Authors' contributions

This work was carried out in collaboration between all authors. Author OAL designed the study, isolation of the oils and wrote part of the manuscript. Author IAO managed the literature searches and wrote the final draft of the manuscript. Author ARO managed the analyses of the GC and GC/MS. All authors read and approved the final manuscript.

Editor(s):
(1) Marcello Iriti, Faculty of Plant Biology and Pathology, Department of Agricultural and Environmental Sciences, Milan State University, Italy.
Reviewers:
(1) Anonymous, National Institute of Pathology", India.
(2) Mokutima Amarachi Eluwa, University of Calabar, Nigeria.
(3) Anonymous, Universidad Nacional de Rosario, Argentina.

ABSTRACT

The chemical compositions of essential oils obtained by hydrodistillation of the leaves and flowers of pink-flower *Plumeria rubra* L., grown in Nigeria were being reported. The chemical analysis was performed by means of gas chromatography-flame ionization detector (GC-FID) and gas chromatography-mass spectrometry (GC-MS) techniques. The major leaves oil constituents were (Z)-β-farnesene (16.0%), α-patchoulene (13.0%), limonene (12.1%), (E)-β-farnesene (10.8%), α-copaene (7.2%) and phytol (6.3%). However, the quantitative significant compounds of the flowers oil were (E)-non-2-en-1-ol (15.7%), limonene (10.8%), phenyl acetaldehyde (9.0%), n-tetradecanal (8.8%), γ-elemene (6.5%) and (E,E)-α-farnesene (6.1%). This is the first report on the volatile constituents from the leaves of *Plumeria rubra*.
Aims: The aim of the of the present study was to examine the constituents of the leaves and flowers oils of *P. rubra* grown in Southwest Nigeria in details, and to compare the results obtained

Corresponding author: E-mail: jumobi.lawal@lasu.edu.ng

with those reported earlier.
Study Design: Isolation of essential oils from the leaves and flowers of *Plumeria rubra* and determination of their chemical constituents.
Place and Duration of Study: Fresh plant materials of *P. rubra* (flowers and leaves) were collected from a location within the Campus of Lagos State University, Ojo, Lagos State, Nigeria, in October 2013.
Methodology: Fresh leaves and flowers were hydodistilled in an all glass Clevenger apparatus and their chemical constituents were analyzed by GC and GC/MS.
Results: A total of twenty six compounds were identified in the leaves and the major ones were (*Z*)-β-farnesene (16.0%), α-patchoulene (13.0%), limonene (12.1%), (*E*)-β-farnesene (10.8%), α-copaene (7.2%) and phytol (6.3%) while the flowers had twenty seven compounds with (*E*)-non-2-en-1-ol (15.7%), limonene (10.8%), phenyl acetaldehyde (9.0%) and *n*-tetradecanal (8.8%) occurring in higher percentages.
Conclusion: The chemical composition of the volatile compounds differed from each other and from data reported previously from other parts of the world.

Keywords: Plumeria rubra; Apocynaceae; essential oil composition; fatty acids; terpenes.

1. INTRODUCTION

Plumeria rubra L. (Apocynaceae) grows as a spreading shrub or small tree to a height of 2-8 m and similar width. It has a thick succulent trunk and sausage-like blunt branches covered with a thin grey bark. The large green leaves can reach 30 to 50 cm long and are arranged alternately and clustered at the end of the branches. The flowers are terminal, appearing at the ends of branches over the summer. Often profuse and very prominent, they are strongly fragrant, and have five petals. The colours range from the common pink to white with shades of yellow in the centre of the flower. They produce seed of about 20-60 winged seeds [1]. The decoction of *P. rubra* has traditionally been used to treat asthma, constipation, promote menstruation and reduce fever. The fruit was reported to be been used as an abortifacient [2]. The flowers are aromatic and are used for the control of diabetes mellitus while the leaves are used to ameliorate ulcers, leprosy, inflammation and rubifacient. The milky sap of the stem and leaf has been applied to skin diseases such as herpes and scabies [2]. Extracts of the plants are known to possess some biological activities of importance such as antimicrobial, anti-inflammatory, analgesic, anthelmintic, antioxidant, antipyretic, abortifacient, antiulcer, antifertility, antitumor, anticancer and hypolipidemic [2-7].

Phytochemical screening showed that *P. rubra* contained several biologically active compounds such as plumericin and isoplumericin that displayed molluscicidal, cytotoxic and antibacterial activities as well as cyanidin 3-*O*-β-(2″-glucopyranosyl-*O*-β-galactopyranoside) and cyanidin-3-*O*-β-galactopyranoside [8] which were responsible for the attractive colours of the flowers of red *P. rubra*. Antimicrobial iridoids plumeridoids A-C, epiplumeridoid C [9] and cytotoxic iridoids, fulvoplumierin, allamcin, plumericin and allamandin were the other constituents of *P. rubra* [2].

Literature reports on the essential oil contents of *P. rubra* have focussed mostly on the flowers. The essential oils of *P. rubra* and its cultivars exhibited high chemical variations depending on the origin. Alkanes, terpene hydrocarbons, oxygenated terpenes, aromatic compounds, alcohols and fatty acids were the main classes of compounds present in the analysed oils from different parts of the world [10-22].

Although the composition of the flower oils of *P. rubra* from Nigeria [10] and other parts of the world have been substantially investigated (Table 1), much less is known about the composition of the leaf oil. The objective of the present study was to examine the chemical constituents of the leaves and flowers oils of *P. rubra* grown in Southwest Nigeria in details, and to compare the results obtained with those reported earlier. The chemical analysis of essential oil of some plant species of Nigeria flora has been reported [23].

2. MATERIALS AND METHODS

2.1 Plant Materials

Fresh plant materials of *P. rubra* (flowers and leaves) were collected from a location within the

Table 1. Major compounds identified in the essential oils of *P. rubra* from literature

Parts	Origin	Major constituents	References
Flower (ro)[hy]	Nigeria	heneicosane (19.15%) nonadecane (15.63%), citronellol (14.63%), geraniol (9.17%)	10
Flower (ro)[hy]	Malaysia	phenylethyl benzoate (12.3%), dodecanoic acid (11.8%), hexadecanoic acid (9.3%)	11
Flower (red)[hy]	Malaysia	hexadecanoic acid (27.2%), linoleic acid (20.7%), tetradecanoic acid (18.9%), dodecanoic acid (10.6%)	11
Flower (pink)[hy]	Malaysia	dodecanoic acid (30.8%), tetradecanoic acid (17.4%), hexadecanoic acid (9.8%), nonadecane (8.2%)	12
Flower (or)[hy]	Malaysia	benzyl salicylate (20.9%), (*E*)-nerolidol (14.1%), benzyl benzoate (8.6%)	12
Flower [mw]	China	9-hexacosene (14.6%), *n*-octadecanal (11.5%), *n*-octadecanol(8.4%), lupeol acetate (8.3%), *n*-hexadecanoic acid (7.9%)	13
Flower [a, b, std]	China	d-nerolidol, farnesol, benzyl benzoate, geranyl benzoate, neryl linalool isomer, terpinyl isovalerate	14
Flower [a, std]	China	d-nerolidol, farnesol, benzyl benzoate, geranyl benzoate	15
		palmitic acid, tetradecanoic acid	16
Flower [a, b, scde]		1,2-benzenedicarboxylic acid (66.11%)	17
Flower [b, sde]	Hawaii	β-phenylethyl alcohol, phenyl acetaldehyde, methyl cinnamate	18
Flower [b, sde]	Hawaii	linalool, phenylacetaldehyde, *trans,trans*-farnesol, phenylethyl alcholo, geraniol, α-terpineol, neral,geranial	19
Flower [b, std]	Egypt	α-pinene, 2-carene, β-pinene, α-phellandrene, p-cymene, linalool, phenylalcohol, citral	20
Leaf [a, b, hy]	Egypt	farnesol, geraniol, phenylethyl benzoate, methyl pentadecane, terpinolene	21
Flower [b, std]	Cuba	butyl oleate (13.8%), butyl palmitate (11.5%), methyl palmitate (9.7%), methyl oleate (9.3%), linalool (8.2%)	22

[a]*Plumeria rubra var. acutifolia;* [b] *quantitative data not available to authors; hy, hydrodistillation; mw, microwave extraction; sdce, supercritical carbon dioxide fluid extraction ; sde, steam distillation and extraction; std, steam distillation; ro, red-orange; or, orange*

Campus of Lagos State University, Ojo, Lagos State, Nigeria, in October 2013. Identification of the plant materials was carried out at the Department of Botany, University of Lagos. A voucher specimen (LUH 5805) was deposited at the University Herbarium.

2.2 Oil Isolation

Fresh flowers (50 g) and leaves (300 g) were separately subjected to hydrodistillation in a Clevenger-type glass apparatus for 3 h in accordance with the established specification [24]. The distilled oils were preserved in sealed sample tubes and stored under refrigeration until analysis.

2.3 Gas Chromatography (GC) Analysis

GC analysis of the oil was carried out on a Hewlett Packard HP 6820 Gas Chromatograph equipped with a FID detector and HP-5MS column (30 m x 0.25 mm id), film thickness was 0.25 μm and the split ratio was 1:25. The oven temperature was programmed from 50°C (after 2 min) to 240°C at 5°C/min and the final temperature was held for 10 min. Injection and detector temperatures were maintained at 200°C and 240°C respectively. Hydrogen was the carrier gas at a flow rate of 1 mL/min. An aliquot (0.5 µL of the diluted oil) was injected into the GC. Peaks were measured by electronic integration. A homologous series of *n*-alkanes were run under the same conditions for determination of retention indices. Each analysis was performed thrice.

2.4 Gas Chromatography-Mass Spectrometry (GC-MS) Analysis

GC-MS analyses of the oils were performed on a Hewlett Packard Gas Chromatograph HP 6890 interfaced with Hewlett Packard 5973 Mass spectrometer system equipped with a HP-5MS capillary column (30 m x 0.25 mm id, film thickness 0.25 µm). The oven temperature was programmed from 70-240°C at the rate of 5°C/min. The ion source was set at 240°C and electron ionization at 70 eV. Helium was used as the carrier gas at a flow rate of 1 mL/min. Scanning range was 35 to 425 amu. Diluted oil in *n*-hexane (1.0 µL) was injected into the GC/MS.

2.5 Identification of Compounds

The constituents of the essential oils were identified by comparing their retention indices with an analysis done under the same temperature-programmed conditions for *n*-alkanes and the oil on a HP-5 MS column under the same chromatographic conditions. Individual compounds were identified by comparing their mass spectra with the internal reference mass spectra library or with authentic compounds. Confirmation of identity was done by comparing their retention indices with the GC-MS library data [25] and with the mass spectra from literature data [26,27].

3. RESULTS AND DISCUSSION

The identities and the percentage composition of compounds present in *P. rubra* are presented in Table 2. The yields of the volatile oils were 0.12% and 0.23% (v/w) respectively for the leaves and flowers. Sesquiterpene hydrocarbons (54.1%) and monoterpene hydrocarbons (13.9%) were the main classes of compounds identified in the leaves oil. The major constituents of the leaves oil were (Z)-β-farnesene (16.0%), α-patchoulene (13.0%), limonene (12.1%) and

Table 2. Chemical composition of essential oils of *Plumeria rubra*

Compounds[a]	RI (Cal.)	RI (Lit.)	% composition		MI
			Flower	Leaf	
α-Pinene	938	932	0.4	-	RI, MS
β-Pinene	979	974	2.9	-	RI, MS
n-Ocotanal	1007	998	2.0	-	RI, MS
(*E,E*)-2,4-Heptadienal	1016	1005	2.0	-	RI, MS, CI
Limonene	1032	1024	10.8	12.1	RI, MS, CI
3,5,5-Trimethylhexanol	1037	1041	-	1.2	RI, MS
Phenyl acetaldehyde	1046	1049	9.0	3.1	RI, MS, CI
γ-Terpinene	1063	1054	0.8	-	RI, MS
1-Octanol	1076	1063	1.1	1.8	RI, MS
Terpinolene	1089	1086	-	1.8	RI, MS
(*E*)-Non-2-en-1-ol	1097	1097	15.7	-	RI, MS, CI
Linalool	1101	1099	-	1.7	RI, MS
n-Nonanal	1105	1100	4.3	3.3	RI, MS
n-Nonanol	1175	1165	-	0.3	RI, MS
β-Cyclocitral	1217	1217	-	1.1	RI, MS
Citronellol	1231	1223	-	0.3	RI, MS
Geraniol	1254	1249	-	0.5	RI, MS, CI
Geranial	1260	1264	-	0.3	RI, MS, CI
n-Tridecane	1300	1300	-	1.1	RI, MS
Eugenol	1364	1356	1.2	1.1	RI, MS
α-Copaene	1378	1374	30	7.2	RI, MS, CI
β-Elemene	1389	1389	0.7		RI, MS
α-Cedrene	1416	1410	1.2		RI, MS

Compounds[a]	RI (Cal.)	RI (Lit.)	% composition		MI
			Flower	Leaf	
β-Caryophyllene	1420	1417	1.5		RI, MS
γ-Elemene	1432	1434	6.5	0.2	RI, MS
(Z)-β-Farnesene	1440	1440	2.0	16.0	RI, MS, CI
α-Patchoulene	1457	1454	-	13.0	RI, MS, CI
(E)-β-Farnesene	1465	1454	-	10.8	RI, MS, CI
γ-Muurolene	1476	1478	-	1.4	RI, MS
(E,E)-α-Farnesene	1500	1505	6.1	-	RI, MS, CI
B-Bisabolene	1510	1505	-	3.5	RI, MS
δ-Cadinene	1523	1522	1.9	-	RI, MS
β-Sesquiphellandrene	1526	1525	-	2.0	RI, MS
Spathulenol	1575	1577	0.7	-	RI, MS
Caryophyllene oxide	1586	1582	1.6	0.3	RI, MS
Viridiflorol	1593	1592	-	0.6	RI, MS
Ledol	1608	1602	1.5	3.4	RI, MS
n-Tetradecanal	1614	1612	8.8	-	RI, MS, CI
Hexadecanal	1812	1817	2.2	-	RI, MS
n-Hexadecanol	1879	1874	1.6	-	RI, MS
n-Octadecanal	2017	2012	5.0	-	RI, MS
Phytol	2125	2122	-	6.3	RI, MS, CI
cis-9-Tricosene	2298	2299	4.4	-	RI, MS, CI
Total			**98.9**	**94.6**	
Monoterpene hydrocarbons			**14.9**	**13.9**	
Oxygenated monoterpenes			**1.2**	**5.0**	
Sesquiterpene hydrocarbons			**22.9**	**54.1**	
Oxygenated sesquiterpenes			**3.8**	**4.3**	
Fatty acids			**22.0**	**-**	
Diterpenes			**-**	**6.3**	
Aliphatic compounds			**25.1**	**7.7**	
Aromatic compounds			**9.0**	**3.1**	

[a]Elution order on HP-5MS column; RI (Cal.) Retention indices relative to n-alkanes on HP-5MS column; RI (Lit.) Literature retention indices; - Not identified; MI, Mode of identification; MS, Mass spectrum; CI, Co-injection with an authentic sample

(E)-β-farnesene (10.8%). Also present in significant amounts were α-copaene (7.2%) and phytol (6.3%). The minor compounds include β-bisabolene (3.5%), ledol (3.4%), n-nonanal (3.3%) and phenyl acetaldehyde (3.1%).

The chemical classes of compounds present in the flowers oil were aliphatic compounds (25.1%), sesquiterpene hydrocarbons (22.9%), fatty acids (22.0%) and monoterpene hydrocarbons (14.9%). The quantitatively significant compounds of the flower oil were (E)-non-2-en-1-ol (15.7%), limonene (10.8%), phenyl acetaldehyde (9.0%) and n-tetradecanal (8.8%), with significant quantities of γ-elemene (6.5%), (E,E)-α-farnesene (6.1%), octadecanal (5.0%), cis-9-tricosene (4.4%), n-nonanal (4.3%) and α-copaene (3.0%).

Few compositional variations were observed between the studied oil samples. (E)-Non-2-en-1-ol, the main compound of the flower oil was not detected in the leaf while α-patchoulene and (E)-β-farnesene, present in leaves oil were not identified in the flowers oil. In addition, while fatty acids were conspicuously absent in the leaves oil, none of the diterpene compound could be detected in the flower. However, compounds such as limonene, phenyl acetaldehyde and (Z)-β-farnesene were identified in both samples though with varying proportion. These observations may be based on the fact that different parts of the same plant may contain different chemical substances [23].

Although heneicosane and nonadecane were previously identified as the major compounds of P. rubra flowers oil from Nigeria [10], these compounds were not present in this study which also has low contents of citronellol and geraniol. The main compounds of essential oil of pink-flower P. rubra from Malaysia namely dodecanoic acid, tetradecanoic acid, hexadecanoic acid and nonadecane, were not identified in this oil sample from Nigeria. Moreover, the main constituents of the present oil samples namely non-2-en-1-ol, limonene, phenyl acetaldehyde, γ-elemene and (E,E)-α-farnesene, were conspicuously absent in the Malaysian oil sample [12]. It was noted that non-2-en-1-ol and limonene were not previously reported to be main compounds of previously investigated P. rubra oils (Table 1). Although, phenyl acetaldehyde was present in the Nigeria, Egypt [20,21] and Hawaii [18,19] samples, other variations were observed in the compositions of these samples. Some compounds such as 1,2-benzenedicarboxylic acid 9-hexacosene, n-octadecanal, n-octadecanol, lupeol acetate, palmitic acid, tetradecanoic acid and n-hexadecanoic acid commonly observed from China oil samples [13-17] were not detected in the Nigeria grown P. rubra oils. The chemical compounds present in the essential oil of P. rubra from Cuba [22] were not identified in the Nigerian samples. The origin, environmental conditions, handling procedure, extraction methods, age and nature of the plant etc are some of the factors that may be responsible for the variations in the chemical composition of essential oils of P. rubra from different parts of the world.

The components present in the essential oils may be of economic importance. For example, limonene among others posses antimicrobial activity [28] while (E)-β-farnesene was used as an insecticide for the control of aphids [29]. On the other hand, (E)-non-2-en-1-ol is a scent material and also useful as an acaricide [30].

4. CONCLUSION

For the first time the compositions of essential oil from the leaf of P. rubra grown in Nigeria are being reported. In addition qualitative and quantitative differences were observed between the oil compositions from Nigeria and other parts of the world. These differences may be probably due to ecological and geographical conditions between Nigeria and other parts of the world as well as the age and nature of the plant, handling procedure etc.

CONSENT

Not applicable.

ETHICAL APPROVAL

Not applicable.

COMPETING INTERESTS

Authors have declared that no competing interests exist.

REFERENCES

1. Botanica. The Illustrated AZ of over 10000 garden plants and how to cultivate them. Könemann. 2004;2.
2. Shinde PR, Patil P, Bairagi VA. Phytopharmacological review of Plumeria species. Sch Acad J Pharm. 2014;3(2):217-227.
3. de Freitas CD, de Souza DP, Araújo ES, Cavalheiro MG, Oliveira LS, Ramos MV. Antioxidative and proteolytic activities and protein profile of laticifer cells of Cryptostegia grandiflora, Plumeria rubra and Euphorbia tirucalli. Braz J Plant Physiol. 2010;22(1):11-22.
4. Misra V, Sheikh MU, Vivek S, Umashankar S. Antipyretic activity of the Plumeria rubra leaves extract. Int J Pharm. 2012;2(2):330-332.
5. Misra V, Yadav G, Uddin SM, Shrivasatav V. Determination of antiulcer activity of Plumeria rubra leaves extracts. Int Res J Pharm. 2012;3(9):194-197.
6. Ramaiyan D, Vijaya RJ, Gupta M, Sarathchandiran I. Ovarian antisteroidogenic effect of three ethnomedicinal plants in prepubertal female mice. Int J Biol Pharm Res. 2012;3(1):30-36.
7. Rekha JB, Jayakar B. Anti cancer activity of ethanolic extract of leaves of Plumeria rubra (Linn). Curr Pharm Res. 2011;1(2):175-179.
8. Byamukama R, Jane N, Monica J, Øyvind MA, Bernard TK. Anthocyanins from ornamental flowers of red frangipani, Plumeria rubra. Scient Horticul. 2011;129(4):840-843.
9. Kuigoua GM, Kouam SF, Ngadjui BT, Schulz B, Chaudhary MI, Krohn K. Minor secondary metabolic products from the stem bark of Plumeria rubra Linn. displaying antimicrobial activities. Planta Med. 2010;76(6):620-625.
10. Obuzor GU, Nweke HC. Analysis of essential oil of Plumeria rubra from Port Harcourt, Nigeria. J Chem Soc Nig. 2011;36(1):56-60.
11. Tohar N, Awang K, Mustafa AM, Ibrahim J. Chemical composition of the essential oils of four Plumeria species grown on

Peninsular Malaysia. J Essent Oil Res. 2006;18(6):613-617.

12. Tohar N, Mustafa AM, Ibrahim J, Awang K. A comparative study of the essential oils of the genus Plumeria Linn. from Malaysia. Flav Fragr J. 2006;21(6):859-863.

13. Yan-Qing L, Hong-Wu W, Shou-Lian W, Zijun Y. Chemical composition and antimicrobial activity of the essential oils extracted by microwave-assisted hydrodistillation from the flowers of two Plumeria species. Anal Lett. 2012;45(16):2389-2397.

14. Zhang L, Liu H, Chen J. Essential oil extracted from Plumeria rubra L. cv. acutifolia and analysis of its constituents. Huagong Jishu Yu Kaifa. 2010;39(6):39-40.

15. Zhang L, Zhang B, Chen F. Effects of different drying methods on the components of essential oil in Plumeria rubra var. actifolia. Zhongguo Xiandai Yingyong Yaoxue. 2012;29(12):1097-1100.

16. Peng Y, Zhang Y, Guo C, Huang A. Analysis of volatile oil from Flos Plumeria rubera LCV by GC-MS. Zhongguo Yashi. 2013;16(7):980-982.

17. Xiao X, Cui L, Zhou X, Wu Y, Ge F. Research of essential oil of Plumeria rubra var. acutifolia from Laos by supercritical carbon dioxide extraction. Zhong Yao Cai. 2011;34(5):789-794.

18. Omata A, Shoji N, Seiji H, Kiyoshi F. Volatile components of Plumeria flowers. Part 2.[1] Plumeria rubra L. cv. 'Irma Bryan'. Flav Fragr J. 1992;7(1):33-35.

19. Omata A, Yomogida K, Nakamura S, Hashimoto S, Arai T, Furukawa K. Volatile components of Plumeria flowers. Part 1. Plumeria rubra forma acutifolia (Poir.) Woodson cv. 'Common Yellow'. Flav Fragr J. 1991;6(4):277-279.

20. Mahran GH, Abdel-Wahab SM, Ahmed MS. Volatile oil of flowers of Plumeria rubra and Plumeria rubra Alba. Egypt J Pharm Sci. 1974;15(1):43-49.

21. Sengab AN, Meselhy KM, Fahmy HA, Sleem AA. Phytochemical and biological studies of Plumeria rubra L. var. acutifolia grown in Egypt. Bull Fac Pharm (Cairo University). 2009;47(3):147-160.

22. Pino JA, Ferrer A, Alvarez D, Rosado A. Volatiles of an alcoholic extract of flower from Plumeria rubra L. var. acutifolia. Flav Fragr J. 1994;9(6):343-345.

23. Lawal OA, Opoku RA, Ogunwande IA. Phytoconstituents and insecticidal activity of different leaf solvent extracts of Chromolaena odorata against Sitophilus zeamais. Eur J Med Pl. 2015;5(3):237-247.

24. British Pharmacopoeia. HM Stationary Office. 1990;2.

25. National Institute of Standards and Technology. Chemistry web book. Data from NIST Standard Reference Database. 2011;69.

26. Adams RP. Identification of Essential Oil Components by Ion Trap Mass spectroscopy. Academic Press, New York; 2007.

27. Joulain D, Koenig WA. The Atlas of Spectral Data of Sesquiterpene Hydrocarbons. E.B. Verlag, Hamburg, Germany; 1998.

28. Hosuna AB, Hamdi N, Halima NB, Abdelkafi S. Characterisation of essential oil from Citrus auranticum L., flowers: antimicrobial and antioxidant activities. J Oleo Sci. 2013;62(7):762-773.

29. Xiuda Y, Zhang YG, Ma YZ, Xu Z, Wang PG, Xia L. Expression of an (E)-β-farnesene synthase gene from Asian peppermint in tobacco affected aphid infestation. The Crop Journal. 2013;1(1):50-60.

30. Gfeller A, Laloux M, Barsics F, Kati DE, Haubruge E, du Jardin P, Verheggen FJ, Lognay G, Wathelet JP, Fauconnier ML. Characterization of volatile organic compounds emitted by barley (Hordeum vulgare L.) roots and their attractiveness to wireworms. J Chem Ecol. 2013;39(8):1129-1139.

15

Volatile Constituents of Essential Oils from the Leaves, Stems, Roots and Fruits of Vietnamese Species of *Alpinia malaccencis*

Le T. Huong[1], Tran D. Thang[2] and Isiaka A. Ogunwade[3*]

[1]Faculty of Biology, Vinh University, 182-Le Duan, Vinh City, Nghệ An Province, Vietnam.
[2]Faculty of Chemistry, Vinh University, 182-Le Duan, Vinh City, Nghệ An Province, Vietnam.
[3]Natural Products Research Unit, Department of Chemistry, Faculty of Science, Lagos State University, Badagry Expressway Ojo, P.M.B. 0001, LASU Post Office, Ojo, Lagos, Nigeria.

Authors' contributions

This work was carried out in collaboration between all authors. All authors read and approved the final manuscript.

<u>Editor(s):</u>
(1) Sabyasachi Chatterjee, Biotechnology Department, Burdwan university, India.
(2) Marcello Iriti, Department of Agricultural and Environmental Sciences, Milan State University, Italy.
<u>Reviewers:</u>
(1) Anonymous, France.
(2) Tonzibo Zanahi Félix, Laboratory of Biological Chemistry, Faculty SSMT, University of Cocody, Abidjan, Ivory Coast.

ABSTRACT

The essential oils obtained from different parts of *Alpinia malaccencis* (Burm f.) (Zingiberaceae) collected from Kỳ Sơn Districts, Nghệ An Province, Vietnam, has been studied. Determination of essential oil components from the leaves, stems, roots and fruits of *A. malaccencis* was performed by gas chromatography-flame ionization detector (GC-FID) and gas chromatography mass spectrometry (GC-MS). β-Pinene (leaf: 56.%; stem: 46.0%; root: 31.7% and fruit: 18.5%) and α-pinene (leaf: 10.3%; stem: 9.8%; root: 6.3% and fruit: 5.9%) were the major constituents of the oils. In addition, β-phellandrene was present in the amount of 12.1%, 12.9% and 12.9% in the stem, root and fruit oils but absent in the leaf. Methyl cinnamate (27.8%) was identified in higher quantity only in the fruit oil but absent in the leaf while α-phellandrene (5.7%) was present in the stem and α-selina-6-en-4-ol (5.5%) was a significant compound of the root oil. The compositions of the root and fruit essential oils were reported for the first time.

Corresponding author: E-mail: isiaka.ogunwade@lasu.edu.ng

Aims: The aim of the research is to investigate for the first time the volatile constituents from *A. malaccencis* collected from Kỳ Sơn Districts, Nghệ An Province, Vietnam.
Study Design: Extraction of essential oils from the air-dried leaves, stems, roots and fruits samples of *A. malaccencis* and investigation of their chemical constituents.
Place and Duration of Study: Leaves, stems, roots and fruits of *A. malaccaencis* were collected from plants growing in Kỳ Sơn Districts, Nghệ An Province, Vietnam, in May 2014.
Methodology: Air-dried and pulverized samples were hydrodistilled in a Clevenger-type apparatus according to Vietnamese Pharmacopoeia to obtained volatile oils whose chemical constituents were analyzed by GC and GC/MS.
Results: Monoterpene hydrocarbons were the dominant class of compound in the leaf oil (74.0%) and stem oil (81.3%) of *A. malaccencis*. Sesquiterpene compounds (21.5%) were identified in appreciable quantity in the roots oil, although monoterpene hydrocarbons (59.3%) are abundant. Oxygenated monoterpenes (31.1%) and monoterpene hydrocarbons (46.7%) constituted the main classes of compounds identified in the fruit oil.
Conclusion: The literature about the oils of *A. malaccencis* indicates a high variability in the chemical composition of the essential oils.

Keywords: Alpinia malaccencis; essential oil composition; monoterpenes; sesquiterpenes.

1. INTRODUCTION

Alpinia is a rather large genus of plants, with more than 230 species. *Alpinia malaccensis* (Burm. f.) R., is a plant in the Zingiberaceae family cultivated for ornamental and medicinal purposes. It grows to over 4 m tall. It has long lush green leaves, which have fragrance. In November and December the flowers emerge above the leaves enclosed in a conical sheath, which splits to reveal a sumptuous cluster of fat pink and white buds [1]. It is a native of Indonesia and Malaysia. It has many medicinal properties. *Alpinia malaccensis* is used to cure wounds and sores [2]. It is chewed to make the voice strong and clear and used for bathing feverish people [3,4]. The leaf extracts was shown to possess antimicrobial [5], antioxidant [5,6] and potent cytotoxic [7] activities. Phytochemical investigation has led to the isolation of 5,6-dehydrokawain, coronarin E, coronarin A, (E)-8(17), 12-labdadiene-15,16-dial, hedyforrestin B, cardamonin, pinocembrin and alpinetin [8].

The volatile compositions of *A. malaccencis* grown in few countries have been reported. The rhizome oil from Bangladesh had α-phellandrene (31.80%), eucalyptol (13.76%), *o*-cymene (11.45%) and β-pinene (11.34%) as its major compounds [1]. The essential oil from the rhizome of Malaysia grown *A. malaccencis* contained methyl (*E*)-cinnamate (78.2%) as the major constituent [9]. The oil sample analysed from Kerala, India [10] was rich in α-phellandrene (36.4%) and *p*-cymene (14.9%). The major constituents of the rhizome oil collected from Phulbani, Odisha, India were α-phellandrene

(43.9%), *p*-cymene (31.7%) and β-pinene (4.6%). The essential oil displayed significant antioxidant and antimicrobial activities [11]. The presence of 1,8-cineole (21.14%), camphor (18.7%) and sabinene (11.64%) have been reported in the rhizome oil from kottayam, India [12]. The leaf oil from Indonesia contained an abundant of α-pinene (30.57%), β-pinene (11.41%), 1, 8-cineole (21.39%) and methyl cinnamate (9.24%) while methyl cinnamate (30.24%), α-pinene (13.04%), β-pinene (12.38%) and 1, 8-cineole (16.58%) were present in the stem with methyl cinnamate (64.4%), α-pinene (14.90%), β-pinene (12.44%) and 1, 8-cineole (9.89%) identified in the rhizome [13]. The rhizome had stronger locomotor inhibition activity compare to the stem and leaf oils [13]. However, 1,8-cineole (11.9%), linalool (9.0%), fenchyl acetate (8.6%) and *trans*-nerolidol (5.7%) were present in the sample from Thailand [14]. The leaf oil of sample from Guandong, China was rich in methyl cinnamate (75%) while the seed oil contained 1,8-cineole, citronelllol, 4-phenyl-3-buten-2-one, decanoic acid, geranyl acetate, nerolidol, lauric acid, α-farnesol, β-farnesol, myristic acid and palmitic acid [15]. The essential oil was thought to contained hydrocarbon which belongs to the pinene group [16]. (*E*)-Methyl cinnamate (64.4%-88.0%) was the main compound in the leaf, rhizome and stem oils of *Alpinia malaccencis* var. *nobilis* from Malaysia [17].

There are no previous references in literature about the essential oil of this plant from Vietnam. The objective of the present study was to examine the constituents of the leaf, stem, root and fruit oils of *A. malaccencis* in details, and to compare the results obtained with those reported earlier.

2. MATERIALS AND METHODS

2.1 Plant Collection

Leaves, stems, roots and fruits of *A. malaccaencis* were collected from randomly selected plants growing in Kỳ Sơn Districts, Nghệ An Province, Vietnam, in May 2014. A voucher specimen, LTH 428, was deposited at the Botany Museum, Vinh University, Vietnam. Plant samples were air-dried prior to extraction.

2.2 Isolation of Volatile Oils

Aliquots of 0.5 kg each of air-dried plant samples were subjected to separate hydrodistillation for 4 h at normal pressure, according to the Vietnamese Pharmacopoeia [18]. The yields of essential oils were 0.25%, 0.19%, 0.32% and 0.25% (v/w, calculated on dry weight basis). Oil samples were light yellow in colouration.

2.3 Gas chromatography (GC) Analysis

Gas chromatography (GC) analysis was performed on an Agilent Technologies HP 6890 Plus Gas chromatograph equipped with a FID and fitted with HP-5MS column (30 m x 0.25 mm, film thickness 0.25 μm, Agilent Technology). The analytical conditions were: carrier gas H_2 (1 mL/min), injector temperature (PTV) 250°C, detector temperature 260°C, column temperature programmed from 60°C (2 min hold) to 220°C (10 min hold) at 4°C/min. Samples were injected by splitting and the split ratio was 10:1. The volume injected was 1.0 μL. Inlet pressure was 6.1 kPa. The relative amounts of individual components were calculated based on the GC peak area (FID response) without using correction factors.

2.4 Gas Chromatography- mass Spectrometry (GC/MS) Analysis

An Agilent Technologies HP 6890N Plus Chromatograph fitted with a fused silica capillary HP-5 MS column (30 m x 0.25 mm, film thickness 0.25 μm) and interfaced with a mass spectrometer HP 5973 MSD was used for the gas chromatography- mass spectrometry (GC/MS) analysis, under the same conditions as those used for GC analysis. Helium (1 mL/min) was the carrier gas. The MS conditions were as follows: ionization voltage 70 eV; emission current 40 mA; acquisitions scan mass range of 35-350 amu at a sampling rate of 1.0 scan/s.

2.5 Identification of the Constituents

The identification of constituents was performed on the basis of retention indices (RI) determined with reference to a homologous series of *n*-alkanes, under identical experimental conditions, co-injection with standards or known essential oil constituents from home made library and by comparing with MS literature data [19-21].

3. RESULTS AND DISCUSSION

The identities and percentages of the compounds present in the studied oil samples could be seen in Table 1. Monoterpene hydrocarbons (74.0%) were the dominant class of compound in the leaf oil of *A. malaccencis*. The sesquiterpene compounds occurred in lesser amount (15.2%). β-Pinene (560%) and α-pinene (10.3%) were the main oil constituents. The abundance of β-pinene and α-pinene makes the oil similar to the leaf sample from Indonesia [12]. However, the oil differs from the Indonesian [13] and China [15] samples to its low content of methyl cinnamate. Moreover, 1,8-cineole a significant component of Indonesian sample was absent in the present study.

Also, monoterpene hydrocarbons (81.3%) predominate in the stem oil while the sesquiterpene compounds occurred in the amount of 10.4%. The compounds occurring in higher quantities were β-pinene (46.0%), β-phellandrene (12.1%), α-pinene (9.8%) and α-phellandrene (5.7%). This compositional pattern differs from data obtained from Indonesia [13] and Malaysia [17] oil samples where methyl cinnamate, 1,8-cineole, α-pinene and β-pinene predominates. The proportion of methyl cinnamate in our oil sample was insignificant (0.5%) while 1,8-cineole was not detected.

Sesquiterpene compounds (21.5%) were identified in appreciable quantity in the roots oil, although monoterpene hydrocarbons (59.3%) are abundant. The main constituents were β-pinene (31.7%), β-phellandrene (12.9%), α-pinene (6.3%) and α-selina-6-en-4-ol (5.5%). This data may represent the first analysis of the root oil.

Table 1. Constituents of *Alpinia malaccencis* oil samples from Vietnam

Compounds[a]	MI	RI[b]	RI[c]	Percent composition (%)			
				Leaf	Stem	Root	Fruit
α-Thujene	MS, RI	930	921	0.2	0.3	0.2	0.2
α-Pinene	MS, RI, Co	939	932	10.3	9.8	6.3	5.9
Camphene	MS, RI	953	946	0.9	0.7	1.0	1.1
β-Pinene	MS, RI, Co	980	974	56.0	46.0	31.7	18.5
β-Myrcene	MS, RI	990	988	0.9	1.5	1.0	1.1
α-Phellandrene	MS, RI	1006	1002	0.3	5.7	3.0	3.5
δ-3-Carene	MS, RI	1011	1008	3.3	-	-	0.1
α-Terpinene	MS, RI	1017	1014	0.2	0.6	0.4	0.3
o-Cymene	MS, RI	1024	1022	0.4	2.5	1.1	1.3
β-Phellandrene	MS, RI, Co	1028	1025	-	12.1	12.9	12.9
(E)-β-Ocimene	MS, RI	1052	1044	0.2	0.1	0.1	0.8
γ-Terpinene	MS, RI	1061	1054	0.4	1.0	1.0	0.5
α-Terpinolene	MS, RI	1090	1086	0.2	1.0	0.6	0.4
Linalool	MS, RI	1100	1095	-	-	-	0.7
Fenchyl alcohol	MS, RI	1122	1118	-	-	0.1	-
allo-Ocimene	MS, RI	1128	1128	0.7	-	-	0.1
trans-Pinocarveol	MS, RI	1131	1135	0.2	0.1	-	0.1
Camphor	MS, RI	1145	1141	-	-	0.1	0.3
Pinocarvone	MS, RI	1165	1160	0.2	0.4	0.2	-
Borneol	MS, RI	1167	1165	-	-	-	0.3
Terpinen-4-ol	MS, RI	1177	1174	-	0.3	0.2	0.5
α-Terpineol	MS, RI	1189	1186	-	0.2	0.2	0.4
Myrtenal	MS, RI	1209	1195	0.9	0.4	0.4	0.2
trans-Carveol	MS, RI, Co	1217	1215	-	-	0.3	-
exo-Fenchyl acetate	MS, RI, Co	1228	1229	-	-	3.7	0.3
Cumin aldehyde	MS, RI	1236	1238	-	0.1	-	-
(Z)-Citral	MS, RI, Co	1240	1242	0.2	0.1	-	0.2
Methyl hydrocinnamate	MS, RI	1280	1276	-	-	-	0.3
Myrtenyl acetate	MS, RI	1334	1324	0.4	-	-	-
Bicycloelemene	MS, RI, Co	1327	1338	-	0.2	-	0.3
δ-Elemene	MS, RI, Co	1340	1335	-	-	0.2	-
α-Cubebene	MS, RI	1351	1345	-	0.1	-	0.2
α-Copaene	MS, RI	1377	1374	0.3	0.2	-	0.7
(E)-Methyl cinnamate	MS, RI, Co	1379	1376	2.2	0.5	1.3	27.8
β-Cubebene	MS, RI	1386	1387	0.8	0.7	2.3	0.3
β-Elemene	MS, RI	1391	1389	0.4	0.5	0.3	-
Longifolene	MS, RI	1404	1407	-	-	-	0.2
α-Gurjunene	MS, RI	1412	1409	0.3	0.2	-	0.2
β-Caryophyllene	MS, RI	1419	1417	0.8	0.7	0.5	1.9
Widdrene	MS, RI	1430	1430	0.3	0.5	-	-
β-Gurjunene	MS, RI	1434	1431	-	0.4	-	0.5
Aromadendrene	MS, RI	1441	1439	0.7	-	-	-
α-Humulene	MS, RI	1454	1452	0.5	0.5	-	0.7
Selina-4(15),7(11)-diene	MS, RI, Co	1473	1470	-	-	3.1	-
γ-Gurjunene	MS, RI, Co	1477	1475	-	-	-	0.4
Germacrene D	MS, RI	1485	1484	-	-	-	1.4
α-Amorphene	MS, RI	1485	1487	-	-	-	0.2
β-Selinene	MS, RI	1489	1489	-	-	-	0.2
Zingiberene	MS, RI	1494	1493	1.0	1.9	-	-
Cadina-1,4-diene	MS, RI	1496	1496	-	-	-	0.1
Bicyclogermacrene	MS, RI	1500	1500	-	-	-	1.0
β-Bisabolene	MS, RI	1506	1505	-	0.8	-	0.4
γ-Cadinene	MS, RI, Co	1513	1513	-	0.2	-	-

Compounds[a]	MI	RI[b]	RI[c]	Percent composition (%)			
				Leaf	Stem	Root	Fruit
trans-γ-Bisabolene	MS, RI, Co	1516	1514	-	0.3	-	-
β-Agarofuran	MS, RI, Co	1520	1516	0.9	-	1.7	-
β-Sesquiphellandrene	MS, RI	1524	1521	-	-	0.7	-
δ-Cadinene	MS, RI, Co	1525	1522	0.7	1.1	1.4	0.8
Calacorene	MS, RI	1546	1544	0.3	-	-	-
Selina-3,7(11)-diene	MS, RI	1547	1545	-	-	0.6	-
α-Agarofuran	MS, RI	1548	1548	0.2	-	0.6	-
Germacrene B	MS, RI	1561	1559	-	-	-	0.4
(E)-Nerolidol	MS, RI	1563	1561	-	0.2	-	0.1
1,5-Epoxysalvial-4(14)-ene	MS, RI, Co	1564	1557	-	-	-	0.1
Spathulenol	MS, RI	1578	1577	0.2	-	-	2.0
Caryophyllene oxide	MS, RI	1583	1581	0.6	0.4	4.1	2.3
Globulol	MS, RI	1585	1590	2.1	-	-	-
Viridiflorol	MS, RI	1593	1592	2.3	-	-	-
Guaiol	MS, RI	1601	1600	-	0.4	0.4	-
Aromadendrene epoxide	MS, RI	1623	1639	-	-	-	0.5
τ-Muurolol	MS, RI, Co	1646	1640	0.4	0.5	-	0.6
α-Selina-6-en-4-ol	MS, RI, Co	1648	1650	0.5	-	5.5	-
α-Cadinol	MS, RI	1654	1652	0.8	0.6	-	0.9
10-nor-Calamenen-10-one	MS, RI, Co	1702	1702	-	-	-	0.2
Vulgarol A	MS, RI, Co	1708	1708	-	-	-	0.2
Valerenol	MS, RI	1711	1711	-	-	-	0.2
Farnesyl acetate	MS, RI	1726	1722	1.0	-	-	-
Benzyl benzoate	MS, RI	1760	1759	1.3	-	0.2	-
Benzyl salicylate	MS, RI	1866	1864	-	-	0.9	-
8,9-Dehydro-9-formyl-cycloisolongifolene	MS, RI, Co	2082	2082	-	-	1.3	-
Phytol	MS, RI	2125	2122	-	-	1.2	0.2
Total				**94.6**	**93.8**	**90.8**	**94.8**
Monoterpene hydrocarbons				74.0	81.3	59.3	46.7
Oxygenated monoterpenes				4.1	2.1	6.5	31.1
Sesquiterpene hydrocarbons				7.3	8.3	11.4	9.7
Oxygenated sesquiterpenes				7.9	2.1	10.0	7.1
Diterpenes				-	-	2.5	0.2
Aromatic esters				1.3	-	1.1	-

[a] Elution order on HP-5 MS column; [b] Retention indices on HP-5MS column; [c] Literature retention indices; - Not identified; MI, Mode of identification; MS, Mass spectrum; RI, Retention indices; Co, Co-injection with authentic sample

Oxygenated monoterpenes (31.1%) and monoterpene hydrocarbons (46.7%) constituted the main classes of compounds identified in the fruit oil. This oil had its quantitatively significant compounds to be methyl cinnamate (27.8%), β-pinene (18.5%) and β-phellandrene (12.9%).

This paper reports for the first time, the composition of the root and fruit oils of A. malaccencis. Although, β-pinene, α-pinene and methyl cinnamate were identified previously in A. malaccencis, some other compositional variations were observed. The present data were devoid of 1, 8-cineole, p-cymene, 13,14,15,16-tetranor-8(17)-labden-12-al and (E)-labda-8(17),12-diene-15,16-dial that were identified in

the oils of A. malaccencis from Bangladesh [1], Malaysia [9], India [10-12], Indonesia [13], Thailand [14] and China [15]. α-Phellandrene, a major compound of Bangladesh [1] and India [10,11] oil samples occurred in much lower amounts (3.0%) in this study while fenchyl acetate was only identified in the root and fruit oil at lower amounts when compared with oil from Thailand [14]. Both β-phellandrene and α-selina-6-en-4-ol present in this result of A. malaccencis were not identified in the previous studies. Moreover, all the main compounds found in the seed oil of the plant from China [15] were not detected in the present investigated oils. The low content of camphor in these oil samples and the absence of sabinene were the other major differences between the Vietnam and Indian [12] oils.

Although, it is well known that different parts of a plant could contain different chemical constituents [18], the observed compositional pattern may indicate that there is no homogeneity in the oil compositions of *A. malaccencis,* which exhibit chemical variability. The compositional variations between the same plant parts may be attributed to differences in the ecological and climatic conditions between Vietnam and other parts of the world as well as the age and nature of the plant, chemotype, handling procedure etc. [18].

4. CONCLUSION

For the first time the compositions of essential oils from the leaf and stem of *A. malaccencis* grown in Vietnam were being reported. The volatile constituents of the root and fruit oils from Vietnam and elsewhere were also being reported for the first time. It was noted that some compound such as β-pinene, α-pinene and methyl cinnamate were identified in this study as well as previous ones from other parts of the world. However, some other constituents such as sabinene, 1, 8-cineole, *p*-cymene, 13,14,15,16-tetranor-8(17)-labden-12-al, (*E*)-labda-8(17),12-diene-15,16-dial, citronelllol, 4-phenyl-3-buten-2-one, decanoic acid, geranyl acetate, nerolidol, lauric acid, α-farnesol, β-farnesol, myristic acid and palmitic acid that were identified in the oils of *A. malaccencis* from previous studies were absent in the present result. Also, the low camphor content in the oils conferred another compositional variation between the Vietnam oil samples and previous ones. A noteworthy observation was that both β-phellandrene and α-selina-6-en-4-ol present in this result of *A. malaccencis* were not identified in the previous studies.

CONSENT

It is not applicable.

ETHICAL APPROVAL

It is not applicable.

COMPETING INTERESTS

Authors have declared that no competing interests exist.

REFERENCES

1. Bhuiyan MZI, Chowdhury JU, Begum J, Nandi NC. Essential oils analysis of therhizomes of *Alpinia conchigera* Griff. and leaves of *Alpinia malaccensis* (Burm. f.) Roscoe from Bangladesh. Afr J Pl Sci. 2010;4(6):197-201.

2. Ravindra KA, Ravi U. Ethnomedicinal studies of tubers of Hoshangabad. Bullet Environ Pharmacol Life Sci. 2011;1(1):57-59.

3. Smith RM. *Alpinia* (Zingiberaceae): A proposed new infrageneric classification. Edinburgh J Bot. 1990;47:37.

4. Kress WJ, Ai-Zhong L, Mark N, Qing-Jun L. The molecular phylogeny of *Alpinia* (Zingiberaceae): a complex and poltphyletic genus of gingers. Amer J Bot. 2005;92(1):167-178.

5. Habsah M, Amran M, Mackeen MM, Lajis NH, Kikuzaki H, Nakatani N, Rahman AA, Ghafar A, Ali AM. Screening of Zingiberaceae extracts for antimicrobial and antioxidant activities. J Ethnopharmacol. 2000; 72(3): 403-410.

6. Sahoo S, Ghosh G, Nayak S. Evaluation of *in vitro* antioxidant activity of leaf extract of *Alpinia malaccensis*. J Med Pl Res. 2012; 6(23):4032-4038.

7. Thu NB, Trung TN, Ha DT, Khoi NM, Hung TV, Hien TT, Yim NM, Bae KH. Screening of Vietnamese medicinal plants for cytotoxic activity. Nat Prod Sci. 2010; 16(1):43-49.

8. Nuchnipa N, Suksamrarn A. Chemical constituents of the rhizomes of *Alpinia malaccensis*. Biochem System Ecol. 2008; 36(8):661-664.

9. Sirat MH, Basar N, Jani NA. Chemical compositions of the rhizome oils of two *Alpinia* species of Malaysia. Nat Prod Res. 2011;25(10):982-986.

10. Raj G, Pradeep DP, Yusufali C, Mathew D, Sabulal B. Chemical profiles of volatiles in four *Alpinia* species from Kerala, South India. J Essent Oil Res. 2013;25(2):97-102.

11. Sahoo S, Shikha S, Sanghamitra N. Chemical composition, antioxidant and antimicrobial activity of essential oil and extract of *Alpinia malaccensis* Roscoe (Zingiberaceae). Int J Pharm Pharmaceut Sci. 2014;6(7):183-188.

12. Joseph R. Karyomorphometrical analysis and exploration of major essential oil constituents in Zingiberaceae. Mahatma

Gandhi University, Kottayam: PhD Thesis. 1999;136-137.

13. Muchtaridi M, Ida M, Subarnas A, Rambia I, Suganda H, Nasrudin ME. Chemical composition and locomotors activity of essential oils from the rhizome, stem and leaf of *Alpinia malaccencis* (Burm F.) of Indonesian spices. J Appl Pharm Sci. 2014;4(1):52-56.

14. Pripdeevech P, Nuntawong N, Wongpornchai S. Composition of essential oils from the rhizomes of three Alpinia species grown in Thailand. Chem. Nat. Comp. 2009;45(4):562-564.

15. Oyen LPA, Nguyen XD. Essential-oil plants. In: Faridah HI, van der Maesen LJG (eds). Plant Resources of South-East Asia (PROSEA). (Pl Res SEAs). 1999;19:60–64.

16. van Romburgh P. On the Essential Oil from the Leaves of *Alpinia malaccensis*

Rosc. In: KNAW, Proceedings, 3, 1900-1901, Amsterdam. 1901;451.

17. Nor AMA, Sam YY, Mailina J, Chua LSL. (*E*)-Methyl cinnamate: the major component of essential oils of A*lpinia malaccensis* var. nobilis. J Trop For Sci. 2005;17(4):631-633.

18. Vietnamese Pharmacopoeia. Medical Publishing House, Hanoi, Vietnam; 1997.

19. Adams RP. Identification of Essential Oil Components by ion trap mass spectroscopy. Academic Press, New York; 2007.

20. Joulain D, Koenig WA. The Atlas of Spectral Data of Sesquiterpene Hydrocarbons. E. B. Verlag, Hamburg, Germany; 1998.

21. National Institute of Standards and Technology. Chemistry web book. Data from NIST Standard Reference, Database 69; 2011. Available: http://www.nist.gov/

16

Assessement of Aqueous Plant Extract for the Control of Kola Weevils (*Balanogastris kolae* & *Sophrorhinus* spp) (Coleoptera: Curculionidae) in Stored *Cola nitida*

E. U. Asogwa[1*], T. C. N. Ndubuaku[1], O. O. Awe[2] and I. U. Mokwunye[1]

[1]*Kola Research Programme, Cocoa Research Institute of Nigeria, Ibadan, Oyo State, Nigeria.*
[2]*Biology Department, Adeyemi College of Education, Ondo, Ondo State, Nigeria.*

Authors' contributions

Everything about this work was done together by all the Authors.

Editor(s):
(1) Sanjib Ray, Department of Zoology, University of Burdwan, West-Bengal, India.
(2) Marcello Iriti, Faculty of Plant Biology and Pathology, Department of Agricultural and Environmental Sciences,
Milan State University, Italy.
Reviewers:
(1) Anonymous, Brazil.
(2) Suleiman M, Department of Biology, Umaru Musa Yar'adua University, Nigeria.
(3) Anonymous, Nigeria.
(4) Prapassorn Bussaman, Department of Biotechnology, Faculty of Technology, Mahasarakham University, Thailand.

ABSTRACT

Kola nuts do not undergo any other additional form of post harvest processing before storage and consumption, hence there is an urgent need to develop new post harvest storage pest control strategies that are safe, of low cost, convenient to use, and environmentally / user friendly. Water extracts from seven (7) medicinal plants including *Nicotiana tabacum* L., *Vernonia amygdalina* Delile, *Eucalyptus camaldulensis* Dehnh, *Hyptis sauvolens* Poit, *Cymbopogon citrtus* Stapf, *Lantana camara* L. and *Musa paradisiaca* L., were evaluated for their toxicity on kola we evils development and emergence in storage. The *Balanogastris kolae* development and emergence from treated stored kolanuts at the various treatment levels decreased with increased concentration of the extracts applied at 25% (7.08 – 14.63), 50% (6.70 – 12.70) and 100% (4.95 – 8.75). The mean numbers of adult *Sophrorhinus* spp emergence at 25% treatment level (0.33 – 0.40) was not significantly different ($p > 0.05$) from their control treatment (0.85). However, at 50% and 100% treatment levels, all the seven plant extracts achieved a low level of *Sophrorhinus* spp emergence

Corresponding author: E-mail: ucheasogwa1@yahoo.com

(0.15 – 0.25) and (0.13 – 0.18) respectively, which was significantly (p < 0.05) different from their control (0.85). The mean number of weevil exit holes recorded for extracts of the various plants decreased with increased concentrations of the extracts applied 25% (30.85 – 41.67), 50% (21.93 – 30.60) and 100% (16.83 -28.10). The few colour changes recorded in the stored kola nuts did not increase with the increased concentration of the extracts 25% (0.75 – 3.05), 50% (0.23 – 3.35) and 100% (0.95 – 2.48). The 7 aqueous extracts can be used at 50% and 100% treatment levels to minimally reduce the menace of kola weevils.

Keywords: Kola nuts; development; emergence; treatments; concentrations.

1. INTRODUCTION

Kola production in Nigeria is beset by a number of problems, principal among these are very low yield and inconsistent pattern of fruit bearing [1]. Thus the role of insect pests, which are capable of destroying more than half of the little produced fruits, cannot be overemphasized [2]. These insect pests include *Balanogastris kolae*, *Sophrorhinus* spp, *Characomasti ctigrapta*, *Phosphorous virescens* etc [3,4]. Among these pests, the kola weevils *Balanogastris kolae* and *Sophrorhinus* spp happen to be the most serious pests of kola in Nigeria. They are referred to as "field – to – store" pests as their infestation is initiated in the field and persists in storage [5]. The females lay eggs 1cm deep in the kola nuts or in other parts of the fruit through wounds and holes made by other insects such as *Ceratitis colae* or through cracks on the husk, which occurs when the follicles dehisce before harvest. The average period from oviposition to the emergence of the adults of *B. kolae* is between 29 to 31 days [6]. The two weevil species cause serious losses to kola nuts in storage every year. The weevils feed mainly on the kola nut cotyledon and develop inside the nuts. Continuous and undetected infestation of kola nuts by these weevils in storage may result in considerable high losses, which sometimes is as high as 60% of the total production in a year [7].

The use of synthetic fumigants such as methyl bromide and aluminum phosphide are perhaps one of the most effective method of protecting stored products against insect degradation [8]. However, use of chemical fumigants in stored products protection is gradually being phased out worldwide because of their adverse effects on the environment, which includes ozone depletion [9] and the development of insect pest resistance [10]. Other negative effects of using synthetic chemicals includes; the development of toxic residues in food commodities and increasing the cost of production. As a result of these limitations, better and more economical methods such as using local alternatives (botanicals) are being developed for the control of storage pests.

Generally, many plant parts with insecticidal, antifeedant and repellant properties have been employed and found effective [11,12,13,14,15,16]. These plant-derived insecticides are believed to be safer, less expensive and more readily available (Jackai and Daoust, 1986). Thus, there is an urgent need to develop new fumigants for post-harvest pest control that are safe, of low cost, convenient to use and environmentally / user friendly [17,18]. Moreover, kola nut do not undergo any other additional form of processing before storage and consumption, hence the use of synthetic chemical for its storage should be discouraged.

There is therefore an urgent demand for effective and eco-friendly plant derived protectants in developing countries like Nigeria for the control of kola nut storage weevils. There are vast amount of secondary metabolites in higher plants: acids, alcohols, aldehydes, alkaloids, esters, fatty acids, flavones, glycosides, hydrocarbons, lactones, nitrogen-containing compounds, sterols, phenols, and terpenoids, which confer pesticidal activity on them [19]. Generally, plants have evolved highly elaborate chemical defenses against insect attack and they have therefore provided a rich source of biologically active chemical compounds, which may be used as crop protecting agents. Fortunately, the tropics are well endowed with numerous flora which are currently not fully exploited. Essential or volatile oils extracted from plants have been shown to possess good potential for use as fumigants against stored products insects, including storage bruchids [20,21,18,22].

This study evaluated the effectiveness of aqueous plant extracts of seven local and common plants in protecting kola nuts in storage against kola nut weevils and to determine if such extracts have any adverse effects on the physical

Assessement of Aqueous Plant Extract for the Control of Kola Weevils...

145

properties of the kola nuts especially with respect to colour changes and exit holes on the kola nuts.

2. MATERIALS AND METHODS

2.1 Collection of the Plant Materials

The leaf samples of seven common plants (Table 1) were collected within the estate of Cocoa Research Institute of Nigeria, Ibadan. The identity of each sample was confirmed at the herbarium of the Forestry Research Institute of Nigeria (FRIN), Ibadan.

2.2 Plant Extraction Procedures

The collected leaf samples of *Nicotiana tabacum* L., *Vernonia amygdalina* Delile, *Eucalyptus camaldulensis* Dehnh, *Hyptis sauvolens* Poit, *Cymbopogon citrtus* Stapf, *Lantana camara* L. and the base trunk of *Musa paradisiaca* L. were chopped into bits and blended with a high-speed mill blender. A range of serial dilutions was made with water to obtain solutions of three doses of 1,000 g/L (100% w/v), 500 g/L (50% w/v) and 250 g/L (25% w/v) by soaking the blended samples in 1 litre of water. This was adapted and modified from earlier methods used by [23,24,25]. The solutions were left 48 hours and then filtered to obtain the aqueous extracts.

2.3 Collection of Kola Samples

Two fresh baskets of kola nuts (unskinned nuts) for this experiment were purchased from Ogumakin market in Ogun State. The kola nuts were skinned, washed and cured (aerated) for 72 hours in the Entomology laboratory before use.

2.4 Application of Treatments

Twenty (20) cured kola nuts were randomly sorted out into three transparent plastic bowls of 1 litre volume each, containing the various concentrations (25% w/v, 50% w/v and 100% w/v) of the extracts. The kola nuts were soaked in these various concentrations for 12 hours. The control treatment (0% w/v) was soaked in distilled water for the same period of time and each of the treatments was replicated four [4] times in a completely randomized design (CRD). The kola nuts were removed after the soaking period and placed in small flat baskets and cured (aerated) in the laboratory for a period of 72 hours to reduce the moisture content to a minimal level.

2.5 Storage of the Nuts

Each set of the twenty (20) cured kola nuts were placed in a black light gauge polythene bag of dimension 42.5 cm x 21.0 cm and tied up. All the treatments were stored under laboratory conditions of temperature and relative humidity (28±3°C and 75±5%) respectively with a space of 20 cm maintained between replicates.

2.6 Post Storage Assessment

The various treatment levels in separate polythene bags were sieved every fortnight (2 weeks) to determine the progress of adult *B. kolae* and *Sophrorhinus* spp development and emergence by direct counting of newly emerged adult weevil until 140 days post treatment period (DPTP). The efficacy and suitability of the various treatments were also considered by determining the number of weevil exit holes on the kola nuts and the number of kola nuts with colour change in each treatment. Data obtained were subjected to the analysis of variance and significant means were separated using the Tukey's Honestly Significance Difference (HSD) Test.

Table 1. Medicinal plants screened for effectiveness in the control of *B. kolae* & *Sophorhinus* spp infesting kola nut

Scientific name	Common name	Family	Parts used
Nicotiana tabacum L.	Tobacco	Solanaceae	Leaf
Vernonia amygdalina Dalile	Bitter leaf	Compositae	Leaf
Eucalyptus camaldulensis Dehnh	Eucalyptus	Myrtaceae	Leaf
Hyptis sauvolens Poit	Hyptis	Labiatae	Leaf
Musa paradisiaca L.	Plantain	Musaceae	Stem
Cymbopogon citrtus Stapf	Lemon grass	Poaceae	Leaf
Lantana camara L.	Lantana	Verbanaceae	Leaf

3. RESULTS

The effect of the various aqueous plant extract treatments on the rate of *B. kolae* and *Sophrorhinus* spp development and emergence from treated stored kolanuts are shown in Tables 2 and 3. All the seven plant extracts were able to suppress the rate of *B. kolae* development and emergence from treated stored kola nuts at the various treatment levels as their emergence decreased with increased concentration 25% (7.08 – 14.63), 50% (6.70 – 12.70) and 100% (4.95 – 8.75). However, the mean number of adult *B. kolae* emergence from the various treatment levels (25%, 50% and 100%) of all the plant extracts were not significantly different (p > 0.05) from each other but differed from their control (Table 2). The mean numbers of *Sophrorhinus* spp emergence at 25% treatment level (0.33 – 0.40) was not significantly different (p > 0.05) from their control treatment (0.85). However, at 50% and 100% treatment levels, all the seven plant extracts achieved a low level of *Sophrorhinus* spp emergence (0.15 – 0.25) and (0.13 – 0.18) respectively, which was significantly (p < 0.05) different from their control (0.85) (Table 3).

The mean number of weevil exit holes observed per treatment decreased with increased concentrations of the extracts application 25% (30.85 – 41.67), 50% (21.93 – 30.60) and 100% (16.83 -28.10). At 50% treatment level, the mean number of exit holes recorded for the seven plant extracts did not differ significantly (p > 0.05) from each other ranging from 21.93 for *V. amygdalina* to 33.10 for *H. saovolens*. However, the mean number of exit holes observed on the nuts differed significantly (p < 0.05) from their control treatments (Table 4).

The few colour changes recorded in the stored kola nuts did not follow any definite pattern, as the changes did not increase nor decrease with the increased concentration of the extracts applied at 25% (0.75 – 3.05), 50% (0.23 – 3.35) and 100% (0.95 – 2.48). For instance, at 50% treatment level, all the plant extracts (2.05 – 3.35) with the exception of *Musa* spp and *Lantan camara* (0.23 and 0.98) showed higher mean colour changes of the nuts than what was obtained at their corresponding 100% treatment level (1.88 – 2.48) (Table 5). Therefore, the colour changes observed could have been as a result of physiological factors associated with storing fresh kola nuts in polythene bags and not from the plant extracts used.

Table 2. Effect of various aqueous plant extract treatments on the development and emergence of *B. kolae* from stored kola nuts

	Mean number of adult *B. kolae* emergence (n = 80)*			
	0%	25%	50%	100%**
N. tabacum	27.83 ± 22.0^a	9.10 ± 14.5^b	7.38 ± 12.5^b	5.88 ± 11.0^b
V. amygdalina	27.83 ± 22.0^a	7.08 ± 13.2^b	6.80 ± 13.1^b	4.95 ± 9.5^b
E. camaldulensis	27.83 ± 22.0^a	9.88 ± 11.9^b	8.40 ± 9.7^b	7.55 ± 6.8^b
H. sauvolens	27.83 ± 22.0^a	11.50 ± 18.8^b	8.83 ± 12.2^b	8.35 ± 9.8^b
M.paradisiaca	27.83 ± 22.0^a	14.63 ± 19.7^b	12.70 ± 18.7^b	8.75 ± 14.5^b
C. citrtus	27.83 ± 22.0^a	11.46 ± 10.1^b	7.30 ± 6.4^b	6.25 ± 7.2^b
L. camara	27.83 ± 22.0^a	13.20 ± 16.1^b	6.70 ± 6.2^b	7.85 ± 7.9^b

*Means with the same superscript down the column are not significantly different (P > 0.05) by Tukey's test
**Each value represents mean of four replicates

Table 3. Effect of various aqueous plant extract treatments on the development and emergence of *Sophorhinus* spp from stored kola nuts

	Mean number of adult *Sophorhinus* spp emergence (n = 80)*			
	0%	25%	50%	100%**
N. tabacum	0.85 ± 1.2^a	0.38 ± 0.6^{ab}	0.23 ± 0.4^b	0.13 ± 0.3^b
V. amygdalina	0.85 ± 1.2^a	0.40 ± 0.6^{ab}	0.25 ± 0.5^b	0.18 ± 0.3^b
E. camaldulensis	0.85 ± 1.2^a	0.35 ± 0.6^{ab}	0.15 ± 0.3^b	0.15 ± 0.3^b
H. sauvolens	0.85 ± 1.2^a	0.33 ± 0.6^{ab}	0.23 ± 0.4^b	0.15 ± 0.3^b
M.paradisiaca	0.85 ± 1.2^a	0.35 ± 0.6^{ab}	0.25 ± 0.4^b	0.15 ± 0.3^b
C. citrtus	0.85 ± 1.2^a	0.33 ± 0.6^{ab}	0.18 ± 0.3^b	0.15 ± 0.3^b
L. camara	0.85 ± 1.2^a	0.33 ± 0.5^{ab}	0.23 ± 0.4^b	0.13 ± 0.3^b

*Means with the same superscript down the column are not significantly different (P > 0.05) by Tukey's test
**Each value represents mean of four replicates

Table 4. Effect of various aqueous plant extract treatments on the number of weevil exit holes on stored kola nuts

	Mean number of weevil exit holes per treatment (n = 80)*			
	0%	25%	50%	100%**
N. tabacum	47.10±23.9[a]	40.35±22.9[ab]	30.33±17.0[bcdefg]	28.10±16.1[bcdefg]
V. amygdalina	47.10±23.9[a]	30.85±16.1[bcdefg]	21.93±11.2[fg]	16.83±9.3[g]
E. camaldulensis	47.10±23.9[a]	41.28±24.2[ab]	28.53±15.9[bcdefg]	23.20±14.6[efg]
H. sauvolens	47.10±23.9[a]	41.67±22.3[ab]	33.10±17.3[abcdef]	23.93±13.0[defg]
M.paradisiaca	47.10±23.9[a]	37.93±18.9[abcd]	30.60±17.4[bcdefg]	22.63±13.4[fg]
C. citrtus	47.10±23.9[a]	37.30±18.5[abcde]	28.55±14.3[bcdefg]	24.45±13.1[cdefg]
L. camara	47.10±23.9[a]	38.60±15.5[abc]	29.13±15.5[bcdefg]	22.58±13.0[fg]

*Means with the same superscript down the column are not significantly different (P > 0.05) by Tukey's test
**Each value represents mean of four replicates*

Table 5. Effect of various aqueous plant extract treatments on the number of stored kola nuts with colour change

	Mean number of kola nuts with colour change (n = 80)*			
	0%	25%	50%	100%**
N. tabacum	1.00±0.0[j]	2.53±0.6[bcde]	3.35±0.3[a]	2.48±0.1[cdef]
V. amygdalina	1.00±0.0[j]	1.60±0.3[j]	2.80±0.6[abcd]	2.25±0.6[defgh]
E. camaldulensis	1.00±0.0[j]	0.20±0.1[k]	2.05±0.6[efghi]	1.88±0.3[ghi]
H. sauvolens	1.00±0.0[j]	3.05±0.5[ab]	2.85±0.3[abc]	1.95±0.1[fghi]
M.paradisiaca	1.00±0.0[j]	0.88±0.3[j]	0.23±0.1[k]	0.95±0.2[j]
C. citrtus	1.00±0.0[j]	0.75±0.0[jk]	2.83±0.4[abc]	2.13±0.4[efghi]
L. camara	1.00±0.0[j]	1.70±0.1[hi]	0.98±0.1[j]	2.43±0.2[cdefg]

*Means with the same superscript down the column are not significantly different (P > 0.05) by Tukey's test
**Each value represents mean of four replicates*

4. DISCUSSION

The kola nut quality (colour) was only slightly affected by the extracts at all the treatment levels, suggesting that such treated produce will have general acceptability by consumers. Most of the plants screened in this toxicity tests against kola weevils had earlier been reported to be efficacious to one species of insect pest or the other. For instance Nicotiana tabacum aqueous extracts (tobacco decoction) controls insects like caterpillars, beetles, stem borers, leaf miners, aphids and thrips [26]. Also aqueous extracts of Nicotiana tabacum, Cymbopogon citrtus and other plants have been found effective in reducing the number of Podagrica beetles damage on okra [27].

The minimal protection of the kola nuts observed in this study was attributed to lower weevil oviposition and reduced progeny emergence due to the effects of the plant extracts. However, the increased number of exit holes and high population of the weevil emergence recorded as the storage progressed was a confirmation of the quick breakdown of the plant extracts in nature. Plant extracts are slow acting and degrades

easily in the environment. There is therefore the need for high rates of their application at an increased frequency to achieve very effective weevil control, which is in line with earlier research findings [28,29,30,31]. The hardy nature of the kola weevils may have also contributed to the low protection conferred on the kola nuts by the extracts.

Although the aspect of the real active constituents of each of the plant extracts was not investigated in the present study, it is logical to suggest that the reduction in population of kola weevil with these aqueous extracts may have been imparted by their water soluble bioactive chemical components.

5. CONCLUSION AND RECOMMENDATIONS

The results of this study have provided additional evidence for insect controlling activity of aqueous extracts of known medicinal plants. The work has also extended the range of possible control agents for kola weevils beyond Tetrapleura tetraptera, as previously reported by [32]. Any of the seven plant extracts used in this study can be successfully applied at 50% or 100% treatment level to minimally reduce the menace of kola weevils on stored kola nuts. However, there is the need for a more extensive work to be done on the control of kola weevils using materials of plant origin.

CONSENT

It is not applicable.

ETHICAL APPROVAL

It is not applicable.

COMPETING INTERESTS

Authors have declared that no competing interests exist.

REFERENCES

1. Odegbaro OA. Regeneration of old kola trees. *Cola nitida* (vent) Schott and Endl. by coppicing. *Turrialba*, 1973;23(3):334-3340.
2. Daramola AM. Common pests of Kola and Cacao with special reference to *Characoma stictigrapta* Hmps and *S. singularis* Hagl. damage to kola in Nigeria. Paper presented at the 6th W. Afr. Cocoa Entomologists Conference. CRIN Ibadan; 1978.
3. Ndubuaku TCN. Economic insect pests of kola. In: Progress in Tree Crop Research. 2nd edition. CRIN, Ibadan. 1989;111-114.
4. Asogwa EU, Ojelade KTM, Anikwe JC, Ndubuaku TCN. Insect pests of cocoa, kola, coffee, cashew tea and their control. Answers Communication Concepts. Apapa. Lagos, Nigeria. 2006;130.
5. Daramola AM, Ivbijaro MF. The distribution and ecology of kola weevils in Nigeria. Nig J Pl Prot. 1975;1(1):5-9.
6. NRI (Natural Resources Institute). A Guide to Insect Pests of Nigerian Crops, Identification, Biology and Control. Fed. Min. of Agric. & Nat. Res., Nig. & the Overseas Devlpt. Admin. UK. 1996;253.
7. Daramola AM. The bionomics of kola weevils *Sophrorhinus* spp (Coleoptera: Curculionidae). PhD Thesis, University of Ibadan. 1973;325.
8. Lale NES. Stored-product entomology and acarology in tropical Africa Mole Publications, Maiduguri, Nigeria. 2002;204.
9. WMO. Scientific assessment of ozone depletion: World Meteorological Organization global ozone research and monitoring project. Report No. 37. WMO, Geneva, Switzerland; 1995.
10. Zettler JL, Halliday WR, Arthur FH. Phosphine resistance in insects infesting stored peanuts in the Southeastern United States. J. Economic Entomol. 1989;82: 1508–1511.
11. Adu OO. Evaluation of seven fumigants as possible cowpea grains protectants. Rep. Nig. Stored Prod. Res. Inst. 1979/80 Tech. Rept. 1983;5:57–62.
12. Whitehead L, David B, William S. Natural Products for innovative pest. Pargamon Press, Great Britain. 1983;586.
13. Chander H, Ahmed S. Laboratory evaluation of natural embelin as grain protectant against some insects of wheat in storage. Indian J. Stored Prod. Res. 1987;23(1):41-46.
14. Ivbijaro MF. Preservation of cowpea (*Vigna unguiculata* L) Walp with the neem seed (*Azadirachta indica* Juss). Protection Ecology. 1983;5:177–182.
15. Pereira J. The effectiveness of six vegetable oils as protectants of cowpea and bambara groundnuts against infestation by *Callosobruchus maculatus* (F). J. Stored Prod. Res. 1982;19:57–62.
16. Jackai LEN, Daoust RA. Insect pest of cowpea. Ann. Rev. of Entomology. 1986; 39:95-119.
17. Zettler JL, Leesch JG, Gill RF, Mackey, BE. Toxicity of carbonyl sulfide to stored product insects. J. Economic Entomol. 1997;90(3):832-836
18. Papachristos DP, Stamopoulos DC. Toxicity of three essential oils to immature stages of *Acanthoscelides obectus* (Say) (Coleoptera: Bruchidae). J. Stored Prod. Res. 2002;38:365-373.
19. Dales MJ. A review of plant materials used for controlling insect pest of stored products. Natural Resource Institute, Chatham, Kent (UK). NRI Bulletein. 1996; 65:84.
20. Don-Pedro KN. Fumigant toxicity of citrus peal oils against adult and immature stages of storage insect pests. Pesticide Science. 1996;47:213-223.
21. Shaaya E, Kostjukovski M, Eilberg J, Sukprakarn C. Plant oils as fumigants and contact insecticides for the control of stored product insect. J. Stored Prod. Res. 1997;33:7-15.

Assessement of Aqueous Plant Extract for the Control of Kola Weevils...

149

22. Tapondjou LA, Adler C, Bouda H, Fontem DA. Efficacy of powder and essential oil from *Chenopodium ambrosioides* leaves as post-harvest grain protectants against six-stored product beetles. J. Stored Prod. Res. 2002;38:395-402.

23. Adewumi MA, Ofuya TI, Folorunso DO. Comparative effectiveness of some aqueous medicinal plant extracts in the control of post-flowering insect pests of cowpea in a rain forest area of Nigeria. In. Medicinal Plants in Agriculture: The Nigerian Experience. Proceedings 3rd Ann. Conf., School of Agric & Agric Tech. (eds.G.E. Onibi, S.O. Angele; V.A.J. Adenkule and M.O. Olufayo). FUTA, Nigeria. 2007;48-51.

24. Folorunso DO, Ofuya TI, Adewumi MA. Effect of some aqueous medicinal plant extracts on *Podagrica* (Coleoptera: Chrysomelidae) infestation and yield of okra in a rain forest area of Nigeria. In. Medicinal Plants in Agriculture: The Nigerian Experience. Proceedings 3rd Ann. Conf., School of Agric & Agric Tech. (eds. G.E. Onibi, S.O. Angele; V.A.J. Adenkule and M.O. Olufayo). FUTA, Nigeria. 2007;52-55.

25. Ameh SA, Ogunwolu EO. Comparative effectiveness of aqueous plant extracts and lambda cyhalothrin in controlling post flowering insect pests of cowpea in the southern guinea savannah of Nigeria. E.S.N. Occassional Publication. 2000; 32:175-180.

26. Stoll G. Natural Crop Protection in the Tropics. 2nd Ed. Margrav Verlog, Weikersheim. 2000;376.

27. Folorunsho DO, Ofuya TI, Adewumi MA. Mortality and repellence of *Podagrica* (Coleoptera: Chrysomelidae) by some aqueous plant extracts in the laboratory. Proc. 2nd Ann. Conf. of School of Agric & Tech., FUTA, Nigeria. 2006;28-30.

28. Golob P, Mwambula JM, Mhango V, Ngulube F. The use of locally available materials as protectants of maize grains against insect infestation during storage in Malawi. J. Stored Prod. Res. 1982;18:67 –74.

29. Sharaby A. Evaluation of some Myrtaceae plant leaves as protectants against the infestation by *Sitophilus oryzae* L and *S. granarius* L. Insect Science and its Application. 1988;9(4):465-468.

30. Ofuya TI, Okoye BC, Olola AS. Efficacy of crude extract from seed of *Monodora myritica* (Gaetrn) as a surface protectant against *C. maculatus* attacking legume seeds in storage. J. Plant Deasese and Protection. 1992;99(5):528-532.

31. Ewete FK, Arnason JT, Larson J, Philogene BJR. Biological activities of extracts from traditionally used Nigerian plants against the European corn borer, *Ostrinia nubilalis*. Entomologia Experimentalis et Applicata. 1996;80:531-537.

32. Anikwe JC, Ojelade KTM. Evaluation of *Tetrapleura tetraptera* (Schum & Thonn) fruit for the control of *Balanogastris kolae* (Desbr) infesting stored kola nuts. Ife J. of Sc. 2005;7(1):27–30.

17

Acaricidal Activities of *Hyptis suaveolens* and *Ocimum sanctum* Against African Dog Tick (*Rhipicephalus sanguinneus*)

Elijah I. Ohimain[1*], Tariwari C. N. Angaye[1], Sunday E. Bassey[1] and Sylvester C. Izah[1]

[1]*Department of Biological Sciences, Ecotoxicology and Environmental Safety Research Unit, Niger Delta University, Bayelsa State, Nigeria.*

Authors' contributions

This work was carried out in collaboration between all authors. Authors EIO and TCNA designed the Study and wrote the protocol. Authors TCNA and SCI wrote the first draft of the manuscript and performed the statistical analysis. Authors EIO and SEB revised the manuscript. All authors managed the literature searches and wrote the first draft of the manuscript. All authors read and approved the final manuscript.

Editor(s):
(1) Shanfa Lu, Institute of Medicinal Plant Development, Chinese Academy of Medical Sciences & Peking Union Medical College, China.
(2) Marcello Iriti, Faculty of Plant Biology and Pathology, Department of Agricultural and Environmental Sciences, Milan State University, Italy.
Reviewers:
(1) Dorota Wojnicz, Department of Biology and Medical Parasitology, Wroclaw Medical University, Poland.
(2) Justin Kabera, Pharmacology, TUTCM, Tianjin, China.

ABSTRACT

Aim: To determine the acaricidal activities of some solvent extracts (chloroform, methanol and n-hexane) and crude extracts of *Hyptis suaveolens and Ocimum sanctum* against African dog tick (*Rhipicephalus sanguinneus*).
Study Design: The study design involves a 24 h LC_{50} dose-mortality static non-renewal bioassay.
Place and Duration of Study: The study was carried out at Rohi Biotechnology Toxicity Laboratory, Port-Harcourt, Rivers State Nigeria, between August and November 2014.
Methodology: The solvent extracts were assessed against the ticks at varying concentrations in a 2-phased rapid and final screening test.
Results: All extracts showed moderate activities during the bioassay, except the crude extract

Corresponding author: E-mail: eohimain@yahoo.com

which was not active beyond the rapid screening phase (i.e. $LC_{100} > 500$ ppm). The chloroform, methanol and n-hexane extracts of *H. suaveolens* induced LC_{50} values of 175.00, 81.25 and 225.00 ppm respectively. On the other hand *O. sanctum* induced mortalities of 200.00, 137.50 and 287.50 ppm for chloroform, methanol and n-hexane extracts respectively. Meanwhile, the positive control was lethal at 1ppm, while the tick survived in the negative control.

Conclusion: The result demonstrates that solvent extracts of *H. suaveolens* and *O. sanctum* can be used as acaricides for the control of dog tick.

Keywords: Acaricide; solvent extracts; tick; Hyptis suaveolens; Ocimum sanctum.

1. INTRODUCTION

In the recent years, the use of synthetic pesticides has attracted global attention due to its toxic impacts on the applied organisms and the environment at large. Notwithstanding, the active sites of the attack by the pesticides depend on the type of pesticides under use. Due to the environmental effects and high cost of synthetic pesticides to indigent disease endemic areas [1], the application of plant-derived pesticides have attracted the attentions of ecotoxicology and parasitology researchers. In Africa, some plants have been reported for their therapeutic applications as pesticides against a variety of animal vectors and parasites. Some plants have found applications as curative agents due to the diverse phytochemicals they produce. Both *H. suaveolens* and *Ocimum sanctum* vital therapeutic components with diverse applications. For instance, *Ocimum* species has been widely reported to possess repellent properties against mosquito [2] and lymphatic filariasis [3]. *H. suaveolens* have also been reported to contain diverse metabolites which have found application as antimicrobial, anti-diarrhoeal, anti-inflammatory, anthelmintic, anti-diabetic, anticancerous, wound-healing and insecticidal agents [4].

In many part many parts of the world, several people domesticate dogs (*Cannis* species) and use them as pets, for food and security. Parasites such as *Rhipicephalus sanguineus* (dog tick), are obligate haematophagous external parasites of some domestic and wild animals; which cause discomfort on infected hosts [5]. Tick infestation often results to loss of appetite by the dog and results to death in cases of poor and inappropriate treatment. Generally, ticks rank second to mosquito amongst parasites of infectious diseases [6,7]. It has been estimated, in literature that 80% of 1.2 million domestic tick-prone animals are at risk of contracting tick-borne diseases, thereby causing a global annual loss of about US$ 7000 million [6]. For instance, literature exist by several authors which reported the incidence of tick-borne diseases for cattle with 7.6% infestation rate, 55.4% for goats and 13.2% for pigs [8-10].

R. sanguineus are controlled by physical and chemical methods and to a lesser extent by biological control. The physical approach involves hand picking of the tick from the skin of the infected animal. Chemical approach involves the use pesticides that contain chemicals in the eradication of the *R. sanguineus*. Some of the common chemical pesticides used for the control of tick in general are delta methrin and amitraz [5,11,12]. The constant use of chemical acaricides could lead to environmental contamination, food toxicity, etc. Hence, the use of plant extracts for the eradication of *R. sanguineus* has gained prominence over physical and chemical methods. Some of the plants species that have been reported to have acaricidal potentials include *Annonas quamosa*, *Centella asiatica*, *Gloriosa superba*, *Mukiamader aspatensis*, *Pergularia daemia*, *Phyllanthusem blica*against adult cattle tick (*Haemaphysalis bispinosa*) [6]. Fernandes and Freitas, [13] also reported the acaricidal activity of *Copaifera reticulate* against *R. microplus* larva. Basedon the prospects of using plant-derived extracts for the control of parasitic vectors, the acaricidal potentials of *H. suaveolens* and *O. sanctum* from Nigeria is hereby evaluated.

2. MATERIALS AND METHODS

2.1 Collection of Plant Materials

The leaf of *H. Suaveolens* and *O. Sanctum* were collected from, Igarra, Edo State, Nigeria in August 2014. The taxonomic identification of both plants was carried out identification keys as described by Ogunkunle [14].

2.2 Plant Extraction/ Phytochemical Analysis

The leaves were shade-dried for 7 days at ambient environmental temperatures (31±2°C).

The dried leaves were powdered using domestic electrical blender and the powdered leaves (400 g) were macerated for 72 h in n-hexane (700 ml, Fisher Scientific international Company), chloroform (700 ml, BHD Chemical Ltd. Poole England) and methanol (700 ml, BHD Chemical Ltd. Poole England); meanwhile for the crude extraction, the juice of the fresh leaves of both plants were used. The active ingredients in the filtrates were respectively extracted in a rotary evaporator (60°C), leaving no trace of solvent. The residue obtained was stored at 4°C until it was ready for use. Phytochemical screenings of the plants were carried out following standard protocols [15].

2.3 Parasite Collection

The attached adults of *R. sanguinneus* were collected from the ears and foot of the dog. The parasites were identified using identification keys as described by Dantas-Torres [16].

2.4 Experimental Setup

The applied experimental setup of this investigation to verify the acaricidal activity of different solvent plant extracts against adult of *R. sanguinneus* was developed following standard protocol [17,18], with slight modifications incorporating rapid and final screening as described by several authors [19-21]. The bioassay was set up with different concentrations of the extracts impregnated with series of prepared filter paper envelopes (Whatman filter paper No. 1), inoculated with a minimum of ten ticks.

The treated envelopes inoculated with adult ticks was tagged and sealed with metallic clip in order to prevent escape. The envelopes were incubated at laboratory conditions (28-30°C and 80–90% relative Humidity for 24 h), as described by Begavan et al. [6]. The envelopes were opened sequel to the incubation period (24 h),

and the mortality rates (%), were recorded. The positive control was impregnated with Zimitraz 12.5% (Zampharm Limited, London-England), while the negative control was set up with distill water.

2.5 Rapid Screening and Final Screening

The rapid screening was set up with their respective replicates at concentrations of 1000 and 500 ppm of the extracts. Furthermore, only extracts active at 500 ppm (i.e. extracts with an LC_{100} of 500 ppm within 24 h), were sanctioned for the final screening.

2.6 Statistical Analysis

The mean mortality and standard deviation of data from the bioassay were calculated, after which they were further subjected to concentration-mortality curve using statistical analysis (Microsoft Excel, 2013 version, with 5% error), to estimate the median lethal concentration.

3. RESULTS

The phytochemical screening and general acaricidal activities of different solvent extracts (chloroform, methanol and n-hexane), of *H. suaveolens and O. sanctum* is presented in Tables 1-3 and Fig. 1. The result of the phytochemical analysis indicated higher amount of phenol in all extracts of *H. suaveolens* compared to *O. sanctum*. On the other hand, higher amount of flavonoid was found in extracts of *O. sanctum* compared to *H. suaveolens*. Tannins and steroids were absent in all extracts of *O. sanctum*. Solvents extracts of *H. suaveolens* witnessed higher amount of steroids compared to tannins. On the other hand, tannins and steroids were absent in the extracts of *O. sanctum*, as well as alkaloids and saponins in all extracts of the plant.

Table 1. Phytochemical analysis of various leaf solvent extracts of the plants

Plants	Extracting medium	Phytochemicals					
		Phenol	Alkaloid	Tannin	Steroid	Saponin	Flavonoid
H. Suaveolens	chloroform	++	-	+	++	-	+
	methanol	++	-	+	++	-	+
	n-hexane	++	-	+	++	-	+
	crude extract	++	-	+	+	-	+
O. Sanctum	chloroform	+	-	-	-	-	++
	methanol	+	-	-	-	-	++
	n-hexane	+	-	-	-	-	++
	crude extract	+	-	-	-	-	++

++: present in abundance; +: present; -: absent

Table 2. Rapid screening results

Plants	Extracting medium	% Mortality ± SD	
		1000 ppm	**500 ppm**
H. Suaveolens	chloroform	100±0.000	100±0.000
	methanol	100±0.000	100±0.000
	n-hexane	100±0.000	100±0.000
	Crude extract	100±0.000	83±1.314
O. Sanctum	chloroform	100±0.000	100±0.000
	Methanol	100±0.000	100±0.000
	n-hexane	100±0.000	100±0.000
	crude extract	100±0.000	67±1.0403

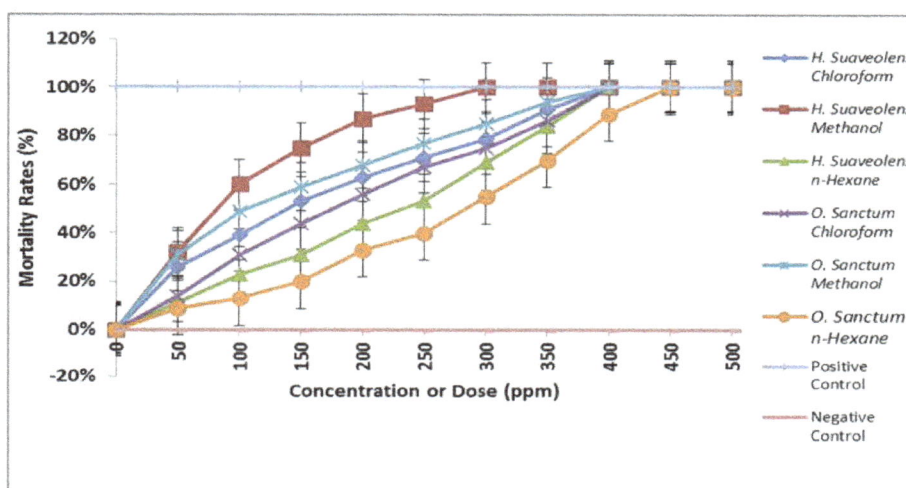

Fig. 1. Dose-mortality graph (5% error ± SD)

Compared to other extracts, results of the rapid screening (Table 2), shows that the crude extracts (for both plants), had total mortality rates (i.e. 100% mortality), at a higher concentration (above 500 ppm). Hence the crude extracts of both plants were not regarded for the final screening.

Results of the final screening (Table 3), shows that the solvent extracts of *H. suaveolens* had minimal total mortality rates (*MTMrt*), at concentrations of 400, 300 and 450 ppm for chloroform, methanol and hexane extracts respectively. While the *O. sanctum* extracts were toxic to the parasites with *MTMrt* at 400 ppm for both chloroform and methanolic extracts compared to the hexane extract with *MTMrt* at 450 ppm.

The median lethal dose (LC_{50}) was statistically determined. Results (Fig. 1) show that, the chloroform, methanol and n-hexane extracts of *H. suaveolens* induced LC_{50} values of 175.00, 81.25 and 225.00 ppm respectively. On the other

hand *O. sanctum* induced mortalities of 200.00, 137.50 and 287.50 ppm for chloroform, methanol and n-hexane extracts respectively. Meanwhile, the positive control was lethal at 1 ppm, while the tick survived in the negative control.

4. DISCUSSION

Compared to the crude extracts (LC_{100}>500 ppm), the solvent extracts of both plants (*H. suaveolens* and *O. sanctum*), were effective against African dog tick, *R. sanguinneus*. The higher rates of acaricidal activities observed amongst the solvent extracts (The *H. suaveolens*-chloroform extract =175.00 ppm, *H. suaveolens*-methanol extract =81.25 and *H. suaveolens*-Hexane extract = 225.00 ppm; *O. sanctum* extracts 200.00, 137.50 and 287.50 ppm for Chloroform, methanol and n-hexane extracts respectively) had been demonstrated from the foregoing. There are several literature demonstrating the acaricidal activities of plant solvent extracts by other researchers.

Table 3. Final screening results

Plant-extracts		% MORTALITY RATES ± SD						
		450 ppm	400 ppm	350 ppm	300 ppm	250 ppm	200 ppm	150 ppm
H. suaveolens	Chloroform	100±0.00%	100±0.00%	91±1.31%	79±1.14%	68±2.134%	57±0.41%	44±0.11%
	Methanol	100±0.00%	100±0.00%	100±0.00%	100±0.00%	93±1.099%	87±3.03%	75±1.40%
	n-hexane	100±0.00%	97±0.44%	84±1.33%	69±1.13%	53±1.34%	44±2.30%	31±0.31%
O. Sanctum	Chloroform	100±0.00%	100±0.00%	82±1.44%	71±2.03%	67±1.33%	50±0.43%	39±2.20%
	methanol	100±0.00%	100±0.00%	89±1.11%	80±2.02%	77±0.42%	61±1.10%	51±1.13%
	n-hexane	100±0.00%	89±1.13%	70±0.73%	55±3.04%	40±1.10%	33±1.11%	20±0.42%
CONTROLS								
Positive control		100±0.00%	100±0.00%	100±0.00%	100±0.00%	100±0.00%	100±0.00%	100±0.00%
Negative control		0±0.00%	0±0.00%	0±0.00%	0±0.00%	0±0.00%	0±0.00%	0±0.00%

Bagavan et al. [6] investigated the acaricidal activities of several plants against cattle tick (Haemaphysalis bispinosa) and results demonstrates that the leaf from the hexane extract of Annona squamosal induced LC_{50} value of 145.39 ppm, while the acetone and methanolic extracts of Gloriosa superb leaf against had LC_{50} value of 419.83 ppm and 225.57 ppm respectively. The authors further reported that methanolic and ethyl acetate leaf extracts of Pergularia daemia and Phyllanthus emblica had LC_{50} values of 294.46 and 256.08 ppm respectively. Zaman et al. [22] reported the synergicidal efficacy of the aqueous extract of several plants (Azadirachta indica leaves, Nicotiana tabacum leaves, Calotropis procera flowers and Trachyspermum ammi seeds) against cattle tick and reported fecundity suppression index of 0.371404, reduced hatching of 22.35% as well as mortality and reduced tick intensity of 50 mg/ml and detachability of 45%. A recent research with the oil of Camellia sasanqua seed against the Rhipicephalus microplus (cattle tick) and the dog tick (R. sanguineus), showed LD_{50} and LD_{100} values of 4.61% and 9.18% for R. microplus and 5.43% and 9.50% with R. sanguineus [23]. Politi et al. [24] showed that 70% ethanolic extract of T. patula was toxic to adult female dog tick with an immersion time of 5 minutes at a concentration of 50.0 mg/ml. The authors also reported a decrease infecundal (21.5%) and mortality (99.78%) rates of larvae. Fernandes et al. [25], reported the acaricidal activity of crude ethanol extract of Magonia pubescens stem bark against Rhipicephalus sanguineus with an LC_{50} value of 1503 ppm.

Some phytochemicals indicated in our study have also been reported by several authors [4, 26,27]. For instance, Cook and Samman, [26] reported that the antimicrobial activities of O. sanctum was attributed to phytochemical like phenol, flavonoid and other carotenoid compounds. Sikkema et al. [27] reported the activity of H. suaveolens was due to the presence of monoterpene constituents which could exert membrane disruption. Cox et al. [28] also reported that H. suaveolens could stimulate cellular leakage of potassium ions, and further results to mortality. Mandal et al. [29], observed higher microbial activity in steam distillation and petroleum ether extracts of H. suaveolens than that of ethanolic extract. Our finding validates previous observations, documented in literature.

Furthermore, earlier studies have shown that extracts belonging to the genus, Ocimum, induced various degrees of activities against ticks [30,31] and even malaria [2] and elephantiasis [3] vectors. As such, this line of research should be encouraged, including phytochemical fractionation, purification as well as mode of action (chemistry), of the plant .Also, the evaluation of the actual bioactive components which was lethal to the ticks should be assayed. Notwithstanding, much attention has been given to ongoing multifaceted and integrated approach exploring eco-friendly alternatives in the control of this tick and other pathogenic arthropods.

5. CONCLUSION

Ticks are important parasite and vectors of human and animal diseases due to their devastating morbidity rate. The control of tick commonly involves the use of synthetic acaricides, which constitute various degrees of environmental toxicity. This article investigated the acaricidal efficacy of H. suaveolens and O. sanctum against dog tick. Solvent extracts of both plants induced moderate mortality rates against the tick. This study justifies the indigenous application of H. suaveolens and O. sanctum which are known for their insecticidal activities. We also recommend the ex-situ trial of these plant in order to actualize their eco-tolerant dose against non-targeted species.

CONSENT

It is not applicable

ETHICAL APPROVAL

It is not applicable

ACKNOWLEDGEMENTS

The authors wish to acknowledge ROHI Biotechnologies Limited, Port-Harcourt, Nigeria for providing the platform for this research work.

COMPETING INTERESTS

Authors have declared that no competing interests exist.

REFERENCES

1. Angaye TCN, Ohimain EI, Zige DV, Didi B, Biobelemoye N. Biocidal activities of Solvent extracts of Azadirachta indica

against Some Endemic Tropical Vector-borne Diseases. International Journal of Tropical Disease & Health. 2014;4(11):1198-1208.

2.   Egunyomi A, Gbadamosi IT, Osiname KO. Comparative effectiveness of ethnobotanical mosquito repellents used in Ibadan, Nigeria. Journal of Applied Biosciences. 2010;36:2383-2388.

3.   Malebo HM, Imeda C, Kitufe NA, Katani SJ, Sunguruma R, Magogo F, et al. Repellence effectiveness of essential oils from some Tanzanian *Ocimum* and *Hyptis* plant species against afro-tropical vectors of malaria and lymphatic filariasis. Journal of Medicinal Plants Research. 2013;7(11):653–660.

4.   Ngozi LU, Ugochukwu N, Ifeoma PU, Charity EA, Chinyelu IE. The Efficacy of Hyptis Suaveolens: A Review of Its Nutritional and Medicinal Applications. European Journal of Medicinal Plants. 2014;4(6):661-674.

5.   Adarsh KTP, Ajeesh KTP, Chithra ND, Deepa PE, Darsana U, Sreelekha KP, et al. Acaricidal Activity of Petroleum Ether Extract of Leaves of Tetrastigmal eucostaphylum (Dennst.) Alston against *Rhipicephalus* (Boophilus) annulatus. The Scientific World Journal. 2014;1–6.

6.   Begavan A, Kamaraj C, Elango G, AbduzZhar A, Abdul Rahuman A, Adulticidal. Larvicidal efficacy of some medicinal plant extracts against tick, fluke and mosquitoes. Veterinary Parasitology. 2011;166(3-4):286-92.

7.   Sonenshine DE, Lane RS, Nicholson WL. Ticks (Ixodida), in: Mullen G, Durden L, (Eds.). Medical and Veterinary Entomology, Academic Press, San Diego. 2002:517–558.

8.   Van den Broek AH, Huntley JF, Halliwell RE, Machell J, Taylor M, Miller HR. Cutaneous hypersensitivity reactions to Psoroptes ovis and Der p 1 in sheep previously infested with P. ovis—the sheep scab mite. Vet. Immunol. Immunopathol. 2003;91:105–117.

9.   Wall R. Ectoparasites: Future challenges in a changing world. Vet. Parasitol. 2007;1481:62–74.

10. Ghosh S, Bansal GC, Gupta SC, Ray D, Khan MQ, Irshad H, et al. Status of tick distribution in Bangladesh, India and Pakistan. Parasitol. Res. 2007;101(2):207–216.

11. Davey RB, Miller RJ, George JE. Efficacy of amitraz applied as a dip against an amitraz-resistant strain of *Rhipicephalus* (*Boophilus*) microplus (Acari: *Ixodidae*) infested on cattle. Veterinary Parasitology. 2008;(1-2):127–135.

12. Barre N, Li AY, Miller RJ, Gaia H, Delathiere JM, Davey RB, et al. *In vitro* and *in vivo* evaluation of deltamethrin and amitraz mixtures for the control of *Rhipicephalus* (*Boophilus*) microplus (Acari: *Ixodidae*) in New Caledonia. Veterinary Parasitology. 2008;(1-2):110–119.

13. Fernandes FF, Freitas EPS. Acaricidal activity of an oleoresinous extract from Copaifera reticulate Leguminosae: Caesalpinoideae against larvae of the southern cattle tick, *Rhipicephalus microplus* Acari: *Ixodidae*. Veterinary Parasitology. 2008;147(1-2):150-154.

14. Ogunkunle ATJ. Properties, users' assessment and applicability of nine types of taxonomic keys in diagnosing some Nigerian species of *Ocimum* L. *Hyptis* Jacq. And *Ficus* L. African Journal of Plant Science. 2014;8(1):6-24.

15. Association of Official Analytical Chemists, AOAC—Official methods of analysis. 16th edition. Arlington, V. A. USA; 1995.

16. Danta-Torres F. Biology and Ecology of the Brown dog tick, *Rhipcephalus sanguineus*. Parasites & Vectors. 2010;3:26-37.

17. World Health Organisation (WHO). Report of the WHO Information Consultation on the evaluation on the testing of insecticides CTD/WHO PES/IC96. 1996;1:96.

18. FAO (Food and Agriculture Organization of the United Nations). Ticks: Acaricide resistance: Diagnosis management and prevention. In: Guidelines Resistance Management and Integrated Parasite Control in Ruminants, FAO Animal Production and Health Division, Rome. 2004;Module 1.

19. Agboola IO, Ajayi GO, Adesegun SA, Adesanya SA, Comparative Molluscicidal activity of fruit pericarp, leaves, seed and stem Bark of *Blighiauni jugata* Baker. Pharmacology Journal. 2011;3:63-66.

20. Bassey SE, Ohimain EI, Angaye TC. The Molluscicidal Activities of Methanolic and Aqueous Extracts of *Jatropha curcas* leaves against *Bulinus globosus* and *Bulinus rholfsi*, Vectors of Urinary

Schistosomiasis. Journal of Parasitology. 2013;103:115-122.

21. Angaye TCN, Ohimain EI, Siasia EP, Asaigbe PI, Finomo OA. Larvicidal activities of the leaves of Niger Delta mangrove plants against *Anopheles gambiae*. Sky Journal of Microbiology Research. 2014;2(7):032-036.

22. Zamana MA, Iqbalb Z, Abbasb RZ, Khanb MN, Muhammad G, Younusa M, et al. *In vitro* and *in vivo* acaricidal activity of herbal extract. Veterinary Parasitology. 2012;186(3-4):431-6.

23. Hai NT, Atsushi M. Evaluation acaricidal efficacy of *Camellia sasanqua* thumb seed oil against the cattle tick *Rhipicephalus (Boophilus) microplus* and the dog tick *Rhipicephalus sanguineus*. International Journal of Medicinal Plant Research. 2014;3(3):284-289.

24. Politi FAS, Figueira GM, Araújo AM, Sampieri BR, Mathias MIC, et al. Acaricidal activity of ethanolic extract from aerial parts of Tagetes patula L. (Asteraceae) against larvae and engorged adult females of *Rhipicephalus sanguineus* (Latreille, 1806). Parasites & Vectors. 2012;5:295.

25. Fernandes FF, D'alessandro WB, Freitas EPS. Toxicity of Extract of Magonia pubescens (Sapindales: Sapindaceae) St.

Hil. To Control the Brown Dog Tick, Rhipicephalus sanguineus (*Latreille*) (Acari: *Ixodidae*). Neotropical Entomology. 2008;37(2):205-208.

26. Cook NC, Samman S. Flavonoids-chemistry, metabolism, cardio protective effect and dietary sources. J Nutr Biochem. 1996;7(2):66-76.

27. Sikkema J, De Bont JAM, Poolman B. Interactions of cyclic hydrocarbons with biological membranes. J. Biol. Chem. 1994;269:8022-8028.

28. Cox SD, Gustafson JE, Mann CM, Markham JL, Liew YC, Hartland RP, et al. Tea tree oil causes K+ leakage and inhibits respiration in *Escherichia coli*. Lett. Appl. Microbiol. 2008;26(5):355-358.

29. Mandal SM, Mondal KC, Dey S, Pati BR. Antimicrobial activity of the leaf extracts of *Hyptis suaveolens* (L.) Poit. Indian J Pharm Sci. 2007;69:568-569.

30. Del Fabbro S, Nazzi F. Repellent effect of sweet basil compounds on Ixode sricinus ticks, Exp. Appl. Acarol. 2008;45:219–228.

31. Mwangi EN, Hassanali A, Essuman S, Myandat E, Moreka L, Kimondo M. Repellent and acaricidal properties of *Ocimum* suave against *Rhipicephalus appendiculatus* ticks, Exp. Appl. Acarol. 1995;19:11–18.

18

In vivo Effect of Cassava Flakes Mixed with *Euphorbia heterophylla* against *Salmonella typhi*

F. O. Omoya[1*], A. O. Momoh[1] and O. A. Olaifa[1]

[1]*Department of Microbiology, Federal University of Technology, P.M.B. 704, Akure, Ondo State, Nigeria.*

Authors' contributions

This work was carried out in collaboration between all authors. Author FOO designed the study and experimental protocol, Authors AOM and OAO performed the experiments, managed the literature searches and analyses of the study. Authors FOO and AOM wrote the first draft of the manuscript and critically revised the manuscript. All authors read and approved the final manuscript.

Editor(s):
(1) Thomas Efferth, Department of Pharmaceutical Biology, Institute of Pharmacy and Biochemistry, Johannes Gutenberg University, Germany.
(2) Marcello Iriti, Department of Agricultural and Environmental Sciences, Milan State University, Italy.
Reviewers:
(1) Ary Fernandes Junior, Microbiology and Immunology, Bioscienes Institute, UNESP, Brazil.
(2) Anonymous, USA.
(3) Anonymous, Pakistan.
(4) Anonymous, Portugal.

ABSTRACT

Aims: The therapeutic effect of *Euphorbia heterophylla* and cassava flakes mixture in treatment of Salmonellosis was studied *in vivo*.
Methodology: Antibacterial activity of aqueous extract of *Euphorbia heterophylla* was first evaluated using agar well diffusion method by measuring the diameters of zones of inhibition on *Salmonella typhi in vitro*. The test organism was susceptible to *Euphorbia heterophylla* extract. Albino rats were infected with *Salmonella typhi* and confirmed using WIDAL test.
Results: The result showed that the infectivity dose was 2.0×10^2 cfu/ml for an albino rat of average weight 110 g. The qualitative analysis of the phytochemical of the plant showed that anthraquinone, glycosides and alkaloid are present. The analysis of the pH of the white cassava flakes used was 3.83 while that of the red cassava flakes was 5.62. The titre value of the infected rats increased significantly from 1:20 to 1:160 three days after infection. Administration of *Euphorbia heterophylla* with cassava flakes mixture was found to effectively treat and reduce the titre value to 1:20 after

Corresponding author: Email: fomoya@yahoo.com

treating for 7 days. The infection caused a decreasing effect on the haematological parameters such as PCV and WBC. The histopathological analyses of the organs of the infected rats caused mild to severe pathological changes varying from widespread vascular damage, haemorrhage, vasculitis, cellular degeneration and necrosis of the organs. The therapeutic effect of the treatment administered using the *Euphorbia heterophylla* – cassava flakes mixture showed recuperating cells of the organs analysed histopathologically.

Conclusion: The results obtained in this work showed that *Euphorbia heterophylla* mixed with cassava flakes is an effective therapeutic agent for Salmonellosis and that the *Euphorbia heterophylla* with white cassava flakes mixture is more effective in the treatment of Salmonellosis.

Keywords: Cassava flakes; Euphorbia heterophylla; Salmonella typhi; therapeutic.

1. INTRODUCTION

Salmonella is a member of the family *Enterobacteriaceae* [1]. Salmonella spp. causes wide range of diseases such as enteric fever, gastroenteritis and bacteraemia. *Salmonella* is a leading cause of food borne illness [2,3]. Food borne infections caused by *Salmonella* serotypes occurs at high frequency in industrialized nations and developing countries and is an important public health problem worldwide. Salmonellosis is a common disease caused by numerous *Salmonella* serovars with clinical manifestations that vary from severe enteric fever to mild food poisoning [4] both in animals [5] and humans [6]. It is characterized by diarrhoea, headache, abdominal pain, fever, and vomiting, beginning 6 to 72 hours after infection. There are many different kinds of these bacteria causing salmonellosis in which *Salmonella* serotype Typhimurium and *Salmonella* serotype Enteritidis are the most common types [7].

Euphorbia heterophylla is an important medicinal herb, belongs to the family *Euphorbiaceae* that has been widely used in traditional medicine in various parts of Africa [8,9] including Nigeria. *E. heterophylla* has been used for the treatment of constipation, bronchitis and asthma. The plant has also been used as purgative [10,11]. The desire to scientifically validate the medicinal properties of these plants has resulted in the investigation of their various biological activities. There are dearth of information on the antimicrobial potentials of *E. heterophylla* although [12] reported the antibacterial activities of leaves extract against strains of typed culture organisms.

Cassava (*Manihot esculenta*) is an important root crop in the tropics [13]. In West Africa, this crop is usually fermented using various methods before consumption [14]. One of the most popular foods derived from fermented cassava is cassava flakes popularly known as *garri*, which is consumed by nearly 200 million people in West Africa [15]. Cassava is the staple food of 250 million of Africans [15]. Different kinds of foods result from cassava processing, e.g. "*garri* and *fufu*", which are fermented cassava derived foods consumed at least once a day by West African people.

Cassava flakes is a dry granular meal made from moist, lactic acid fermented product of cassava roots. Cassava flakes can be processed with carotenoid-rich palm oil (yellow *garri*) or without palm oil (white *garri*). This product is widely acceptable and consumed by both the rich and poor in Nigeria. Many of the fermented products consumed by different ethnic groups have therapeutic values, some of the most widely known are fermented milks (that is, yoghurt, curds) which contain high concentrations of probiotic bacteria that can lower the cholesterol level [16], Improvement of nutrients absorption and digestion, restores the balance of bacteria in the gut to hinder constipation, abdominal cramps, asthma, allergies, lactose and gluten intolerance [17]. The slurries of carbohydrate based fermented Nigerian foods such as ogi, fufu and wara have been known to exhibit health promoting properties such as control of gastroenteritis in animals and human [18,19].

Some microorganisms involved during the fermentation produce antimicrobial products [20] that are beneficial. Previous study on *Euphorbia heterophylla* and folk medicinal believe of the Ife people (Yoruba speaking people of Nigeria) is that when *Euphorbia heterophylla* is mixed with garri, it cures typhoid and some are even of the opinion that it is more effective with red garri. This research is therefore focused on the *in vivo* effect of cassava flakes mixed with *euphorbia heterophylla* against *Salmonella typhi*.

2. MATERIALS AND METHODS

2.1 Collection of *Euphorbia heterophylla*

Fresh intact leaves of *Euphorbia heterophylla* were obtained from a local garden in Iyana church area of Ibadan, Oyo State, Nigeria.

2.2 Collection of Test Organism

Pure isolate of *Salmonella typhi* was obtained from the Microbiology research laboratory of the University of Technology, Akure, Ondo State, Nigeria.

2.3 Antimicrobial sensitivity Test of the *Euphorbia heterophylla* extract

The antimicrobial test was carried out using the agar diffusion method described by [21]. The test organism was inoculated on already prepared Nutrient agar plate and spread uniformly with sterile glass spreader. Cavities of 1 cm diameter were made on the nutrient agar using a sterile cork borer. 0.1 ml of the plant extract was introduced into each of the cavities. Sterile distilled water was introduced into one of the cavities as positive control. The plates were allowed to stand for 1 hour on the bench for diffusion to occur. sPlates were thereafter incubated at 37°C for 24 to 48 hours. The diameter of zones of inhibition were then observed and recorded.

2.4 Laboratory Experimental Rats

Eight to ten weeks old albino rats of weights ranging from 124 g to 180 g were used for the experiment. These rats were obtained from Animal Production and Health Laboratory, Federal University of Technology Akure, Ondo State. Nigeria. The rats were fed with grower's mash throughout the period of the experiment.

2.5 Treatment of infected Animals

Twenty one albino rats of both sexes were classified into three with each group having seven animals each, the animals were allowed free access to water and food pellets. The animals in (a) and (b) were infected with *Salmonella typhi* orogastrically, those in group (a) were treated with *Euphorbia heterophylla* mixed with yellow cassava flakes and those in group (b) were treated with *Euphorbia heterophylla* mixed with white cassava flakes.

The animals in the control group (c) were fed with only the grower's mash throughout the period of the experiment.

2.6 Culturing and Harvesting of *Salmonella typhi* Cells

Two loopful of *Salmonella* pure culture was inoculated into 500 ml of sterile nutrient broth and incubated at a temperature of 37°C for 24 hours. After incubation, it was centrifuged for 15 minutes at a speed of 3000 rpm. The pellets were rinsed into a sterile flask. Serial dilution was prepared by aseptically pipetting 1 ml of the *Salmonella* stock culture into 9 ml of distilled water in a test tube and thoroughly mixed to give a dilution of 10^{-1}, 1 ml of 10^{-1} dilution was pipetted into another test tube containing 9 ml of sterile distilled water using a fresh pipette to make a dilution of 10^{-2} and subsequently to dilution 10^{-7}.

2.7 Feeding of Albino Rats with *Salmonella typhi*

Two ml of *Salmonella typhi* from the 10^{-7} dilution was orogastrically ingested using the feeding loop. Observations were made hourly to determine if there would be any infection, time of infection and the number of rats infected.

2.8 Widal Test Analysis

Widal test on the rats' blood samples was done according to the method of [21]. The whole blood was collected into labelled EDTA bottles and centrifuged at 1500 rpm for 10 minutes to separate the serum from the cells. The serum was carefully withdrawn and titrated against standard antisera following the manufacturer's instructions. The results were then recorded with 1:40 taken as significant titre value.

2.9 Preparation of *garri* Using *Euphorbia heterophylla*

One hundred gram of *Euphorbia heterophylla* was weighed into 1000 ml of boiling water, sieved and used to prepare *Eba* using yellow and white cassava flakes in separate sterile plates.

2.10 Histological Studies

Male and female Swiss albino rats (8-10 weeks old) weighing 100-140 g were obtained from the Department of Animal Production and Health, Federal University of Technology, Akure, Nigeria.

The animals were housed in separate cages, kept in a clean environment and fed with food and water *ad libitum* (2 g of the Euphobia-gari mixture for 7 days). The animals were dozed with chloroform and the various organs (heart, kidney, liver) were removed, grossly examined and stained with haematoxylin-eosin before examining under the light microscope if the treatment has any effect on them. The organs were compared with that of the control rats. The histological processing was carried out and interpreted at the Department of Animal Production and Health Laboratory, Federal University of Technology, Akure, Ondo State.

2.11 Statistical Analysis

Analysis of variance (ANOVA) and Duncan's multiple comparison tests among data were carried out using SPSS and MS Office Excel software for the significance of the main effects (factors), and treatments along with their interactions.

3. RESULTS AND DISCUSSION

The results obtained from the analyses showed that the infectivity dose of the animals vary according to their body weight. However the average infectivity dose of the organisms on the animals was 2.0×10^2 cfu/ml. Table 1 showed the result of the antibacterial evaluation of the *Euphorbia heterophylla* extract. Comparatively, the least effective was the aqueous extract of *Euphorbia heterophylla*; while the most effective was *Euphorbia heterophylla* + white cassava flakes. However, ciprotab (a standard commercial antibiotic) was most effective, having the highest diameter of zone of inhibition. The results of the widal test performed on the experimental animals before, during and after infection as well as after treatment for 3 days and 7 days respectively shows that the infection of the animals caused significant increase in the titre values obtained. This is shown in Table 2. For instance, the titre value for *Salmonella typhi* before infection was 1:20, during infection, it rose to 1:160 and treatment began, it dropped gradually to 1:40 and by the 7th day of the inception of treatment it was 1:20 again.

The result of the histopathological studies showed that there were mild to severe pathological changes majorly varying from widespread vascular damage, haemorrhage, vasculitis, cellular degeneration and necrosis. The kidneys of the rats infected with *Salmonella* and treated with both the mixture of *Euphorbia heterophylla* and white or yellow *garri* respectively showed mild interstitial mononuclear cell infiltrations with slight tubular necrosis that resulted in glomerular shrinkage of the Bowman's capsule. The control had normal nephrotic cells without any degeneration. This is shown in plates 1a, b and c respectively. The histopathology of the liver presented showed varying degrees of vacuolar degeneration which appears slightly swollen for the group fed with *Euphorbia heterophylla* mixed with red cassava flakes. Mild microsclerosis and fatty degeneration of hepatic cells leading to necrosis of the hepatocytes, Haemorrhage and widening of blood sinusoids were also observed for the rats fed with *Euphorbia heterophylla* mixed with white cassava flakes. The control group showed mild microsclerosis and fatty degeneration of hepatic cells. This is shown in plates 2a, b and c respectively.

Table 1. Antimicrobial evaluation of the *Euphorbia heterophylla* extract

Extract	Salmonella typhi
Aqueous Extract of Euphorbia heterophylla	12±2.0
Euphorbia heterophylla + Yellow cassava flakes	14±1.0
Euphorbia heterophylla + White cassava flakes	18±0.21
Ciprotab	23±1.4

Values are mean ± SD of three replicates.

The heart of the rat fed with the red /white cassava flakes mixed with *Euphorbia heterophylla* is shown in plates 3a, b and c. Histopathological examination reveals myocardites with fragmentation of myofibrils in the group fed with the mixture of *Euphorbia heterophylla* and red cassava flakes, while the group fed with the mixture of *Euphorbia heterophylla* and white cassava flakes showed vascular degeneration of mononuclear cell infiltration, thrombosis and vasculitis of the cardiac muscles. The control showed normal cardiac muscles with slight cell infiltrations of the striata.

Table 2. Titre values of widal test results obtained from experimental albino rats before, during and after infection

Samples	Salmonella typhi	Salmonella paratyphi A	Salmonella paratyphi B	Salmonella paratyphi C
A1	1:20	1:40	1:20	1:40
A2	1:20	1:20	1:40	1:20
A3	1:20	1:40	1:40	1:40
B1	1:80	1:80	1:40	1:80
B2	1:160	1:160	1:80	1:80
B3	1:80	1:80	1:80	1:160
C1	1:40	1:40	1:80	1:40
C2	1:40	1:20	1:40	1:20
C3	1:40	1:20	1:40	1:20
D1	1:20	1:20	1:40	1:20
D2	1:20	1:20	1:40	1:20
D3	1:20	1:20	1:20	1:20

A: Before infection; B: After infection; C: 3 days after treatment administration; D: 7 days after treatment administration

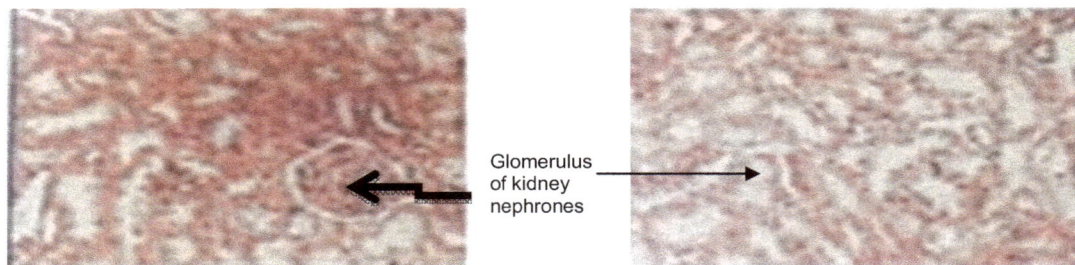

Glomerulus of kidney nephrones

Plate 1a. Kidney of infected rat and treated with white *garri*;   Plate 1b. kidney of the control

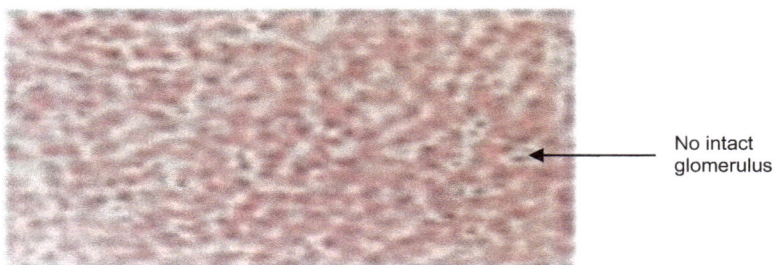

No intact glomerulus

Plate 1c. Kidney of infected rat and treated with yellow *garri*

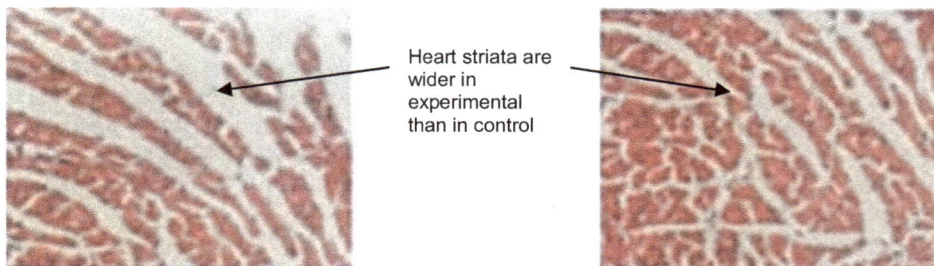

Heart striata are wider in experimental than in control

Plate 2a. Heart of infected rat and treated with white *garri*   Plate 2b. Control

Normal heart striata as in control

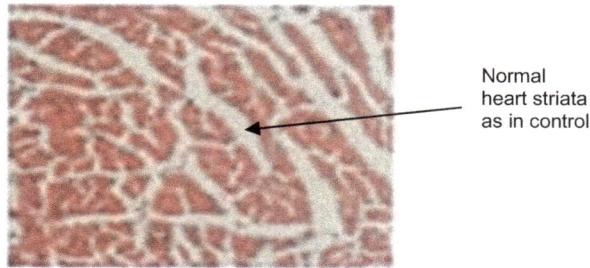

Plate 2c. Heart of infected and treated with yellow *garri*

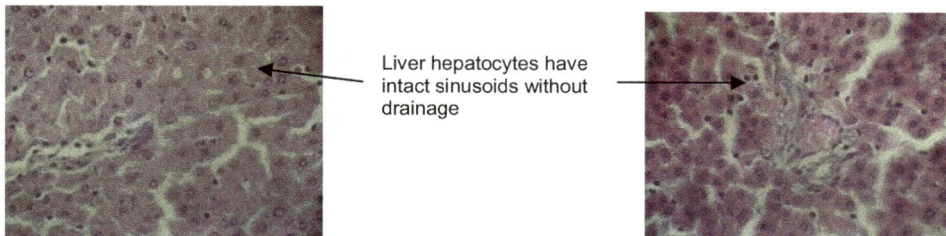

Liver hepatocytes have intact sinusoids without drainage

Plate 3a. Liver of infected rat and treated with white *garri*   Plate 3b. Control

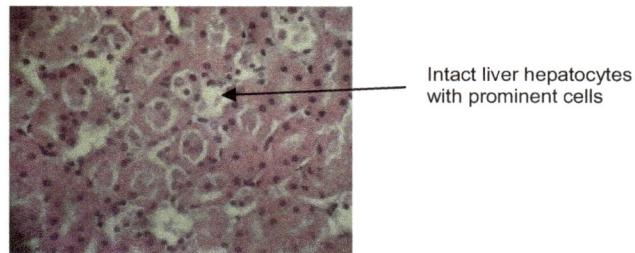

Intact liver hepatocytes with prominent cells

Plate 3c. Liver of infected rat and treated with red *garri*

4. DISCUSSION

From the result obtained in the antibacterial evaluation of the *Euphorbia heterophylla* extract (Table 1) showed that the plant has antibacterial property against S. typhi. According to [22], any substance that is able to exert a zone of inhibition of 6 mm and above has antibacterial activity against such bacteria. The titre values obtained (Table 2) for the WIDAL test carried out on the animals before, during and after infecting as well as after treatment also confirmed that the animals were infected and that the organism caused the infection. Equally, the end result of the titre value of the WIDAL test confirmed the therapeutic efficacy of the *Euphorbia heterophylla* mixture. The histopathological analyses of the organs showed that the treatments caused visible pathological changes of the organs. The kidneys showed mild changes such as wide spread vascular damage, haemorrhage, vasculitis and mild interstitial mononuclear cell infiltration and tubular degeneration. These are probably the damages caused by the organisms according to [23], these signs indicates the infection of *Salmonella typhi*. However, the fact that they are mild indicates the effectiveness of the therapeutic agent being used for treating the infection. The liver sinusoids were found in place and the liver hepatocytes were not spacious as the therapeutic agent contained no detoxicant for the liver to detoxify which means that it is a good therapeutic agent. The heart muscle striata were unaffected and no cardiac puncture as well as heart muscle necrosis. According to [24] any substance introduced into the digestive system or circulatory system that do not exert these effects have therapeutic efficacy. The therapeutic agents therefore contained no deleterious substances that could cause these damages in the organs of the animals. It is conceivable from the results obtained that

Euphorbia heterophylla mixed with yellow and white *garri* can be used in the control of *Salmonella typhi* infections, especially the problems caused in the liver and kidney by the organism. It can be used to treat disruptions in the kidney and liver. The gross result showed that the therapeutic efficacy of these mixtures are outstanding and therefore holds high hope that if adequate purification measures are used and proper harnessing of the therapeutic ingredients are done, it can help in the development of novel antibacterial agents and equally help to combat resistant *Salmonella typhi.*

5. CONCLUSION

The results obtained in this work showed that *Euphorbia heterophylla* mixed with cassava flakes is an effective therapeutic agent for Salmonellosis and that the *Euphorbia heterophylla* with white cassava flakes mixture is more effective in the treatment of salmonellosis.

CONSENT

It is not applicable.

ETHICAL APPROVAL

All authors hereby declare that all experiments have been examined and approved by the appropriate ethics committee and have therefore been performed in accordance with the ethical standards laid down in the 1964 Declaration of Helsinki.

ACKNOWLEDGEMENTS

The authors wish to acknowledge the staff of post graduate Microbiology laboratory, Department of Animal Production and Health Laboratory and Chemistry laboratory of The Federal University of Technology, Akure, Ondo State, Nigeria for their assistance.

COMPETING INTERESTS

Authors have declared that no competing interests exist.

REFERENCES

1.   Wray C, Davies RH. *Enterobacteriaceae.* In Poultry Diseases. 5th edition. EDs F; 2002.
2.   Wales J. A personal appeal from wikipedia foundation, Inc. U.S. 2008;2-7.
3.   World Health Organization (WHO). Salmonellosis Control: The Role of Animal and Product Hygiene, Technical Report Series, 774, WHO, Geneva; 1998.
4.   Egharevba RKA, Ikhatua MI. Ethnomedicinal uses of plants in the treatment of various skin diseases in Ovia North East, Edo State, Nigeria. Nigerian Tribune. 2008;1-4.
5.   Jones WP, Waston RP, Wallis ST. Salmonellosis. Bovine Medicine: Diseases and Husbandry of Cattle. 2nd ed. UK: Blackwell Science. 2004;215-230.
6.   Hohmann EL. Non-typhoidal salmonellosis. Clinical Infectious Diseases. 2001;32:253-269.
7.   Wrebid T. Jordan, Pattison M, Alexander D, Faragherw T, Sanders B. General animal pathology. Living Stone Publisher. 2010;96-109.
8.   Bentancur-Galvis LA, Morales GE, Forero JR. Cytotoxic and antiviral activities of Columbian Medicinal plant extracts of the Euphorbia genus. Mem Inst. Oswaldo Cruz, Riode Janeiro. 2002;97(4):541-546.
9.   Clarke ML, Harvey DG, Humphrey DJ. Veterinary toxicology. 2nd edition. Bailliere Tindall, London. 1991;219.
10. Burkegharevba R. K. ill, H. M. The useful plants of west tropical Africa. Roy. Bot. gard. Ken. 1994;(2):12-15
11. Akobundu I, Okezie A, Agyakwa CW. A handbook of West African Weeds. Second Edition. African Book Builders Ltd. 2 Awosika Avenue, Bodija U.I. P.O. Box 20222 Ibadan. 1998;260-261
12. Brock TD, Madigan TM. Biology of Microorganisms. Fifth edition. Prentice International, Inc. 1988;541-544.
13. Prescott LM, Harley JP, Klein DA. Microbiology. Fifth edition McGraw Hill Publishers, USA. 2002;926-933.
14. Radostits OM, Gay CC, Hinchcliff KW, Vonstable PO. Veterinary medicine, a text book of the disease of cattle, horses, sheep, pigs and goats. 10th ed. London: Saunders Elsevier. 2007;896-921.
15. Al-Burtamani SKS, Fatope MO, Marwah RG, Onifade AK, Al-Said AS. Chemical composition, antibacterial and antifungal activities of the essential oils of tuberculation from Oman. J. Ethnopharm. 96: 107-112Acute toxicity of *Euphorbia heliscopia* in Rats. Pak. J. Nutri. 2005;5(2):135-140.
16. Adedapo AA, Abatan MO, Olorunsogo. Toxic effects of some plant in the genus

Euphorbia on haematological and biochemical parameters of rats. Vdet. Arhic. 2004;74:53-64.

17. Salmonellosis. Topic overview on Salmonellosis; 2012. Available:www.webmd.com/food-recipes/food-poisoning/tc/salmonellosis-topic-overview

18. Upadhyal RR, Zarintan MH, Ansarin M. Isolation of Ingenol from the irritant and cocarcinogenic latex of *Euphorbia seguieriana.* Pl. Med. 1980;30:32-34

19. Morgan HR. Typhoid fever, Microsoft. Student 2007 (DVD) Redmond, W.A. Microsoft Corporation; 2007.

20. Available:http://en.wikipedia.org/wiki/salmonella

21. Walderhand M. Food borne pathogenic microorganisms and natural toxins, handbook U.S. food and drug administration. Centre for Food Safety and Applied Nutrition. 2007;3-5.

22. Trongtokit Y, Rongsriyam Y, Komalamisra N, Apiwathnasorn C. Comparative Repellants of 38 essential oils against mosquito bites. Phytotherapy Research. 2005;19(4):303-9.

23. White DG, Zhao S, Sudler R, Ayers S, Friedman S, Chen S, Mcdermott S, Waner DD, Meng J. The isolation of antibiotic-resistant Salmonella from retail ground meats. New Engl. J. Med. 2001;345(16):1147-1154.

24. Clark MA, Barret EL. The phs gene and hydrogen sulphide production By *Salmonella typhimurium.* J Bacteriology. 1987;169(6):2391-2397.

19

Assessment of Antioxidant and Cytotoxic Activities of Extracts of Some *Ziziphus* Species with Identification of Bioactive Components

Sameera N. Siddiqui[1] and Mandakini B. Patil[1*]

[1]*Department of Biochemistry, Rashtrasant Tukdoji Maharaj Nagpur University, Nagpur-440033, Maharashtra, India.*

Authors' contributions

This work was carried out in collaboration between both the authors. Authors MBP and SNS designed the study, wrote the protocol, performed the statistical analysis and wrote the first draft of the manuscript. Author SNS managed the analysis of the study and the literature searches. Both the authors read and approved the final manuscript.

5/17351
Editor(s):
(1) Marcello Iriti, Faculty of Plant Biology and Pathology, Department of Agricultural and Environmental Sciences, Milan State University, Italy.
Reviewers:
(1) Anonymous, National Research Centre, Egypt.
(2) Mario Bernardo-Filho, Universidade do Estado do Rio de Janeiro, Brazil.
(3) Anonymous, Federal University of Rio de Janeiro, Brazil.

ABSTRACT

Aims: To investigate antioxidant activity of crude extracts and cytotoxic activity of partially purified bioactive compounds of *Ziziphus mauritiana* and *Ziziphus oenoplia* extracts.
Study Design: Experimental study.
Background: Breast and lung cancers are known to cause high morbidity and mortality worldwide. *Ziziphus* plants are wildly grown species known for their folkloric implications with bioactive phytochemicals believed to be responsible for pharmacological activity.
Materials and Methods: Antioxidant action was determined with crude bark extracts and *in vitro* antiproliferation activities were determined by using partially purified fractions obtained from bark extracts of *Z. mauritiana* and *Z. oenoplia* using DPPH and MTT assay, respectively. Possible active ingredients in the potent fractions were identified by Gas Chromatography – Mass Spectrometry (GC-MS).
Results: Considerable antioxidant activity was demonstrated by *Z. mauritiana* methanol extracts

*Corresponding author: E-mail: mbpatil@hotmail.com

(ZMMA); while *Z. mauritiana* alkaloid fraction (ZMA) exhibited highest cytotoxic activity (IC_{50}- 19.35 µg/ml) against human lung carcinoma A549 cells and *Z. oenoplia* alkaloid fraction (ZOA) against human adenocarcinoma mammary gland MDA-MB-231 cells through MTT assay, its further analysis witnessed reduced MMP expression using gelatin zymography. GC-MS technique employed to identify the bioactive compounds of most potent alkaloid fraction ZMA revealed existence of isoquinoline, morphinan, glaucine and pyrazoline compounds.

Conclusion: Our study concludes occurrence of strong antioxidant, antiproliferative and a possible anti-invasive activity to support robust traditional belief in the medicinal properties of *Ziziphus* species.

Keywords: Ziziphus mauritiana; Ziziphus oenoplia; antiproliferative activity; antioxidant activity; anti-invasive activity.

1. INTRODUCTION

Plants contain essential components responsible to cure several ailments, serving as natural source of medicine and play an important role in the development of potent therapeutic agents [1].

The genus *Ziziphus* is one such category known to possess ethnomedicinal properties comprising some important species like *Z. jujuba, Z. mauritiana, Z. spinachristi, Z. lotus, Z. spinosa* etc. *Ziziphus* is a genus that includes about 40 species of spiny shrubs in the buckthorn family as a fruit tree [2]. There are large numbers of traditional benefits of *Ziziphus* plants since ancient times- leaves, fruits, seeds and barks of these plants have been used medicinally. *Z. mauritiana* (ZM) plant parts traditionally used are: kernels - sedative effect, stop nausea, relieves abdominal pain in pregnancy and wounds healing; seeds - for diarrhea and oral contraceptives; leaves - as an astringent, diaphoretic and prescribed for typhoid in children; bark - as an astringent in gingivitis, for the treatment of diarrhoea and dysentery [3,4]. Bark extracts of *ZM* are reported to have antiulcer, spermicidal and antimicrobial properties [5]. According to Ayurveda and traditional knowledge, *Z. oenoplia* (ZO) plant parts are also used to cure diseases: root- wound healing, ulcer, ascaris infection, stomachalgia, gastrointestinal disorder; fruit- stomach ache; root- as an astringent, anthelmintic, digestive and antiseptic property [6].

Normal essential metabolic processes within the cell produce free radicals and other reactive species that can attack important macromolecules leading to cell damage. Natural protective mechanisms against the destructive effect of free radicals are antioxidants, a substance capable to neutralize free radicals or its effects. The term oxidative stress refers to the consequence of imbalance between free radical generation and antioxidant defense. Oxidative stress is assumed to play a crucial role in the aging process and in pathology of age-related diseases. Reactive Oxygen Species (ROS) hampers the normal functioning of a number of biological molecules such as nucleic acids, membrane lipids or enzymes. Hence, plant derived antioxidants might stabilize or neutralize free radicals either by acting as anti-free radical molecules, or by chain-breaking of free radical propagation or by interaction with transition metal ions and show a beneficial role in preventing free radical related diseases [7].

Traditional Chinese Medicine also involves use of *Ziziphus* extract for cancer treatment. The *Ziziphus* extracts have also been reported to possess various therapeutic potential, including cytotoxicity against HCT15, HL-60, Molt-4, Hela and few other cancer cell lines [3,7].

Cancer cells metastasize through the route involving multiple step processes, but the most significant turning point in cancer is the establishment of distant metastasis [8]. Migratory and invasive capabilities help cancer cells invade surrounding tissues and gain direct access into the blood vessels [9]. Motility and invasion of tumor cells into new target tissues results in the formation of a secondary tumor. Degradation of matrix proteins of the basement membrane is essential for the cell to become metastasized. An over-expression of proteolytic enzymes, like zinc-dependent endopeptidases of matrix metalloproteinases (MMPs) family; MMP-2 and MMP-9 (gelatinase A and B) play a crucial role in degrading most extracellular matrix (ECM) components that form the basal membrane [10]. MMP-2 and MMP-9 are associated to tumor invasion and metastasis due to their capacities for tissue remodeling through the extracellular matrix, basement membrane degradation and induction of angiogenesis. Thus, these gelatinases are essential for tumor cell migration, tumor spreading, tissue invasion of tumor cells, and metastasis [11,12]. Hence by monitoring the level of these two proteins in presence of *Ziziphus* fractions could provide a clue for their mechanism of action.

The objective of present study comprises screening for antioxidant activity of different crude extracts and also the investigation for antiproliferative action along with anti-invasive effects shown by active fractions of different extracts of ZM and ZO.

2. MATERIALS AND METHODS

2.1 Reagents and Standards

The MTT salt [3-(4, 5-dimethylthiazol-2-yl)-2, 5-diphenyl-tetrazolium bromide], Dimethylsulphoxide (DMSO), trypan blue, antimycotic antibiotic, all the cultivation media and other additives used for cell culture, also L-ascorbic acid, 1,1-diphenyl-2-picrylhydrazyl (DPPH) were purchased from Himedia (Mumbai, India). All the HPLC grade solvents used were purchased from SRL (Mumbai, India).

2.2 Cell lines and Culture Media

Human adenocarcinoma mammary gland cells MDA-MB-231, human lung carcinoma cells A549 and normal human hepatic cells WRL-68 were purchased from National Centre for Cell Sciences (NCCS), Pune, India. MDA-MB-231 cells were cultured in Leibovitz's L-15 medium with 2 mM L-glutamate (no carbon dioxide), WRL-68 cells were cultured in the same medium as MDA-MB-231 cells (5% carbon dioxide) and A-549 cells were cultured in Ham's F-12 medium with 2 mM L-glutamate (5% carbon dioxide), all supplemented with 10% (v/v) fetal bovine serum (FBS), 100 U/ml penicillin and 100 mg/ml streptomycin.

2.3 Plant Material

Ziziphus mauritiana Lam. and *Ziziphus oenoplia (L)* Mill. Gard. were identified by taxonomist of University Department of Botany, RTM Nagpur University, Nagpur, Maharashtra, India, where a specimen is conserved with the voucher number as RTMNU BD 9138 and 9140, respectively.

2.4 Extract Preparation

Bioactive compounds from the bark of *ZM and ZO* were extracted using ethyl acetate and the extract was designated as ZMEA and ZOEA [13]. Another method followed was initial extraction with ethyl acetate followed by methanol (A) extraction of *ZM* (ZMMA) and *ZO* (ZOMA) using soxhlet apparatus [14]. Isolates were also obtained as brownish crude residue with dichloromethane extract of *ZM* (ZMDCM) and *ZO* (ZODCM). This procedure of extraction was adopted as stated by Perez et al. [15]. Extraction method started with methanol containing ascorbic acid at low temperature [16]. This was followed by ethyl acetate and then with methanol (B) extract of *ZM* (ZMMB) and *ZO* (ZOMB). Last extraction method was performed using a mixture of dioxane-water (96:4, v/v) to isolate aqueous-dioxane extract of *ZM* (ZMAD) and *ZO* (ZOAD) as stated by Ramasamy [17]. All these crude extracts were screened for antioxidant activities.

2.5 Partial Purification

Crude extracts were further processed to isolate specific partially purified compounds. ZMEA and ZOEA extracts were column chromatographed over silica gel (60-120 mesh size) and eluted with benzene:ethyl acetate mixture in 2:1 ratio to obtain *ZM* triterpenoids (ZMT) and *ZO* triterpenoids (ZOT) fractions, as mentioned by Kundu et al. [18]. ZMMA and ZOMA extracts were also passed through silica gel 60-120 mesh size column and eluent of ethyl acetate: methanol (1:3) provided *ZM* flavonoids (ZMF) and *ZO* flavonoids (ZOF) as main fractions during partial purification [14]. Similarly, ZMDCM and ZODCM extracts when subjected to silica gel column chromatography and eluents from CH_2Cl_2-MeOH (1:8) furnished *ZM* alkaloids (ZMA) and *ZO* alkaloids (ZOA) fractions, by the method as mentioned by Perez et al. [15]. In the same way, ZMMB and ZOMB extracts were applied on equilibrated Sephadex LH20 in 80% ethanol and eluted in 50% acetone to get partially purified tannin fractions [16] as *ZM* tannins (ZMTn) and *ZO* tannins (ZOTn). Likewise, ZMAD and ZOAD extracts were further processed in distilled water and then finally in absolute ether to get partially purified fractions of *ZM* lignins (ZML) and *ZO* lignins (ZOL), by the method as stated by Ramasamy [17].

Each extract obtained was phytochemically screened for the determination of constituents using standard methods of analysis [19,20].

2.6 Determination of Antioxidant Activity

2.6.1 DPPH radical scavenging assay

The radical scavenging potential was estimated by DPPH method [21]. When the DPPH solution (1, 1-diphenyl-2-picrylhydrazyl) is mixed with a substance capable of donating a hydrogen atom, it produces a reduced form of compound (diphenylpicrylhydrazine) with loss of violet color. The crude solvent extracts [dicholoromethane (DCM), methanol (M-A), ethyl acetate (EA), methanol (M-B) and aqueous-dioxane (AD)] of both the Ziziphus species were mixed with 1.5 ml freshly prepared DPPH solution (0.05 mM prepared in methanol) at 1, 5 and 10 mg/ml. The change in colour from deep-violet to light-yellow was measured spectrophotometrically at 517 nm after incubation in dark for 30 min at 37°C. DPPH solution was used as negative control and ascorbic acid (250 μM) as reference compound. Tests were carried out in triplicate. The radical scavenging activity was performed to investigate the existence of antioxidant potential of crude Ziziphus bark extracts. By comparing the test results with control (without extract) the DPPH percentage inhibition was calculated by using following formula [21],

$$\text{DPPH radical Scavenging activity} \ \text{or} \ \% \text{ Inhibition} = \left[\frac{A_C - A_S}{A_C} \right] \times 100$$

Where, A_C is the absorbance of DPPH and A_S is the absorbance of extract

2.7 Evaluation of Cell Viability Assay

2.7.1 Cell proliferation assay

Cytotoxic activity of partially purified Ziziphus fractions against WRL-68, MDA-MB-231 and A549 cells was determined by the colorimetric method of MTT reduction [22]. Succinate dehydrogenase present in mitochondria of the cell, reduces tetrazolium salt 3-[4,5-dimethylthiazol-2-yl]-2,5-diphenyltetrazolium bromide (MTT) to insoluble formazan crystals and this activity can be used to estimate functions of viable cells. Five dilutions (10, 25, 50, 75 and 100 μg/ml) of each fraction of both the Ziziphus species were tested against the cancer cell lines for 48 h and analyzed for cell

proliferation by MTT assay. Since reduction of MTT can only occur in metabolically active cells, the level of activity is a direct measure of activity of viable cells [23].

2.7.2 Substrate gel analysis

Gelatinolytic activities for the presence or absence of secreted MMPs were analyzed by gelatin substrate gel electrophoresis or zymography. Using this technique both active and latent species can be visualized. Samples (20 μl) were prepared in 2% (w/v) SDS and 10% (v/v) glycerol. Gelatinase zymography was performed on 10% (w/v) polyacrylamide gel co-polymerised with 0.2% (w/v) gelatin. Following electrophoresis the gels were washed twice in 50 mM Tris-HCl, pH 8.0, containing 5 mM $CaCl_2$, 1 μM $ZnCl_2$ and 2.5% (w/v) Triton X-100 for 15 min to remove SDS, followed by two washes for 5 min each in 50 mM Tris-HCl, pH 8.0, containing 5 mM $CaCl_2$, and incubated overnight in the same buffer at 37°C. The gels were stained for 30 min with Coomassie Brilliant Blue R-250 (0.5%) prepared in a mixture of 50% methanol and 10% glacial acetic acid and destained in 7% acetic acid [24].

2.8 Gas Chromatography – Mass Spectrometry

A Varian 4500 GC coupled with Varian MS240 ion trap mass spectrometer (Varian, Walnut Creek, USA) was employed for the determination of analytes using electron ionization (EI) mode. Aliquotes of 1 μl sample were injected using a split programmable temperature injection (STI) Type 1079 kept at 270°C. The ion trap, manifold and the transfer line were kept at 240, 40 and 250ºC, respectively. Separations were performed on Varian Chrompack Capillary column WCOT Fused Silica (30 m long, 0.25 mm ID) CP-Sil 8CB and helium (Ultra pure 99.99%) was employed as a carrier gas. Compounds were identified by direct comparison of their MS with data from the NIST library.

2.9 Statistical Analysis

The results were expressed as Mean±S.E.M. using GraphPad Prism 5.0 (GraphPad, USA). The differences were determined using one-way ANOVA followed by Dunnett's multiple comparison test. IC_{50} was estimated using non-linear regression method (curve fit) with dose-response inhibition of plots for the percentage of antiproliferation activity against the concentration of tested compounds. Significance level was set at p=0.05.

3. RESULTS AND DISCUSSION

Newman and Cragg [25] reported that more than half of the new chemicals approved by World Health Organization were derived directly or indirectly from natural products. Based on this information, ZM and ZO plants traditionally used for treatments of several diseases were examined for their therapeutic activity and presence of bioactive compounds.

3.1 Antioxidant effects of *Ziziphus* Extracts

3.1.1 DPPH radical scavenging assay

Natural antioxidants from medicinal plants are of increasing interest as they prevent deleterious effects of free radicals in biological system, leading to cure numerous ailments and may replace synthetics by natural ones. Results presented in Table 1 indicate the potential free radical scavenging property of crude extracts in a concentration-dependent manner as evaluated by its ability of trapping the unpaired electrons of DPPH. *Ziziphus* extracts were able to reduce the purple-colored radical DPPH to yellow colored radical DPPH-H at par to the standard ascorbic

acid, expressing stronger reducing power. ZMMA extract showed a high antioxidant activity, with an IC_{50} value of 4.11 ± 0.21 mg/ml compared to Ascorbic acid that produced IC_{50} values of 3.94 ± 0.20 mg/ml, while ZOAD (IC_{50}- 5.20 ± 0.36 mg/ml) exhibited the least activity. However, all the crude extracts exhibited significant antioxidant activity.

Based on previous data, it is shown that the powerful antioxidant activity of polar extracts is due to the presence of substances with free hydroxyls [26]. In this context, flavonoids possess an ideal structure for the scavenging of free radicals, since they present a number of hydroxyls acting as hydrogen-donators which makes them important antioxidant agents [27]. The antioxidant activity of phenolic compounds is mainly due to their redox properties, as key role in neutralizing free radicals, quenching singlet and triplet oxygen species, or decomposing peroxides. Results indicate that ZMMA obtained from *Z. mauritiana* bark holds great capability to donate hydrogen therefore represents effective DPPH scavenging activity. Dahiru and Obidoa [28] have shown flavonoid, tannin and phenolic compounds of *Z. mauritiana* with protective effects against oxidative damage induced by chronic alcohol administration in rats. In addition, strong antioxidant property was also demonstrated *in vitro* by ethanolic bark extract of *Z. mucronata* subsp. *mucronata* [21].

Table 1. Radical scavenging activity of *Z. mauritiana* and *Z. oenoplia* bark extracts

Ziziphus species	Concentration			IC_{50}
	1 mg	5 mg	10 mg	(mg/ml)
Z. mauritiana				
ZMDCM	04.41 ±0.37	29.83 ±0.16	59.17 ±0.34	5.02 ±0.24
ZMM-A	05.70 ±0.18	69.85 ±0.72	74.45 ±0.51	4.11 ±0.21
ZMEA	04.11 ±0.29	30.13 ±0.60	57.58 ±0.36	5.01 ±0.27
ZMM-B	04.54 ±0.53	59.91 ±0.49	67.84 ±0.27	4.69 ±0.22
ZMAD	02.96 ±0.12	06.37 ±0.37	21.29 ±0.54	5.22 ±0.35
Z. oenoplia				
ZODCM	02.99 ±0.50	11.03 ±0.25	38.01 ±0.41	5.17 ±0.34
ZOM-A	04.03 ±0.33	33.42 ±0.51	65.08 ±0.23	5.01 ±0.20
ZOEA	03.98 ±0.18	14.12 ±0.36	43.90 ±0.07	5.15 ±0.37
ZOM-B	03.87 ±0.45	28.53 ±0.21	61.69 ±0.58	5.04 ±0.23
ZOAD	02.87 ±0.28	08.19 ±0.78	29.14 ±0.32	5.21 ±0.36
Ascorbic acid	09.03 ±0.01	84.99 ±0.04	87.95 ±0.03	3.94 ±0.20

Data are presented as Mean ± S.E.M of three replicates. The abbreviations used denote respective species viz., ZM- Z. mauritiana and ZO- Z. oenoplia. Abbreviates also denote the solvents used for extraction viz., DCM- dichloromethane; M-A- methanol; EA- ethyl acetate; M-B- methanol containing ascorbic acid and AD- aqueous-dioxane

3.2 Effect of Active Fractions of *Ziziphus* Extract on Viability of Cultured Cells

3.2.1 MTT assay

Partially purified active fractions of *Ziziphus* bark extracts were analyzed for antiproliferative properties against MDA-MB-231 and A549 cells after checking the effects and concentration of *Ziziphus* fractions on WRL-68 cells. Most potent fractions were investigated for anti-invasive effect to find out their mode of action and further analyzed for the presence of promising bioactive components using GC-MS (Fig. 1).

WRL-68 cells were treated with different concentrations of *Ziziphus* fractions (50, 100, 150, 200 and 250 µg/ml) to study the cytotoxic effects, before analyzing its antiproliferative activity on cancer cells. Data clearly reveals that the partially purified *Ziziphus* fractions are less toxic towards WRL-68 cells even at 250 µg/ml concentration (Fig. 2A).

Results obtained with the active fractions of both the *Ziziphus* species showed significant dose-dependent antiproliferative action on the mentioned cancer cell lines (Fig 2). Several reports in the literature exemplify susceptibility of different tumor cell lines to cytotoxic agents [29]. *ZM* fractions illustrate enhanced antiproliferative activity against A549 cells presenting an order of relative potencies: ZMA > ZMT > ZMF > ZMTn,

while ZML showed no activity (Fig. 2B). Our results are in agreement with literature reporting potent therapeutical effects of *Z. mauritiana* extracts [3,7].

On the contrary, ZO fractions illustrated effectual antiproliferation against MDA-MB-231 cells, as the activity was witnessed in following order: ZOA > ZOT > ZOF > ZOTn, ZOL gave no activity (Fig. 2C). Estimated growth reduction clarifies ZMA (19.35±0.86 µg/ml) and ZOA (25.85±0.47 µg/ml) with highly significant antiproliferation against A549 and MDA-MB-231 cells, respectively (Table 2). A similar previous study had also reported the potent action of extracts of *Z. spina-christi* possessing efficient cytotoxic potency towards Hela and MDA-MB-468 cells [29].

3.3 Identification of Active ZMA Fraction by GC-MS analysis

Most potent bioactive fraction was subjected to compound identification by GC-MS. Based on the mass spectrum comparison with NIST library, ZMA demonstrated the existence of four possible compounds (Fig. 3) as Isoquinolin-6-ol, 7-methoxy-1-methyl- (**1**), Morphinan, 7,8-didehydro-4,5-epoxy-3,6 dimethoxy-17- methyl-, (5α,6α)- (**2**), Glaucine (**3**), 2-Pyrazoline, 5-(1,1-dimethylethyl)-5-hydroxy-3-trifluoromethyl-1-(2-isopropyl-5-methylphenoxyacetyl)- (**4**).

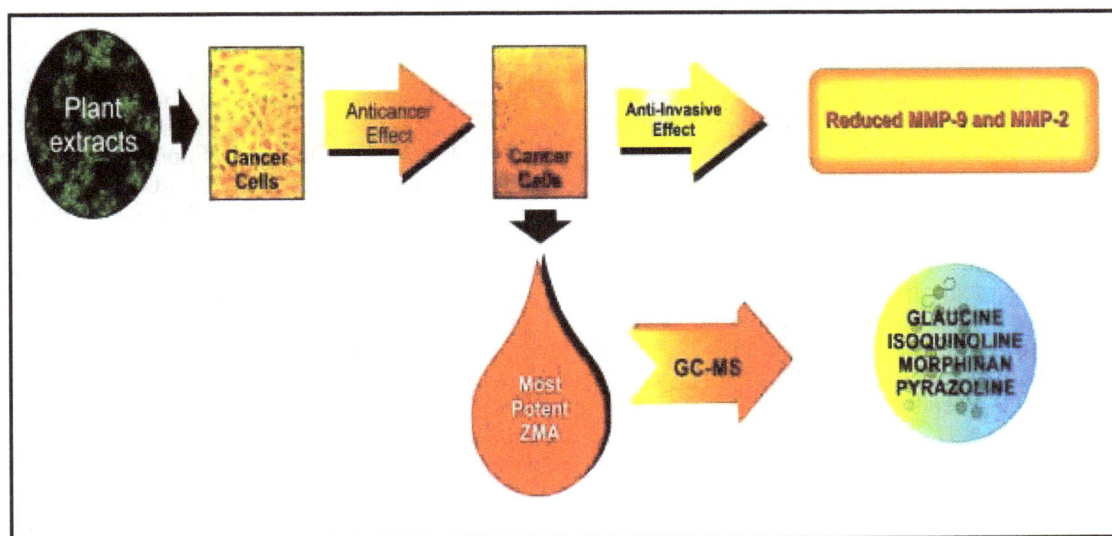

Fig. 1. Schematic representation for the effect of most potent partially purified alkaloid fraction of *Z. mauritiana* (ZMA) bark on A549 cancer cell lines

ZMA - Z. mauritiana alkaloid fraction; MMP – matrixmetallo proteinase; GC-MS – Gas Chromatography – Mass Spectrometry

Table 2. Potent fractions of *Z. mauritiana* and *Z. oenoplia* with IC$_{50}$ values against A549, MDA-MB-231 cancer cell lines and WRL-68 normal cells

Cell lines	*Ziziphus* active fractions	IC$_{50}$ (µg/ml)
A549	ZMA	19.35±0.86
	ZMT	29.96±0.75
	ZMF	34.22±1.91
MDA-MB-231	ZOA	25.85±0.47
	ZOT	37.37±0.16
	ZOF	65.56±0.55
WRL-68	ZMA	73.95±0.93
	ZMT	58.03±1.41
	ZMF	64.31±1.06

IC$_{50}$ is concentration that reduces cell viability of cancer cell lines to 50%
The data is expressed as Mean±S.E.M from the three triplicate experiments. Range of concentrations: A549 and MDA-MB-231 cancer cells (10, 25, 50, 75, 100 µg/ml), WRL-68 cells (50, 100, 150, 200, 250 µg/ml)

Table 3 and Fig. 3 show the chromatogram and chromatographic data. Peak in the respective spectrum at 184 m/z (100%), 146 m/z (65%), 174 m/z (13%), 147 m/z (10%) seems to be isoquinolin-6-ol 7-methoxy-1-methyl- **(1)**. Another peak at 313 m/z (100%), 59 m/z (40%), 229m/z (26%), 282 m/z (21%) corresponds to morphinan,7,8-didehydro-4,5-epoxy-3,6 dimethoxy-17-methyl-, (5α,6α)- **(2)** and the peak 355 m/z (100% relative intensity), 340 m/z (45%), 354 m/z (15%), 297 m/z (10%) was consistent with the occurrence of glaucine **(3)**. Peak at 149 m/z (100%), 400 m/z (20%), 57 m/z (20%) seems to be 2-pyrazoline, 5-(1,1-dimethylethyl)-5-hydroxy-3-trifluoromethyl-1-(2-isopropyl-5-methylphenoxyacetyl)-**(4)**.

Potent antioxidant ZMMA extract was also subjected to identification of possible compounds by GC-MS. Results showed presence of known bioactive compounds like stigmasterol, carotene, flavonoids like kaempferol and luteolin with few other compound derivatives already reported to possess several therapeutic properties including antimicrobial effects [30].

The GC-MS chromatogram analysis of the most effective fraction had revealed 4 compounds (Fig. 3). Isoquinoloine, morphinan, glaucine and pyrazoline compounds identified through GC-MS analysis of ZMA fraction are already reported with pharmacological activity. Some details about these compounds also mention certain

drawbacks such as, glaucine used as antitussive agent, also with anticonvulsant and antinociceptive properties, acts by blocking calcium channels in smooth muscles like human bronchus but with symptoms of nausea, vomiting and dilated pupils [31]. Morphine and some derivatives employed as an opioid analgesic drug to treat acute and chronic pain, however concerns with a prognostic that constipation, addiction, tolerance and hormone imbalance are other multiple actions causing side effects [32,33]. On the contrary isoquinoline alkaloids like berberine along with traditional usage have been experimented to show anti-inflammatory, antidepressant, neuroprotector, antineoplastic effects and also beneficial effects on HIV, diabetes mellitus and cardiovascular system [34,35]. Pyrazoline derivatives have been reported by Sharma [36] quoting references with anti-inflammatory, analgesic, antimicrobial, antifungal, antidepressant and also anticancer activity. Synergistic activity of these compounds conquering the described side effects cannot be overlooked. This forms a matter of further investigation.

3.4 Effect of Potent *Ziziphus* Fractions on MMP-2 and MMP-9 Level of Cultured Cells

3.4.1 Substrate gel analysis

Cancer cells proliferate in defiance of normal control, but can invade and colonize surrounding tissues giving rise to secondary tumors called metastasis [37]. Invasion and metastasis is dependent on degradation of the extracellular matrix (ECM), by proteases, particularly MMP-2 (gelatinase A; 72 kDa type IV collagenase) and MMP-9 (gelatinase B; 92 kDa type IV collagenase) expressions [24]. Any agent or drug which can interfere with any of these steps can significantly reduce the metastatic potential and can be useful in inhibition of tumor metastasis. To investigate the mechanism of cell death induced by *Ziziphus* fractions in cancer cell lines, zymography analysis was performed to confirm the expression of MMPs as a marker to assess anti-invasive action. The ZMA and ZOA fractions of *Ziziphus* species showing high cytotoxic potential were investigated for anti-invasive activity to diagnose the mode of action by gelatin zymogram analysis. In our study, treatment of A549 and MDA-MB-231cells with ZMA and ZOA fractions, respectively, were found to reduce the expression of MMP-9 and MMP-2, while ZMF demonstrated negligible difference in the level of MMPs. Reduction of band intensity and sizes of MMP-9 and MMP-2 compared to the control was observed after developing the gelatin zymograms (Fig. 2D). Previously, we have reported the *in vitro* anticancer activities of *ZM*

bark fractions with apoptotic effects on MDA-MB-231 and A549 cells [38]. Thus, the alkaloids of *ZM* and *ZO* reflect persuasive antiproliferation and anti-invasive effect with their respective cell lines.

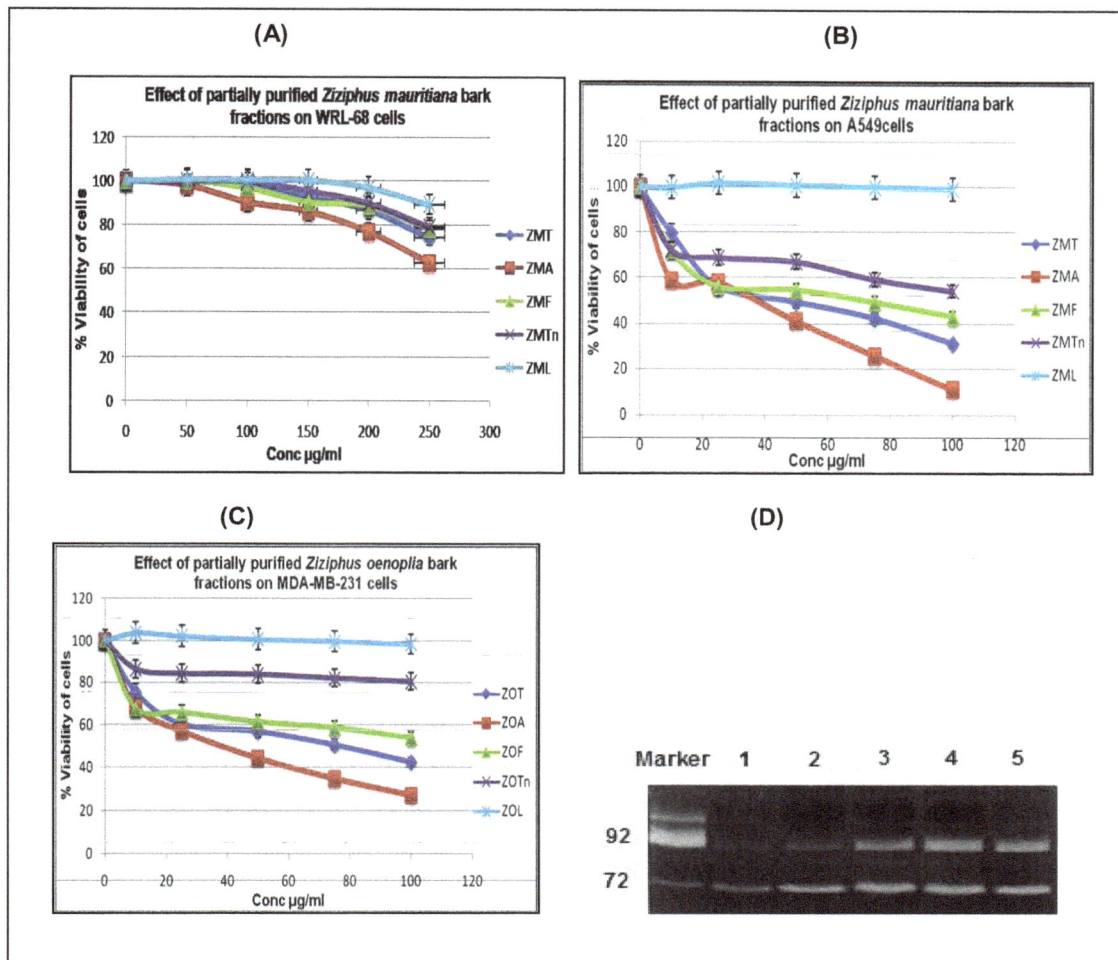

Fig. 2. Proliferation inhibition evaluated for *invitro* cytotoxicity. Effect of: (A) *Z. mauritiana* fractions on WRL-68 cells, (B) *Z. mauritiana* fractions on A549 cells, (C) *Z. oenoplia* fractions on MDA-MB-231 cells. The results are expressed as percent viability of cells determined relative to untreated control cells, values represent *Mean±S.E.M*. (D) Gelatin zymogram analysis for matrix metalloproteinase expression in A549 and MDA-MB-231 cells after respective ZMA and ZOA treatment, showing decrease in the level of MMP-9 (92 KDa) and to a certain extent of MMP-2 (72 KDa) also. The gel shows: Marker; Effect of (1) ZMA on A549 cells; (2) ZOA on MDA-MB-231 cells; (3) ZMT on A 549 cells; (4) Control of A549 cells and (5) Control of MDA-MB-231 cells

Ziziphus mauritiana (ZM), Ziziphus oenoplia (ZO): T- triterpenoids, A- alkaloids, F- flavonoids, Tn- tannins and L- lignins

i) GC-MS Chromatogram of ZMA

ii) Isoquinolin-6-ol, 7-methoxy-1-methyl-

iii) Morphinan, 7,8-didehydro-4,5-epoxy-3,6 dimethoxy-17-methyl-, (5α,6α)-

iv) Glaucine

v) 2-Pyrazoline, 5-(1,1-dimethylethyl)-5-hydroxy-3-trifluoromethyl-1-(2-isopropyl-5-methylphenoxyacetyl)-

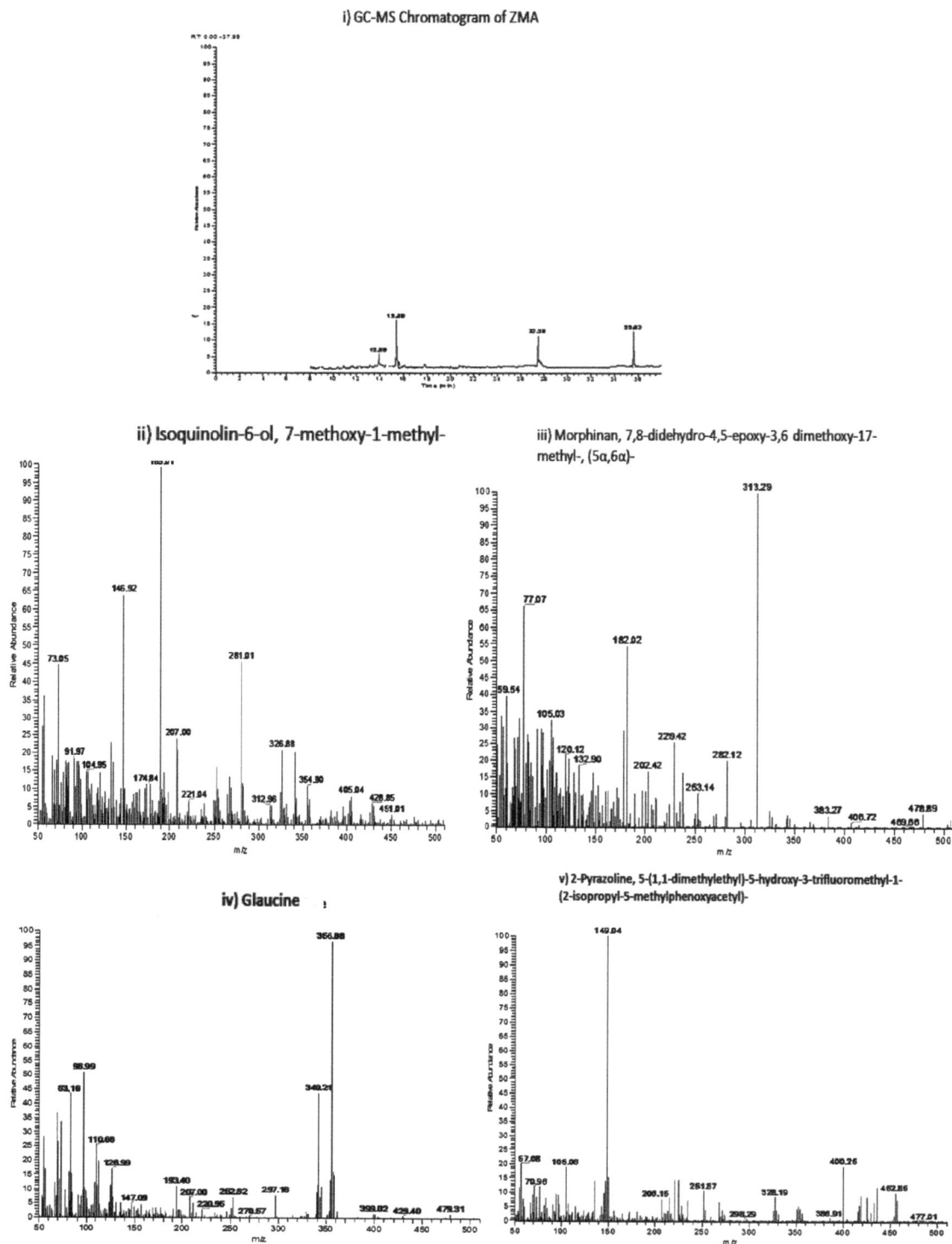

Fig. 3. Gas chromatography – mass spectrometry performed with the most active alkaloid fraction from the bark of *Ziziphus mauritiana*. The compounds identified are shown with its mass spectrum (MS) as isoquinoline, morphinan, glaucine and pyrazoline

Table 3. Identification of chemical constituents of the most effective ZMA fraction by gas chromatography-mass spectrometry (GC-MS)

Compound name	Molecular formula	Molecular weight	Rt (min)	EI-MS m/z (%)	Structure
Isoquinolin-6-ol, 7-methoxy-1-methyl-	$C_{11}H_{11}NO_2$	189	15.40	184(100), 146(65), 174(13), 147(10)	
Morphinan, 7,8-didehydro-4,5-epoxy-3,6 dimethoxy-17-methyl-, (5α,6α)-	$C_{19}H_{23}NO_3$	313	27.39	313 (100), 59(40), 282(21), 229(26)	
Glaucine	$C_{21}H_{25}NO_4$	355	13.90	355 (100), 340 (45), 354(15), 297 (10)	
2-Pyrazoline, 5-(1,1-dimethylethyl)-5-hydroxy-3-trifluoromethyl-1-(2-isopropyl-5-methylphenoxyacetyl)-	$C_{20}H_{27}F_3N_2O_3$	400	35.62	149 (100), 400(20), 57(20), 105(20)	

Rt= Retention time; EI-MS= Electronic Impact-Mass Spectrometry

4. CONCLUSION

In conclusion, the present study highlights the antioxidant and antiproliferative potential of bark extracts of *ZM* and *ZO*. Our results provide promising baseline information for its traditional medicinal property and possibility of *Ziziphus* extracts as a potent agent for development of natural antioxidant and anticancer agents. Purification of active ingredients, their identification and pharmacological, synergistic and toxic activities, if any, certainly needs further investigation.

CONSENT

It is not applicable.

ETHICAL APPROVAL

Present study requires no ethical approval, as it does not deal with any kind of risk. Cancer cell lines usage has already established international ethical considerations.

ACKNOWLEDGEMENTS

Authors thank UGC, New Delhi for financial assistance and Head of the Department of Biochemistry for laboratory facilities and encouragement. Authors are grateful to Dr. Anshuman Khardenavis and Dr. Kashyap from National Environmental Engineering Research Institute, Nagpur, for GC-MS analysis of samples, also to Dr Dhananjay Raje for guidance and statistical analysis of data.

COMPETING INTERESTS

Authors have declared that no competing interests exist.

REFERENCES

1. Feng Y, Wang N, Zhu M, Feng Y, Li H, Tsao S. Recent progress on anticancer candidates in patents of herbal medicinal products. Recent Pat Food Nutr Agric. 2011;3:30-48.

2. Washid K, Argal A. Chromatographic screening of the ethanolic extracts of *Zizyphus xylopyrus* (Retz.) Willd. International Journal of Pharmacy and Life Sciences. 2011;2:625-628.

3. Goyal M, Nagori BP, Sasmal D. Review on ethnomedicinal uses, pharmacological

activity and phytochemical constituents of *Ziziphus mauritiana* (*Z. jujuba* Lam., non Mill). Spatula DD. 2012;2:107-116.

4. Chebouat E, Dadamoussa B, Kabouche A, Allaoui M, Gouamid M, cheriti A, Gherraf N. Gas chromatography-mass spectrometry (GC-MS) analysis of the crude alkaloid extract of *Ziziphus mauritiana* Lam., grown in Algerian. Journal of Medicinal Plants Research. 2013;7:1511-1514.

5. Upadhyay S, Upadhyay P, Ghosh AK, Singh V. *Ziziphus mauritiana*: A review on pharmacological potential of this underutilized plant. Int J Curr Res Rev. 2012;4:141-144.

6. Majumder P. *In vitro* anthelmintic activity of *Zyziphus oenoplia* (L.) Mill root extracts – a promising ethnomedicinal plant. International Journal of Research and Reviews in Pharmacy and Applied Sciences. 2011;1:334-340.

7. Perumal S, Mahmud R, Piaru SP, Cai LW, Ramanathan S. Potential antiradical activity and cytotoxic assessment of *Z. mauritiana* and *Syzygium polyanthum*. International Journal of Pharmacology. 2012;8:535-541.

8. Patel LR, Camacho DF, Shiozawa Y, Pienta KJ, Taichman RS. Mechanisms of cancer cell metastasis to the bone: A multistep process. Future Oncol. 2011;7:1285-1297.

9. American Cancer Society. Cancer facts and figures for African Americans 2013-2014. Atlanta: American Cancer Society. 2013.

10. Halder SK, Osteen KG, Al-Hendy A. Vitamin D3 inhibits expression and activities of matrix metalloproteinase-2 and -9 in human uterine fibroid cells. Hum Reprod. 2013;28:2407-2416.

11. Sun Y, Lu N, Ling Y, Gao Y, Chen Y, Wang L, Hu R, Qi Q, Liu W, Yang Y, You Q, Guo Q. Oroxylin A suppress invasion through down-regulating the expression of matrix metallic proteinase-2/9 in MDA-MB-435 human breast cancer cells. Eur J Pharmacol. 2009;603:22-28.

12. Carlo AD. Evaluation of neutrophil gelatinase-associated lipocalin (NGAL), matrix metalloproteinase-9 (MMP-9) and their complex MMP-9/NGAL in sera and urine of patients with kidney tumors. Oncol Lett. 2013;5:1677-1681.

13. Cordeiro PJM, Vilegas JHY, Lancas FM. HRGC-MS analysis of terpenoids from *Maytenus ilicifolia* and *Maytenus aquifolium* ("Espinheira Santa"). J Braz Chem Soc. 1999;10:523-526.

14. Uddin K, Sayeed A, Islam A, Rahman AA, Ali A, Khan GRMAM, Sadik MG. Purification, characterization and cytotoxic activity of two flavonoids from *Oroxylumindicum* Vent. (Bignoniaceae). Asian J Plant Sci. 2003;2:515-518.

15. Perez E, Saez J, Blair S, Franck X, Figadere B. Isoquinoline alkaloids from *Duguetia vallicola* stem bark with antiplasmodial activity. Lett Org Chem. 2004;1:102-104.

16. Hagerman AE. Tannin Handbook. Miami University, Oxford OH 45056. 2002;78. Available:www.users.muohio.edu/hagermae/

17. Ramasamy K. Ligninase and its Biotechnological applications, Bangalore, India. 1982;170-175.

18. Kundu AB, Barik BR, Mondal DN, Dey AK, Banerji A. Zizyberanalic acid, a pentacyclic triterpenoid of *Zizyphus jujube*. Phytochemistry. 1989;28:3155-3158.

19. Harborne JB. Phytochemical Methods. A guide to modern techniques of plant analysis. 1st Edn., Chapman and Hall, London; 1973. ISBN: 0412572605.

20. Trease GE, Evans WC. Pharmacognosy. 11th Edn. Brailliar Tiridel and Macmillian Publishers, London; 1978.

21. Olajuyigbe OO, Afolayan AJ. Phenolic content and antioxidant property of the bark extracts of *Ziziphus mucronata* Willd. subsp. *Mucronata* Willd. BMC Complement Altern Med. 2011;11:130-137.

22. Liu WK, Ho JCK, Cheung FWK, Liu BPL, Ye WC, Che CT. Apoptotic activity of betulinic acid derivatives on murine melanoma B16 cell line. Eur J Pharmacol. 2004;498:71-78.

23. Yin L-M, Wei Y, Wang Y, Xu Y-D, Yang Y-Q. Long term and standard incubations of WST-1 reagent reflect the same inhibitory trend of cell viability in rat airway smooth muscle cells. Int J Med Sci. 2013;10:68-72.

24. Roomi MW, Monterrey JC, Kalinovsky T, Rath M, Niedzwiecki A. *In vitro* modulation of MMP-2 and MMP-9 in human cervical and ovarian cancer cell lines by cytokines, inducers and inhibitors. Oncol Rep. 2010;23:605-614.

25. Newman DJ, Cragg GM. Natural products as sources of new drugs over the 30 years from 1981 to 2010. J Nat Prod. 2012;75:311–335.

26. Mensor LL, Menezes FS, Leitão GG, Reis AS, Santos TC, Coube CS. Screening of Brazilian plant extracts for antioxidant activity by the use of DPPH free radical method. Phytother Res. 2001;15:27-30.

27. Choudhary RK, Saroha AE, Swarnkar PL. Radical scavenging activity of phenolics and flavonoids in some medicinal plants of India. Journal of Pharmacy Research. 2011;4:712-713.

28. Dahiru D, Obidoa O. Evaluation of the antioxidant effects of Ziziphus mauritiana Lam. leaf extracts against chronic ethanol-induced hepatotoxicity in rat liver. Afr J Tradit Complement Altern Med. 2008;5(1):39–45.

29. Jafarian A, Zolfaghari B, Shirani K. Cytotoxicity of different extracts of aerial parts of Ziziphus spina-christi on Hela and MDA-MB-468 tumor cells. Adv Biomed Res. 2014;3:38-42.

30. Sameera NS, Mandakini BP. Investigations into the antibacterial activity of Ziziphus mauritiana Lam. and Ziziphus xylopyra (Retz.) Willd. International Food and Research Journal. 2015;22(2). (In press).

31. Ujváry I. Psychoactive natural products: Overview of recent developments Ann Ist Super Sanita. 2014;50(1):12-27.

32. The American Society of Health-System Pharmacists. Morphine Sulfate. Retrieved 3 February 2015.

33. Brennan MJ. The effect of opioid therapy on endocrine function. Am J Med. 2013;126(3 Suppl 1):S12–8.

34. Gu J, Gui Y, Chen L, Yuan G, Lu H-Z. Use of natural products as chemical library\for drug discovery and network pharmacology. PLoS ONE. 2013;8(4):e62839. DOI:10.1371/journal.pone.0062839.

35. Zha W, Liang G, Xiao J, Studer EJ, Hylemon PB, Pandak WM, Wang G, Li X, Zhou H. Berberine inhibits HIV protease inhibitor-induced inflammatory response by modulating ER stress signaling pathways in murine macrophages. PLoS ONE. 2010;5(2):e9069.

36. Sharma V. Synthesis and biological evaluation of indolizinyl pyrazoline derivatives for anti-inflammatory and analgesic activity. Dissertation report, Krupanidhi college of Pharmacy, Rajiv Gandhi University of Health Sciences, Bangalore, Karnataka. 2009.

37. Yang J, Lin C, Hsin C, Hsieh, M. Chang Y. Selaginella tamariscina attenuates metastasis via Akt pathways in oral cancer cells. PLoS One. 2013;8:e68035.

38. Patil MB, Siddiqui SN. In vitro evaluation of antiproliferative effect and apoptotic induction on tumor cell lines by Ziziphus mauritiana Lam. International Journal of Applied Biotechnology and Biochemistry. 2011;1(4):439-448.

20

Evaluation of *In-vivo* and *In-vitro* Antioxidant Activities of Methanol Extract of *Salacia lehmbachii* Loes Leaf

Winifred N. Okechi[1], Babatunde A. S. Lawal[1*], Nnabugwu P. Wokota[1] and Jibril Hassan[1]

[1]*Department of Pharmacology, University of Calabar, P.M.B. 1115, Calabar, Cross River State, Nigeria.*

Authors' contributions

This work was carried out in collaboration between all authors. Author BASL designed the study and supervised the work, author WNO performed the experiments and wrote the first draft of the manuscript, authors NPW and JH did extensive literature review and performed the statistical analysis. All authors read and approved the final manuscript.

Editor(s):
(1) Marcello Iriti, Faculty of Plant Biology and Pathology, Department of Agricultural and Environmental Sciences, Milan State University, Italy.
Reviewers:
(1) Anonymous, Kasdi Merbah University, Algeria.
(2) Rafeeq Alam Khan, University of Karachi, Pakistan.

ABSTRACT

Aims: This study was carried out to evaluate the *in-vitro* and *in-vivo* antioxidant activities of methanol extract of *Salacia lehmbachii* leaf (SLLE).
Place and Duration of Study: Department of Pharmacology, University of Calabar, NIGERIA, between October, 2014 and December, 2014.
Methodology: Ability to scavenge 2,2–diphenylpicryl hydrazyl (DPPH) radicals as well as chelate divalent ferrous ions served as paradigms for *in-vitro* methods. On the other hand, cross-clamping of both hepatic artery and hepatic portal veins for 60 min and reperfusion for the next 60 min in rats produces oxidative stress with consequent lipid peroxidation against which the activity of the extract was tested.
Results: SLLE showed considerable potency *in-vitro* in the brine shrimp assay with an IC_{50} of 4.66 µg/ml. At very low concentrations (<10 µg/ml), *SLLE* showed superior activity over that of Vitamin C

Corresponding author: E-mail: syncronig@yahoo.co.uk

in the DPPH assay with IC_{50} of 4.9 µg/ml and 9.6 µg/ml for SLLE and Vit C respectively. At higher concentrations (10-1000 µg/ml), the antioxidant activity was found to be very weak indeed. The FIC assay showed a dose-dependent and significant ($P<.01$) response for both the SLLE (2.199±19.29) and the standard ethylenediaminetetraacetic acid (EDTA) (81.94±5.022); while EDTA showed ability to prevent Fenton-type reaction, SLLE showed a lack of this ability and even a possible enhancement of Fenton-type reactivity. When given at a dose of 100 mg/kg, SLLE also produced significant ($P<.05$) protective activity against hepatic lipid peroxidation in ischaemic / reperfussion injury in rats.

Conclusion: The antioxidant activity of the extract was found to be superior to that of Vit C at low concentrations in the DPPH while not so remarkable at higher concentration and FIC ability. Significant activity in lowering MDA in ischemic-reperfusion model in rats seen at the highest dose (100 mg/kg) ($P<.05$) demonstrated its tissue protective potential.

Keywords: Salacia lehmbachii; antioxidant; DPPH scavenging; ferrous ion chelation; malondialdehyde; methanol extract.

1. INTRODUCTION

The enhanced understanding and the current state-of-the-art in free radicals biology and reactive oxygen species (ROS) has resulted in better management of diseases related to age [1] and degenerative conditions such as cancer, cataracts, cardiovascular diseases, immune system decline and brain dysfunction [2]. Free radicals have been implicated as major contributors to these and various other pathological conditions [2]. Agents that exhibit antioxidant characteristics are therefore capable of potential benefit in these conditions and such antioxidants may exert their effect on biological systems by different mechanisms including, but not limited to, electron donation, metal ion chelation, co-antioxidants, or by gene expression regulation [3].

Plants of the *salacia* genus have been reported to possess antioxidant properties- particularly those that have been used traditionally for the management of diabetes mellitus such as *S. Oblonga* [4]. Other known species of this genus that have shown remarkable antioxidant effect are *S. reticulata*, and *S. chinensis* [5].

Salacia lehmbachii Loes belongs to the plant family Celestraceae and is a plant of west tropical African origin which is also found in the southern part of Nigeria such as Akwa Ibom State and in the Oban hills of Cross River State of Nigeria as well as in Cameroon and the south west province of Bakassi forest reserve. The plant belongs to the Family Celastraceae although little is known about its full biological profile, its use in the treatment of malaria infection locally and other possible biological effects of both the leaf and root bark are currently under investigation.

Because there is no documented report of scientific studies on *S. lehmbachii* regarding the antioxidant activity of the leaves, this study was therefore aimed at investigating the potential antioxidant characteristics of the leaves of this plant by evaluating its ability to modulate the effect of oxidative stress both *in-vivo* and *in-vitro*.

2. MATERIALS AND METHODS

2.1 Chemicals and Reagents

2,2–diphenylpicryl hydrazyl (DPPH), Vitamin C (Vit C), ferrous sulphate ($FeSO_4$), 1,10-phenanthroline, ethylenediaminetetraacetic acid (EDTA), 2,4-diphenylhydrazine, thiobarbituric acid (TBA), and sodium dodecyl sulphate (SDS) were sourced from Sigma Chemical Company Inc., St. Louis, MO, USA. n-hexane, chloroform, methanol, and acetic acid were all of analytical grade and purchased from a reputable chemical store in Calabar, Nigeria.

2.2 Plant Materials

The leaves of *S. lehmbachii* were obtained from the forest region in Akwa Ibom State of Nigeria. The plant material was harvested in the morning and processed for extraction within 24 hours of harvesting. The plant was identified by Mr Abe Noa in Cameroon National Herbarium (CNH), Yaounde, with Voucher No. 40730/SRF/CAM.

2.3 Animals

A total of 24 healthy Sprague-Dawley albino rats of both sexes with an average weight of 100-150 g were used in the study. They were sourced from the animal house, Department of Pharmacology, University of Calabar, Cross River State. The animals were maintained under laboratory condition for two weeks in order to acclimatize.

2.4 Extraction Procedure

The leaves of *S. lehmbachii* were air-dried at room temperature for 2 days, oven-dried at 40°C to dryness and ground to uniform powder using a grinding machine. 50 g of the finely ground powder was soaked with 500 ml of n-Hexane and left for 24 hours after which the solution was filtered through a Whatmann filter paper No 42 (125 mm). The marc from the preceding was further soaked in chloroform for 24 hours, filtered, and soaked finally in methanol for 24 hours and filtered. All the above filtrates were evaporated to dryness in a laboratory oven at 40°C [6] to obtain the n-hexane, chloroform and methanol extracts respectively.

2.5 Brine Shrimp Toxicity Testing

The toxicity potential of the methanolic leaf extracts of *S. lehmbachii* (SLLE) was evaluated using the brine shrimp assay procedure according to Meyer et al. [7]. In brief, the brine shrimp (*Artemia salina*) eggs were hatched in artificial sea water (9.5 g NaCl in 250 ml of distilled water). After 24 hours, the hatched nauplii (brine shrimp larvae) were allowed to stand for 1 hour. The extract was dissolved in the saline solution to varying concentrations vis 0, 5, 10, 20, 40, 50, 60, 80, and 100 µg/ml. Sea water without extract was used as the negative control. Fifteen (15) nauplii were withdrawn through glass capillary and placed in each vial containing 4.5ml of brine solution. A volume of 0.5 ml of the plant extract was added to 4.5 ml of the brine solution and maintained at room temperature for 24 hours under light. The dead larvae were counted after 24 hours and percent mortality for each level of exposure was calculated as follows:

$$\% \, Mortality = \frac{No \, of \, dead \, brine \, shrimps}{Total \, no \, of \, brine \, shrimps} x \, 100$$

Equation 1

The mortality data was fitted to a nonlinear equation of the inverse exponent type from which the LC_{50} was determined. The equation employed is as follows:

$$Y = A * (1\text{-}Exp(\text{-}C*X)) + B$$

Equation 2

2.6 *In-vitro* Antioxidant Assay

The plant extract was analyzed for its free radical scavenging activity using two different methods; the DPPH method of Brand-Williams et al. [8] and modified by Sanchez-Moreno et al. [9] and the ferrous-ion chelating method [10] with modifications.

2.6.1 DPPH free radical scavenging activity

Low concentrations (2 µg/ml-10 µg/ml) as well as high concentrations (12.5 µg/ml-1000 µg/ml) of SLLE and Vit C were prepared for the study. Fresh solution of DPPH (152 µM) was prepared, wrapped in aluminum foil and kept in the dark to prevent autoxidation. To 1 ml each of the SLLE and Vit C solutions was added 1 ml of the DPPH solution, the mixture was shaken vigorously and allowed to stand in the dark for 1 hour and subsequently its absorbance was measured spectrophotometrically at 517 nm. A blank solution containing only the solvent methanol without the SLLE or Vit C was subjected to the same DPPH treatment. All determinations were performed in triplicate and the radical scavenging activities of the test and standard samples expressed as percentage of inhibition were calculated according to the following equation;

$$\% \, Inhibition \, of \, DPPH \, Activity = \frac{[A_b - A_a]}{A_b} x \, 100$$

Equation 3

Where; A_b-absorbance of the blank (solution without the extract or standard); A_a-absorbance of the SLLE or Vit C solution.

2.6.2 Ferrous-ion chelating assay

Concentrations (50 µg/ml, 100 µg/ml, 150 µg/ml, 200 µg/ml) of SLLE and EDTA were prepared for the study. To 1 ml each of these solutions, 3.5 ml of methanol, 0.1 ml of $FeSO_4$ (2 mM) solution and 0.2 ml of 1, 10 phenanthroline (5mM) were added sequentially. The resulting mixtures were allowed to incubate for 10 min at room temperature and the absorbance was read at 562 nm using a spectrophotometer (SpectroVis Plus, Vernier International, 5026 Calle Minorga, Sarasota, FL.,34242 U.S.A). A blank solution containing the test samples without the phenanthroline reagent was subjected to the treatments with the same reagents as above. All determinations were performed in triplicate and the percentage ferrous ion chelating ability was calculated using the following formula:

$$\% \, Ferrous \, ion - chelating \, Activity = [1 - (Ab_s/Ab_c)] \, x \, 100$$

Equation 4

Where Ab_s = Absorbance value of the test sample. Ab_c = Absorbance value of the control.

2.7 Effects of SLLE on Malondialdehyde Levels in Hepatic Ischaemic / Reperfusion Injury in Rats

Twenty four albino rats were randomly allocated to four groups of six rats each as follows: Group I, control (0.5 ml/kg) Phosphate buffered saline {PBS}); Group II, Vit C (100 mg/kg); Group III, SLLE (50 mg/kg); Group IV, SLLE (100 mg/kg). Treatments were administered to the animals daily for 10 days and on the 10th day they were fasted for 12 hrs and anesthetized intraperitoneally with 20% w/v urethane (0.6 ml/100 g). Following anesthesia, warm ischemic injury was induced in their livers by cross clamping the portal vein and hepatic artery for 60 minutes, followed by reperfusion/reflow for another 60 minutes. The liver tissues were rapidly excised and rinsed in ice cold saline.

A 10% w/v homogenate of the liver was prepared using PBS and to 0.1 ml of the homogenate, 1.0 M acetic acid-sodium acetate buffer, pH 4.0 and 1.5 ml of TBA reagent (0.5 g of TBA and 0.3 g of SDS in 100 ml PBS) were added sequentially. The tube was capped in a glass bead and the mixture was heated for 15 min in a boiling water bath, cooled in ice water and 1ml of glacial acetic acid followed by 2 ml of chloroform were added. The mixture was shaken and centrifuged. The optical density of the supernatant was determined at 532 nm using a 1 cm cuvette. The final volume was ca. 4.2 ml, while a reagent blank was run simultaneously. The concentration of the malondialdehyde (MDA) was computed using the molar extinction coefficient was 1.56 x 10^5 in the following equation:

C = A/[e x b]   Equation 5

Where e = molar extinction co-efficient (1.56×10^5 $m^{-1}cm^{-1}$); b = pathway (width of the cuvette, 1 cm); c = concentration of the MDA in the sample and A = Absorbance of the sample read from the spectrophotometer.

2.8 Statistical Analysis

Data obtained from the experiments were analyzed by ANOVA using Statistical Package for Social Sciences (SPSS) software for windows and post-hoc testing was performed for inter-group comparison using Tukey's multiple comparison. Where applicable students t-test was used to compare significant differences between treated and control groups at discreet dose levels. All data were expressed as mean±standard error of mean (SEM). The values of $P<.05$ were considered significant.

3. RESULTS

3.1 Brine Shrimp Toxicity Assay

Lethality of the SLLE was determined by fitting a nonlinear regression curve to the mortality data obtained from the assay as shown in Fig. 1. The parameter values calculated for the inverse exponent equation were 69.99, 25.92 and 0.091 for parameters A, B and C respectively from Equation 2 above. The LC_{50} was then calculated to be 4.66 µg/ml.

3.2 Dpph Stable Radical Scavenging Activity of SLLE

The stable radical inhibitory activities of SLLE and Vit C are presented below (Fig. 2). At low concentrations (<10 µg/mL), The mean percentage inhibition of the SLLE (39±8.8) when compared to that of Vit C. (22±7.3) was found not to be significant after ANOVA. When t-test was carried out across all concentrations below 10 microgram/mL however, some significant difference was seen at some concentrations. At higher concentrations (10-500 µg/mL) also, mean for SLLE (22±6.4), though higher than that for Vit C (10±7.7) was not significantly different. As shown, the SLLE exhibited a much more superior antioxidant effect when compared with Vit C at these two concentration ranges. When comparison was made between SLLE and Vit C at individual concentrations however, it was found that SLLE showed significant difference to Vit C at some concentrations (Figs. 2a. and 2b).

3.3 Ferrous-Ion Chelating Activity of SLLE and EDTA

Table 1. shows the relative ability of SLLE to chelate ferrous ion (Fe^{2+}) compared to EDTA. The mean percentage inhibition of the SLLE (2.199±19.29) when compared to that of EDTA (81.94±5.022) was found to be significant ($P<.01$). Results generally showed that while

EDTA was dose-dependently inhibiting Fe^{2+}, SLLE was showing a reverse activity such that the activity was declining from a positive value at 50µg/mL to a negative value at 200 µg/mL. At the lowest dose employed in this study (50 µg/mL), the extract showed a chelating activity of 51.39±9.7 while the standard (EDTA) showed chelating activity of 70.37±11.26.

Table 1. Ferrous-Ion chelating activity of SLLE and EDTA

Concentration (µg/ml)	Ferrous Ion chelating activity (%)	
	SLE	EDTA
50	51.39±9.7	70.37±11.26
100	3.70±6.07	91.67±6.99***
150	-3.70±5.63	76.85±9.80**
200	-42.59±30.0	88.89±5.56*

Data are presented as mean±SEM. Statistical significance was carried out between SLLE and EDTA at each concentration level using student's t test.* (P<.05); ** (P<.01); *** (P<.001); n = 3

3.4 Effect of SLLE on Hepatic Malondialdehyde Levels of Rats Subjected to Ischaemic / Reperfusion Injury

The result of the treatments on the hepatic MDA levels of ischemic / reperfusion-injured rats showed a reduction by Vit C although the reduction was not significant (Fig. 3). The lower dose of the SLLE (50 mg/kg) resulted in a slightly higher levels of MDA compared with saline-treated animals while the higher dose (100 mg/kg) resulted in a significant (P<.05) reduction of MDA levels. This reduction was also found to be much better than that provided by Vit C.

4. DISCUSSION

The safety potential of the methanol extract of *S. lehmbachii* had earlier been reported for *in-vivo* acute toxicity LD_{50} in rats [11]. While the acute toxicity evaluation in rats showed that the animals could tolerate a dose as high as 5,000 mg/kg, the in-vitro lethality assay in brine shrimps in the current study however resulted in a LC_{50} of 4.66 µg/ml in a 24-hour exposure model. The very low value of this toxicity parameter signifies a very potent activity of the leaves of the plant which could be of benefit in activity-guided fractionalization of the plant extract as well as potent and significant activity on biological systems; this may form the basis for biological screening in the search for potentially useful therapeutic agents from this plant. The relatively high dose tolerated in the whole animals when related to the high potency of *in-vitro* lethality suggested that a significant fraction of the orally administered dose may have been subjected to first-pass metabolism thereby affecting oral absorption and entry of significant amount as to constitute any potential for adverse effects to the animals so exposed.

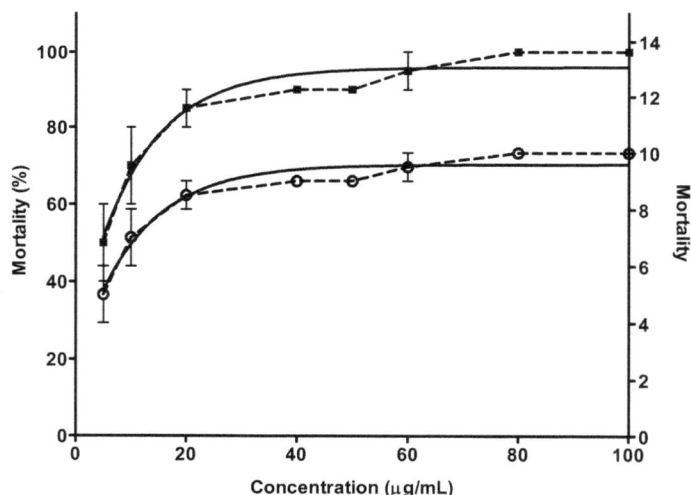

Fig. 1. Concentration vs mortality (right axis, ○) and % mortality (left axis, ■) data for SLLE in Brine Shrimp Assay

LC_{50} was calculated as 4.66 µg/ml. Data was fitted to an inverse exponent equation (Equation 2) with parameter values as follows: A = 69.99; B = 25.92; C = 0.091. Superimposed solid curves are nonlinear curves for the mortality plots. n = 15

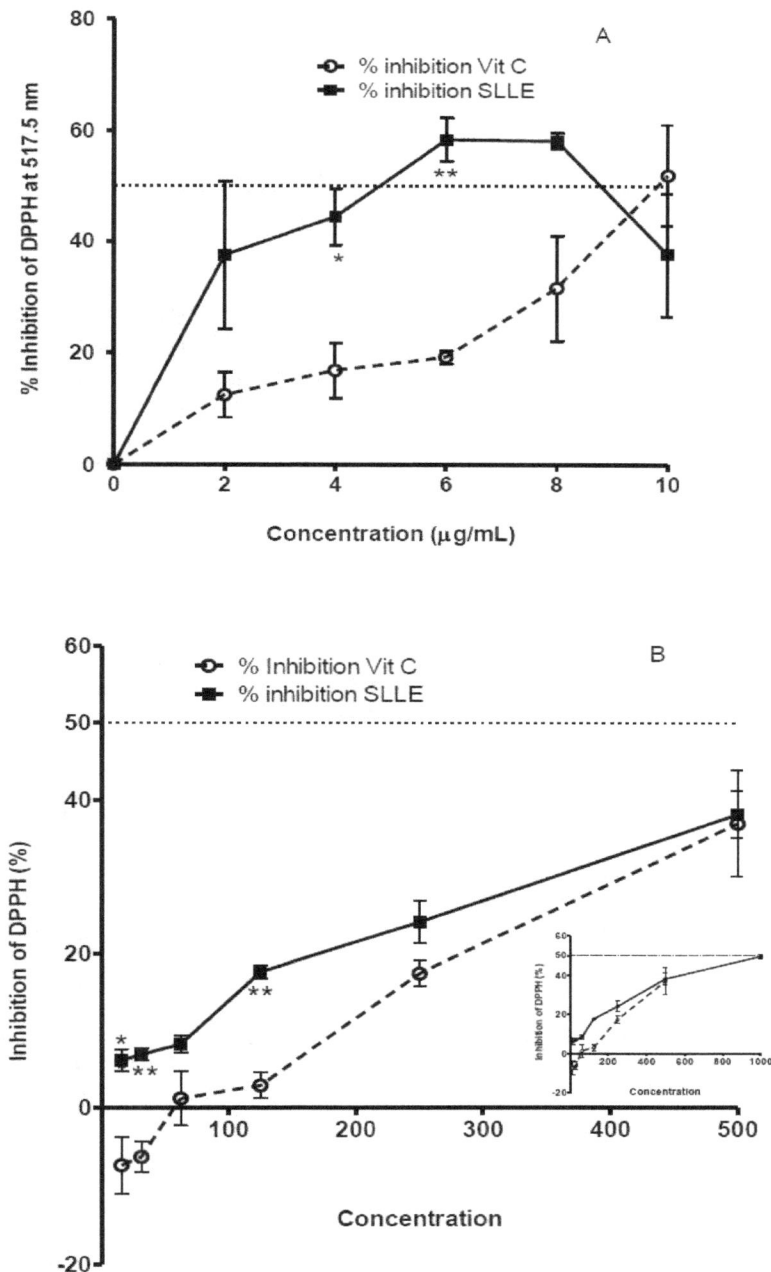

Fig. 2. DPPH radical scavenging activity of SLLE and Vit C at [A] low and [B] high concentrations

Low concentration range was 0-10 μg/mL while high concentration range was between 12.5-1000 μg/mL. Statistical significance was carried out between SLLE and Vit C at each concentration level using student's t test.* (P<.05); ** (P<.01); *** (P<.001); n=3

In the evaluation of antioxidant activity using the DPPH method, SLLE exhibited a much more superior antioxidant effect when compared with Vit C at both the low (0-10 μg/mL) and high (12.5-500 μg/mL) concentration ranges used in the study. When the two treatments were assessed by ANOVA over the entire concentrations in the two concentration ranges, the antioxidant effects of both Vit C and SLLE were found not to be significantly different though

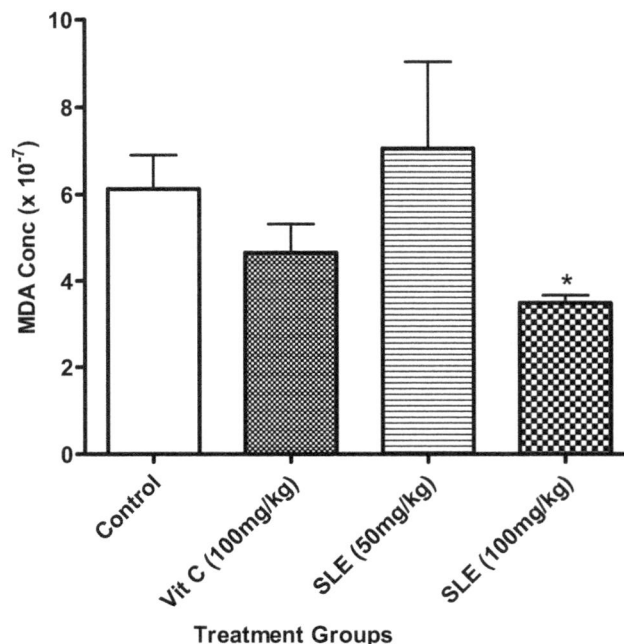

Fig. 3. Effects of SLLE and Vit C treatments on MDA levels in Ischaemic / reperfusion-injured hepatic tissue

*The concentration of the MDA was computed using the molar extinction coefficient of 1.56×10^5. Rats in the groups were subjected to ischemic/reperfusion injury of the liver and control rats were treated with normal saline while the other groups received either Vit C or two different doses of the SLLE. Each drug treated groups were compared with the control group using unpaired student's t-test. *. P<.05; n = 6*

when comparisons were made at individual concentrations using student's t-test, significant differences were found between the SLLE and Vit C. While the effects of the two treatments were easily observed and computed at the low concentration ranges, it was curiously observed that stable radical scavenging activity at higher doses were not as amenable and straightforward and in fact, radical scavenging activity at the higher concentrations were relatively minimal if not completely absent; this can be seen when cognizance is taken of the fact that IC50 of SLLE for DPPH radical scavenging will require a concentration above the maximum 1,000 µg/mL employed in the study (See insert of Fig. 2b).

In the FIC test, it was found that the standard compound, EDTA, was able to exhibit a concentration-dependent inhibition of the Fenton reaction of Fe^{2+} with 1, 10 phenanthroline; an action that is consistent with the known effect of EDTA. For the leaf extract however, there was a consistently decreasing effect of the extract on ion chelation after the increase elicited by 50 µg/ml. At the lower end of the concentration used in the study, both EDTA and SLLE showed

positive chelating activity while at increasing concentrations, unlike EDTA, SLLE activity declined into the negative portion of the curve. Although comparison between the two agents revealed that SLLE was significantly (P<.05) inferior to EDTA, the reason for the decrease of the values of SLLE into the negative domain needs to be addressed. At the very least, total lack of chelating activity ought to limit the SLLE curve towards zero by approaching the x-axis. The fact that (50 ug/mL) of SLLE showed a positive chelating activity suggests that if the concentration range of the study had been extended below 50 ug/mL, we might probably have seen a positive, maybe concentration-dependent chelating activity. One possibility is that the extract may actually possess the ability to trigger a Fenton-type reaction that is capable of generating reactive oxidants. Given the fact that the plant is used indigenously for the treatment of malaria infection and bearing in mind the molecular activity of artemisinin antimalarials which involves oxidant effect on malaria parasites, the relationship between these effects of SLLE needs to be further explored and clarified.

It has been said that the main strategy in avoiding ROS generation that is associated with redox-active metal catalysis involves chelating of metal ions. The reducing power of polyphenols suggests that they will possess potential hydrogen donating abilities [12] which will be made available to the Fe^{2+}, thereby effectively removing them from solution and prevent the Fenton reaction that can generate ROS. Since SLLE was found to have relative abundance of polyphenolic compounds, it was expected to exhibit iron-chelating properties which should confer on it the ability to prevent Fenton-type reaction which is implicated in many diseases and neurodegenerative disorders like Parkinson's and Alzheimer's diseases [13]. The result of this study showed that SLLE lacks this activity and as such any antioxidant property exhibited must be due to other mechanisms. It is not yet known what nature of chemical species is contained in SLLE but phytochemical screening of the plant is ongoing. In terms of general group composition however, *S. lehmachii*, just as other *salacia* species is known to contain polyphenolics [11].

Lipid peroxidation is a well-established mechanism of cellular injury in both plants and animals, and is therefore used as an indicator of oxidative stress in cells and tissues [14]. Measurement of MDA is therefore widely used as an indicator of lipid peroxidation [15] and increased levels of lipid peroxidation products have been associated with a variety of chronic diseases in both human and animal models [16]. In the present study, a significant reduction ($P<.05$) in the production of MDA was observed in the group that was given SLLE 100 mg/kg. This implies the ability of the extract to protect membrane lipids from oxidation. This effect could be related to the presence of polyphenols as indicated in the preliminary phytochemical analysis [11]. Plant phenolic compounds trap chain-initiating radicals at the interface of the membrane, thus, preventing the progression of the radical chain reaction. The group that was given Vit C at a dose of 100 mg/kg showed slight decrease in MDA as compared to the group that was given 50 mg/kg of the extract and the control group that was given only vehicle. The effect of the extract on the MDA concentration, suggests a dose -dependent response, as a higher concentration decreased the MDA concentration significantly. This is also in agreement with similar effects reported for another *Salacia* species. Krishnakumar et al. [17] reported that *S. oblonga* root extracts possess anti-lipid

peroxidative activity in the cardiac tissue of streptozotocin-diabetic rats. *S. oblonga* produced a significant decrease in peroxidation products viz., TBA-reactive substances, conjugated dienes and hydroperoxides. A study had shown that *S. reticulate* reduced the kidney, pancreatic and plasma peroxide levels as well as kidney aldose reductase activity [18] which suggests that it might equally have the same effect on other tissues such as the liver and this has been confirmed in the current study. In addition, Ismail and co-workers [19] reported that increased acid and alkaline phosphatase activity and decreased serum albumin in cotton pellet granulomatous rats were normalized after treatment with 1,000 mg/kg *S. oblonga* root bark powder in a study designed to evaluate the its anti-inflammatory activity. The activity of antioxidant enzymes such as superoxide dismutase, catalase, glutathione peroxidase and glutathione reductase were also increased in the heart tissue of diabetic animals treated with the extract suggesting its antioxidant activity. Also, nitric oxide production from lipopolysaccharide-activated mouse peritoneal macrophage and radical scavenging activities of the methanol extract of *S. chinensis* were reported in addition to potent antioxidant activity [20].

From this study, it can be seen that SLLE possessed robust antioxidant activity at low doses as well as the ability to prevent oxidative damage due to lipid peroxidation in the body; an ability that is shared with other species of the *salacia* genus. At higher concentrations however, its antioxidant activity is very weak or suspect and appears to be counteracted by other phenomena that has not been fully understood and therefore will require further studies to unravel.

5. CONCLUSION

In conclusion, the results showed that SLLE at low concentrations may have great relevance in the prevention and therapies of diseases in which oxidants or free radicals are implicated, and as such, SLLE could serve as an economic source of natural antioxidants. At higher doses or concentration however, the activity of the extract needs to be further clarified.

ACKNOWLEDGEMENTS

This work was partially sponsored by World Bank/STEP-B University of Calabar project grant awarded to Dr. B. A. S. Lawal's UNICAL Antimalarial STEP-B Project Group (UASPG).

CONSENT

It is not applicable.

ETHICAL APPROVAL

All authors hereby declare that "Principles of laboratory animal care" (NIH publication No. 85-23, revised 1985) were followed, as well as specific national laws where applicable. All experiments have been examined and approved by the appropriate ethics committee.

COMPETING INTERESTS

Authors have declared that no competing interests exist.

REFERENCES

1. Aruoma OI. Free radicals, oxidative stress and antioxidants in human health and disease. Journal of American Oil Chemists' Society. 1998;75:199-212.
2. Sies HW. Oxidative stress: Oxidants and antioxidants. London: Academic Press. 1991;4:67-90.
3. Krinsky NI. Mechanism of action of biological antioxidants. Proc Soc. Exp. Biol. Med. 1992;200:248-254.
4. Faizal P, Suresh S, Kumar SR, Augusti KT. A study on the hypoglycemic and hypolipidemic effects of an ayurvedic drug Rajanyamalakadi in diabetic patients. Indian Journal of Clinical Biochemistry. 2009;24(1):82-87.
5. Mohan V, Sandeep S, Deepa R, Shah B, Varghese C. Epidemiology of type 2 diabetes: Indian scenario. Indian J. Med. Res. 2007;125:217–230.
6. Anwa F, Kalsoom U, Sultana B, Mushtaq M, Mehmood T, Arshad HA. Effect of drying method and extraction solvent on the total phenolics and antioxidant activity of cauliflower (Brassica oleracea L.) extracts. International Food Research Journal. 2013;20(2):653-659.
7. Meyer BN, Ferrigni NR, Putnam JE, Jacobsen LB, Nichols DE, McLaughlin JL. Brine Shrimp: A convenient general bioassay for active plant constituents. Journal of Medicinal Plant Research. 1982; 45:31-34.
8. Brand-Williams W, Cuvelier ME, Berset C. Use of free radical method to evaluate antioxidant activity. LWT-Food Science and Technology. 1995;28:25–30.
9. Sanchez–Moreno CA, Larrauri JA, Saura CF. Journal of Science, Food and Agriculture. 1998;(76):270-276.
10. Selvakumar K, Madhan R, Srinivasan G, Baskar V. Antioxidant assays in pharmacological research. Asian J. Pharm. Tech. 2011;1(4):99-103.
11. Takem LP, Lawal BAS, Udoh FV, Abe NP. Anti-Abortificient activities of aqueous root extract of Salacia lehmbachii in sprague-dawley rats. Journal of Pharmaceutical Sciences and Pharmacology. 2014;2:1-5.
12. Mathew S, Abraham TE. Studies on the antioxidant activities of cinnamon (Cinnamomum verum) bark extracts, through various in vitro models. Food Chem. 2006;94:520-528.
13. Decker EA. Strategies for manipulating the pro-oxidative/antioxidative balance of foods to maximize oxidative stability. Trends in Food Science and Technology. 1998;9:241–248.
14. Yildiz HF, Coban RS, Terzi TA, Ates ML, Aksoy NG, Cakir HB, et al. Nigella sativa relieves the deleterious effects of Ischemia reperfusion injury on liver. World Journal of Gastroenterology. 2008;33:5204–5209.
15. Draper HH, Squires EJ, Mahmood HK, Wu J, Agarwal S, Hadley MA. Comparative evaluation of thiobarbituric acid methods for the determination of malondialdehyde in biological materials. Free Radic Biol. Med. 1993;15:353-363.
16. Kosugi HD, Kato TR, Kikugawa KN. Formation of yellow, orange and red pigments in the reaction of alk-2-enals with 2- thiobarbituric acid. Anal Biochem. 1987;165:456-464.
17. Krishnakumar K, Augusti KT, Vijayammal PL. Hypoglycaemic and anti-oxidant activity of Salacia oblonga Wall. extract in streptozotocin induced diabetic rats. Indian J Physiol Pharmacol. 1999;43:510-514.
18. Yoshino K, Yuko M, Takashi K, Yasutaka T, Kunimasa K. Anti-diabetic activity of a leaf extract prepared from Salacia reticulata in mice. Bioscience, Biotechnology, and Biochemistry. 2009;73: 1096-1104.
19. Ismail TS, Gopalakrishnan S, Begum VH, Elango V. Anti-inflammatory activity of Salacia oblonga Wall. and Azima tetracantha Lam. J. Ethnopharmacol. 1997;56:145-152

20. Yoshikawa M, Pongpiriyadacha Y, Kishi A, Kageura T, Wang T, Morikawa T, et al. Biological activities of *Salacia chinensis* originating in Thailand: The quality evaluation guided by alpha-glucosidase inhibitory activity. Yakugaku Zasshi. 2003; 123(10):871-880. Japanese.

21

In vitro Antioxidant Activity and Polyphenolic Content of a Polyherbal Tea and Its Constituents

V. Paddy[1], J. J. van Tonder[1] and V. Steenkamp[1*]

[1]*Department of Pharmacology, Faculty of Health Sciences, University of Pretoria, Private Bag X323, Arcadia 0007, South Africa.*

Authors' contributions

This work was carried out in collaboration between all authors. Author VP conducted experimental work and wrote the first draft of the manuscript. Author JJvT co-supervised the study and edited the manuscript. Author VS designed and supervised the study and reviewed and edited the manuscript. All authors read and approved the final manuscript.

Editor(s):
(1) Marcello Iriti, Faculty of Plant Biology and Pathology, Department of Agricultural and Environmental Sciences, Milan State University, Italy.
Reviewers:
(1) Ana Carolina Oliveira da Silva, Laboratory of Applied Ethnobiology, Rural Federal Univ. of Pernambuco (UFRPE), Brazil.
(2) Anupama Sharma, Biochemistry, G. R. Medical College, Gwalior, India.

ABSTRACT

Aims: Type 2 diabetes mellitus (T2DM) is associated with debilitating co-morbidities, mainly due to chronic hyperglycaemia-induced damage which is mediated by excess reactive oxygen species (ROS). Plant preparations have been shown to contain polyphenolic compounds that function as antioxidants. Various herbal teas have been sold as treatment of diabetes mellitus. The aim of this study was to evaluate a commercial, polyherbal tea, Diabetea and its constituents: *Achillea millefolium* L., *Agathosma betulina* Bartl. & Weidl., *Salvia officinalis*. L., *Taraxacum officinalis* L., *Thymus vulgaris*. L., *Trigonella foenum-graecum* L. and *Urtica urens* L. to assess their antioxidant and polyphenolic content.
Methodology: The polyphenol-linked cell-free and cell-based antioxidant activities of hot water (HW) and dichloromethane (DCM) extracts of Diabetea and its constituents were evaluated for ABTS$^{•+}$ and DPPH$^•$ radical scavenging ability and for ROS scavenging activity using 2',7'-dichlorodihydrofluorescein diacetate (DCFH-DA) in Ea.hy926 endothelial cells, respectively. The phenolic and flavonoid content was also assessed.
Results: All HW extracts were rich in polyphenols. *T. vulgaris* contained the highest amount of flavonoids (760.2±1.3 mg rutin equivalent (RE)/g) of all extracts, followed by *S. officinalis*

(491.7±12.5 mg RE/g). The extracts of *T. vulgaris* were the most active against ABTS$^{\bullet+}$ (~600.0 mg trolox equivalents (TE)/g activity) and DPPH$^{\bullet}$ (535.0 mg TE/g activity). The HW extracts of *T. vulgaris, S. officinalis* and *U. urens* significantly ($p<0.05$) mitigated cellular ROS, whereas none of the DCM extracts had this effect. The HW extracts of the Diabetea, *A. betulina, T. officinalis* and *T. foenum-graecum* and most DCM extracts (exception *A. betulina*) had a significant ($p<0.05$) intracellular pro-oxidant activity. The cell-free antioxidant activity of the HW extracts correlated significantly (r=0.98) with its polyphenolic content.
Conclusion: Diabetea exerted strong cell-free antioxidant activity. The HW extracts contained greater polyphenol-linked antioxidant activity than the DCM extracts. The HW extracts of *T. vulgaris, S. officinalis* and *U. urens* contain bioactive compounds that exert *in vitro* antidiabetic potential. Identification of the compounds responsible for this activity is warranted.

Keywords: Antioxidant activity; diabetea; diabetes mellitus; polyphenolic content; reactive oxygen species.

ABBREVIATIONS

ABTS$^{\bullet+}$	2,2-azinobis-3-ethylbenzothiazoline-6-sulfonic acid free radical
CAM	Complementary and alternative medicine
DCFH$_2$-DA	2',7'-dichlorodihydrofluorescein diacetate
DCM	Dichloromethane
dH2O	Distilled water
DM	Diabetes mellitus
DMEM	Dulbecco's Modified Eagle's Medium
DPPH$^{\square}$	1,1-diphenyl-2-picryl-hydrazyl free radical
EtOH	Ethanol
FCR	Folin-Ciocalteu's reagent
FCS	Fetal calf serum
FPG	Fasting plasma glucose
GA	Gallic acid
GAE	Gallic acid equivalents (mg gallic acid/g extract)
H$_2$O$_2$	Hydrogen peroxide
HW	Hot water
MeOH	Methanol
PI	Polarity index
RE	Rutin equivalents (mg rutin/g extract)
RFI	Relative fluorescence intensity
ROS	Reactive oxygen species
SEM	Standard error of the mean
T2DM	Type 2 diabetes mellitus
TE	Trolox equivalents
TFC	Total flavonoid content
TPC	Total phenolic content

1. INTRODUCTION

Type 2 diabetes mellitus (T2DM) is the most common subtype of diabetes mellitus (DM), affecting between 85 to 95% of all DM patients [1]. T2DM is an increasing global health concern, currently affecting an estimated 387 million individuals [1]. At present there is no cure for T2DM and the search for new and improved treatment is ongoing. T2DM is the consequence of biochemical dysfunctions such as insulin-resistance and -insufficiency, amongst others [2]. This results in defective carbohydrate metabolism in adipocytes, myocytes and hepatocytes; leading to chronic hyperglycaemia, which is the hallmark of T2DM [1]. Chronic hyperglycaemia leads to an overproduction of reactive oxygen species (ROS), a heightened sensitivity of cells to ROS, defective response of the antioxidant defense system, biophysical modification of cells and glucotoxicity [3]. Collectively, these may lead to cellular hypertrophy, apoptosis, necrosis, contractile dysfunction and fibrosis [3], all of which contribute to secondary complications associated with T2DM.

ROS are unstable and highly reactive oxygen derivatives with incomplete orbital electron pairs [4]. These include: singlet oxygen ($O_2^{\bullet}$), superoxide (O_2^-), hydrogen peroxide (H_2O_2), hydroxyl radicals ($OH^{\bullet-}$) and hypochlorous acid (HClO), amongst others [4]. In the natural state, ROS are essential intermediates required for immune reactions, detoxification, signaling cascades and the production of energy [5]. However, excess ROS caused by pathological conditions such as chronic hyperglycaemia, can cause peroxidation of lipids, deoxyribonucleic acid bases, structural proteins and enzymes, which ultimately leads to biofunctional impairment on a cellular level [6].

Antioxidants are substances that significantly delay or prevent the effects of ROS [7]. Several types of antioxidants have been identified according to their function against the damaging consequences of excess ROS [8]. These antioxidants neutralize ROS by means of inhibition, reduction, scavenging, chelation or quenching [5]. Antioxidants are classified as either enzymatic or non-enzymatic. Enzymatic antioxidants such as superoxide dismutase, glutathione peroxidase and catalase are endogenous auto-regulatory agents [5]. Examples of non-enzymatic antioxidants include vitamins, flavonoids, α-lipoic acid, carotenoids, coenzyme Q10, copper, zinc, manganese, selenium and folic acid [9]. Various plant-derived polyphenols are examples of non-enzymatic antioxidant compounds [10] such as thymol, which has been isolated from thyme [11].

The majority of individuals in both developing and developed countries make use of complementary and alternative medicine (CAM) as therapeutic interventions [12]. Traditional medicine forms a major part of CAM. On the African continent approximately 70–95% of individuals make use of herbal remedies [12]. Diabetea, a herbal tea mixture, is one of many commercial teas used as a therapy for DM. Diabetea is comprised of *Achillea millefolium* L. (yarrow), *Agathosma betulina* Bartl. & Weidl. (buchu), *Salvia officinalis*. L. (sage), *Taraxacum officinalis* L. (dandelion), *Thymus vulgaris* L. (thyme), *Trigonella foenum-graecum* L.

(fenugreek) and *Urtica urens* L. (nettle). Although the individual plants comprising Diabetea have been reported as traditionally used to treat diabetes, most of the constituents as well as the polyherbal tea have not been evaluated in depth. The aim of this study was therefore to assess the *in vitro* potential of Diabetea and its constituents to aid in the alleviation of ROS, which is associated with chronic hyperglycaemia.

2. MATERIALS AND METHODS

2.1 Plant Material and Extraction

A. millefolium L. (Asteraceae, whole plant), *A. betulina* Bartl. & Wendl. (Rutaceae, leaves), *S. officinalis* L. (Lamiaceae, leaves), *T. officinalis* L. (Asteraceae, aerial parts), *T. vulgaris* L. (Lamiaceae, leaves and stems), *T. foenum-graecum* L. (Fabaceae, seeds) and *U. urens* L. (Urticaceae, whole plant) were purchased from a local health shop (Pretoria, South Africa). The Diabetea mixture was purchased from Sing-Fefur organic herbs (Robertson, South Africa). All plant material was bought in dried form. Each plant sample was ground into a fine homogenous powder (IKA-Werke Yellowline A10 analytical grinder) before extraction.

Hot water (HW) and dichloromethane (DCM) were used as extraction solvents. The HW extraction was done using a decoction method, whereby 2 g homogenous plant powder was mixed with 20 ml distilled water (dH$_2$O). The solution was left on an electronic shaker (Beckman Coulter, VRN-200) for 1 h and incubated in an ultrasonic bath (Bransonic 52 Cleaning Equipment Co.) for another hour, after which the mixtures were macerated for 24 h at 4°C. The following day the mixtures were left on a shaker for 30 min, to reach room temperature, before they were boiled (Labotec, Büchi Heating Bath, B-490) for 15 min. Mixtures were centrifuged for 30 min at 1000 g (Allegra x-22, Beckman Coulter), filtered (0.22 μm) and kept at 4°C overnight. The following day the mixtures were concentrated via lyophilization (Freezone 6, Labconco) and stored at -70°C. The DCM extraction was performed in a similar fashion to that of the HW extraction up to the centrifugation step, whereafter the supernatant was concentrated by means of *in vacuo* rota-evaporation (Labotec, Büchi Rotavapor) at 60°C. The concentrate was reconstituted in dimethyl sulfoxide and stored at -70°C. Yields were determined gravimetrically.

2.2 Total Polyphenolic Content

2.2.1 Total phenolic content

Total phenolic content (TPC) was determined following a spectrophotometric, 96-well microplate method, using Folin-Ciocalteu's reagent (FCR), as described by Slinkard and Singleton [13], with minor modifications. Gallic acid (GA) was used as the phenolic acid standard to construct a calibration curve at concentrations ranging from 0.1 to 0.8 mM using 20% v/v ethanol (EtOH) as solvent. Experimental wells contained; 50 µl of extract (100 µg/ml), 60 µl of FCR and 100 µl of 3% w/v sodium carbonate (Na_2CO_3) solution. The phytochemical interference was accounted for by wells containing plant extract (50 µl) and dH_2O (160 µl). FCR (60 µl) with dH_2O (150 µl) served as control while wells with dH_2O (210 µl) only, served as blank. The plates were incubated in the dark for 1 h and absorbance was measured at 630 nm using a Bio-tech Instruments ELX800$_{UV}$ plate reader. The TPC was expressed in terms of gallic acid equivalents (GAE) (mg GAE /g extract ± SEM).

2.2.2 Total flavonoid content

Total flavonoid content (TFC) was determined following a spectrophotometric, 96-well microplate method, of Quettier-Deleu [14], with minor modifications. Rutin was used as the flavonoid standard to construct a calibration curve (20 - 200 µg/ml) with methanol (MeOH) as solvent. The reaction mixture consisted of 40 µl plant extract (100 µg/ml), 20 µl of a 3% w/v sodium nitrate (NaNO3) solution, 20 µl aluminium trichloride ($AlCl_3$) (1% w/v) and 100 µl of sodium hydroxide (NaOH) at 2 M. The plates were incubated in the dark for 10 min, after which absorbance was measured at 450 nm (Bio-tech Instruments, ELX800$_{UV}$). The wells containing 40 µl sample and 140 µl distilled water served as background control to eliminate phytochemical interference, whereas wells with 180 µl dH_2O served as blank. The TFC was expressed in terms of rutin equivalents (mg RE/g extract±SEM).

2.3 Cell-free Antioxidant activity

2.3.1 ABTS$^{•+}$ assay

The 2,2-azinobis-3-ethylbenzothiazoline-6-sulfonic acid free radical (ABTS$^{•+}$) neutralization was determined using a spectrophotometric, 96-well microplate method described by Re et al. [15],

with minor modifications. The ABTS$^{•+}$ free radical solution was prepared by incubating a mixture of ABTS (7 mM) and 2.45 mM potassium persulfate ($K_2S_2O_8$) dissolved in dH_2O, in the dark, for 12-16 h at 4°C. Prior to experimentation the ABTS$^{•+}$ solution was diluted with ethanol (EtOH) to a standard absorbance of 0.7±0.02 at 734 nm. The reaction mixture consisted of 50 µl of plant extract (1 - 20 µg/ml) and 150 µl ABTS$^{•+}$. The plates were incubated at room temperature, in the dark, for 15 min and the absorbance was read at 630 nm. The control wells contained 50 µl of dH_2O and 150 µl ABTS$^{•+}$. Phytochemical interference was accounted for by wells containing extract (50 µl) with dH_2O (150 µl), whereas 200 µl dH_2O served as blank. Trolox dissolved in pure MeOH was used as positive control. The antioxidant capacity of each extract was expressed quantitatively in terms of trolox equivalents (TE) (mg TE /g extract) and at the extract concentration where 50% of ABTS$^{•+}$ was neutralized (IC$_{50}$).

2.3.2 DPPH$^{•}$ assay

The 1,1-diphenyl-2-picryl-hydrazyl free radical (DPPH$^{•}$) scavenging activity was determined using a spectrophotometric 96-well microplate method as described by Gyamfi et al. [16], with minor modifications. The DPPH$^{•}$ solution was prepared fresh for every experiment using MeOH. Fifty microliters of plant extract (1 - 20 µg/ml) was added to 150 µl of DPPH$^{•}$ (100 µM). Each plate was incubated at room temperature, in the dark, for 15 min after which absorbance was read at 570 nm. Wells containing MeOH (50 µl) and DPPH$^{•}$ (150 µl) served as control and wells with MeOH (200 µl) only served as blank. Phytochemical interference was accounted for by wells containing extract (50 µl) and MeOH (150 µl). The free radical scavenging activity of each extract was expressed in terms of trolox equivalents (TE) (mg TE/g extract) and at the extract concentration where 50% of DPPH$^{•}$ was attenuated (IC$_{50}$).

2.4 Cellular Antioxidant Activity

2.4.1 Cell culture propagation and maintenance

Cell-based antioxidant activity of each extract was determined in EA.hy926 human umbilical vein cells (ATCC CRL-2922; gift from Dr Edgell, University of North Carolina, USA). Since hyperglycaemia-induced ROS damage to endothelial cells is associated with severe cardiovascular diseases [17], this cell line was used in this study. All cell work was conducted under strict sterile conditions and incubated in a 5% CO_2 incubator at 37°C in Dulbecco's Modified Eagle's Medium (DMEM), which was supplemented with 1% penicillin/streptomycin and 10% fetal calf serum (FCS).

2.4.2 DCFH-DA assay

The ability of crude plant extracts to attenuate p-chloranil-induced ROS was determined using a 96-well microplate method with 2',7'-dichlorodihydrofluorescein diacetate ($DCFH_2$-DA) as described by Boissy et al. [18], with modifications. White plates were pre-seeded with Ea.hy926 cells at 1.5×10^4 cells/well. Eighty microliters of DMEM- (DMEM without FCS), containing 5 µM $DCFH_2$-DA was added to wells and incubated for 1 h at 37°C in 5% CO_2. The wells were carefully aspirated and 80 µl of a p-chloranil solution (40 µM) prepared in Hank's buffered salt solution was added. Eighty microliters of plant extract (1 - 20 µg/ml) was added to the experimental wells and the plates were incubated for 2.5 h at 37°C in a 5% CO_2 atmosphere. Trolox was used as positive control at a final concentration of 20 µg/ml. Wells containing 80 µl of p-chloranil and 80 µl DMEM- served as control wells. Fluorescence was measured at λ_{ex} = 485 nm and λ_{em} = 540 nm, with a gain setting of 750 (FLUOstar Optima, BMG Labotech). The results were expressed in terms of relative fluorescence intensity (RFI).

2.5 Statistical Analysis and Data Representation

All experiments were conducted in technical and biological triplicate. Values are expressed as mean ± standard error of the mean (SEM). Data was analyzed using one-way analysis of variance (ANOVA) tests. If statistically significant differences were detected, individual group comparisons were performed using Tukey's HSD test. Individual extracts were compared to positive and negative controls using Student's t-tests. The Pearson's correlation coefficient was used to measure associations. The significance level was set at $p < 0.05$. GraphPad Prism 6.0 was used to analyze data.

3. RESULTS AND DISCUSSION

The total phenol and flavonoid content of Diabetea and the individual herb extracts is presented in Table 1. The HW extracts were found to be rich in polyphenols, whereas the DCM extracts hardly contained any polyphenols (Table 1). This is not surprising since water has a polarity index (PI) of 9.0, having a strong interaction with electronegative compounds such as polyphenols, whereas DCM has a PI of 3.1 [19].

Cellular antioxidant activity of polyphenols depends on their ability to move across the cell membrane, this action is selective [20]. The HW extracts caused a greater attenuation of $ABTS^{•+}$ (Table 2) than $DPPH^•$. This could be because the $ABTS^{•+}$ assay is aqueous based, favouring hydrophilic compounds, whereas the $DPPH^•$ assay is an organic based assay, favouring hydrophobic phytoconstituents [21]. However, in the present study, none of the DCM extracts were significantly active against $DPPH^•$ (Table 2), indicating that no potent hydrophobic antioxidants were extracted using DCM. This was also evident in the cell-based test results (Fig. 1).

Table 1. Polyphenolic content of diabetea and its individual herbs

Plant	Total phenol content (mg GAE/g)		Total flavonoid content (mg RE/g)	
	HW	DCM	HW	DCM
A. betulina	43.3±2.2	5.4±0.2	194.2±0.9	1.2±0.8
T. officinalis	22.3±0.8	5.9±0.2	188.6±2.5	0.8±0.7
T. foenum-graecum	38.7±0.6	5.6±0.1	147.9±2.6	1.1±0.9
S. officinalis	58.3±1.6	5.0±0.2	491.7±12.5	4.0±0.7
U. urens	31.1±1.3	5.9 ±0.2	234.4±1.3	0.4±1.3
T. vulgaris	101.3±1.7	5.6±0.1	760.2±1.3	5.6±1.3
A. millefolium	41.6±1.2	5.4±0.1	313.1±5.1	3.9±1.4
Diabetea	44.4±1.0	5.2±0.2	256.6±2.6	3.8±1.7

HW: hot water extract, DCM: dichloromethane extract, GAE: gallic acid equivalents, RE: rutin equivalents

Diabetea contained a considerable amount of polyphenols within its HW extract (Table 1) with 44.4±1.0 mg GAE/g and 256.6±2.6 mg RE/g. It also exerted potent cell-free antioxidant activity (Table 2) with an IC_{50} of 85.4 µg/ml for DPPH$^{\bullet}$ and 27.1 µg/ml for ABTS$^{\bullet+}$. Its' chemical antioxidant activity was shown to be independent of its polyphenolic content because of the potent antioxidant activity of its DCM extract (Tables 1 and 2), with an IC_{50} of 25.2 µg/ml against ABTS$^{\bullet+}$. On the other hand, Diabetea was ineffective regarding cellular-ROS neutralization (Figs. 1 and 2). Instead, it caused a significant overproduction of intracellular ROS. It has been shown that herbal remedies can have an antioxidant or pro-oxidant effect depending on their concentration and/or structural properties [22].

The HW extract of T. vulgaris had the highest abundance of polyphenols (101.3±1.7 mg GAE/g and 760.2±1.3 mg RE/g) and the most potent antioxidant activity in both cell-free (IC_{50}: 10.8 µg/ml DPPH$^{\bullet}$, 6.7 µg/ml ABTS$^{\bullet+}$) and cell-based assays (Fig. 1) of all extracts tested. These findings are supported by previous studies [23-25]. Dorman et al. [23] prepared a HW decoction of T. vulgaris for 1 h instead of 15 min, which yielded 95.6 mg GAE/ g extract [23]. The slight difference in phenolic content observed between the present study and that of Dorman et al. [23] could have been caused by the difference in the duration of extraction, resulting in the breakdown of the structural integrity of some phyto-constituents. Rababah et al. [25] only extracted 11.02±49.8 mg GAE/g extract from T. vulgaris

when water extracts were prepared by heating at 60ºC for 1 h, which is approximately a tenth of what was obtained by Dorman et al. [23], who also extracted for 1 h. Rababah et al. [25] reported that more polyphenols were extracted at higher temperatures, which could further explain this discrepancy. Therefore, it could be inferred that extraction temperature has a much greater influence on extraction yield than the duration of the extraction process. Other thyme species have also been found to contain notable polyphenol rutin equivalent activity [26].

Carvacrol and thymol are two polyphenols that have been isolated from T. vulgaris [27-29]. Thymol is a more potent antioxidant phyto-constituent than carvacrol [30,31]. Rababah et al. [25] found both carvacrol and thymol to be active against DPPH$^{\bullet}$. The IC_{50} values were >100 µg/ml [25], which was not considered potent antioxidant activity in the present study. A number of polyphenols have been isolated from T. vulgaris, such as luteolin, quercetin, rutin, catechin, caffeic acid and apigenin [26]. Luteolin is a potent antioxidant [32], with activity reported to be equivalent to that of quercetin [33]. Another group of naturally occurring antioxidants found in T. vulgaris are phenylpropenes (such as eugenol and 4-allylphenol), which also possess antioxidant capacities comparable to known antioxidants such as α-tocopherol and butylated hydroxy toluene [34]. The quantity as well as the quality of the phytoconstituents extracted from T. vulgaris, in the present study, is the most likely cause for its significant ($p < 0.05$) cell-free and cell-based antioxidant activities. The cell-free

Table 2. Antioxidant activity of diabetea and its individual herbs assessed using cell free assays

Plant	DPPH$^{\bullet}$ scavenging (IC_{50}, µg/ml)		ABTS$^{\bullet+}$ scavenging (IC_{50}, µg/ml)		DPPH$^{\bullet}$ scavenging (mg TE/g extract)		ABTS$^{\bullet+}$ scavenging (mg TE/g extract)	
	HW	DCM	HW	DCM	HW	DCM	HW	DCM
A. betulina	>100.0	>100.0	42.1	n.c.	10.0	0.0	215.0	202.5
T. officinalis	>100.0	>100.0	35.0	n.c.	0.0	0.0	247.5	165.0
T. foenum-graecum	>100.0	>100.0	57.0	51.8	0.0	0.0	97.5	240.0
S. officinalis	16.9	>100.0	13.9	82.7	375.0	0.0	460.0	330.0
U. urens	>100.0	>100.0	27.0	>100.0	80.0	0.0	327.5	460.0
T. vulgaris	10.8	>100.0	6.7	17.3	535.0	0.0	600.0	597.5
A. millefolium	40.5	>100.0	20.5	21.1	150.0	0.0	375.0	387.5
Diabetea	85.4	>100.0	27.1	25.2	75.0	0.0	317.5	562.5
Trolox	4.9		4.4					

*Significant $p < 0.05$, HW: Hot water extract, DCM: dichloromethane extract, n.c. not converged, TE: trolox equivalents

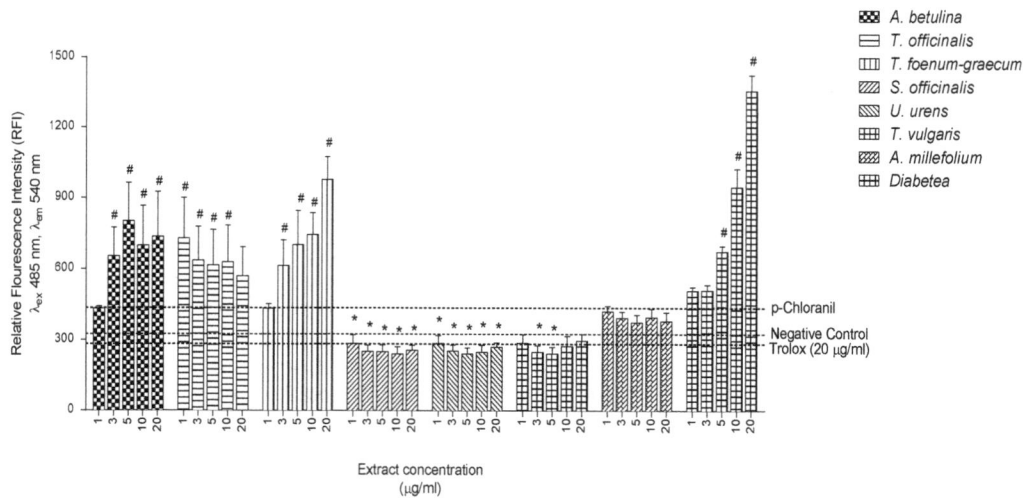

Fig. 1. Cell-based antioxidant activity of hot water extracts tested at 1 to 20 µg/ml. Reactive oxygen species (ROS) were generated from Ea.hy926 endothelium cells using *p*-chloranil (20 µM in reaction). Each bar represents the mean fluorescence intensity ± SEM of triplicate (n = 9) tests. Significant (*p*<0.05) antioxidant activity of plant extracts tested against *p*-chloranil (*) and overproduction of ROS compared to *p*-chloranil (#) was determined using the student's *t*-test. *p*-Chloranil, negative control and trolox are represented by dotted lines

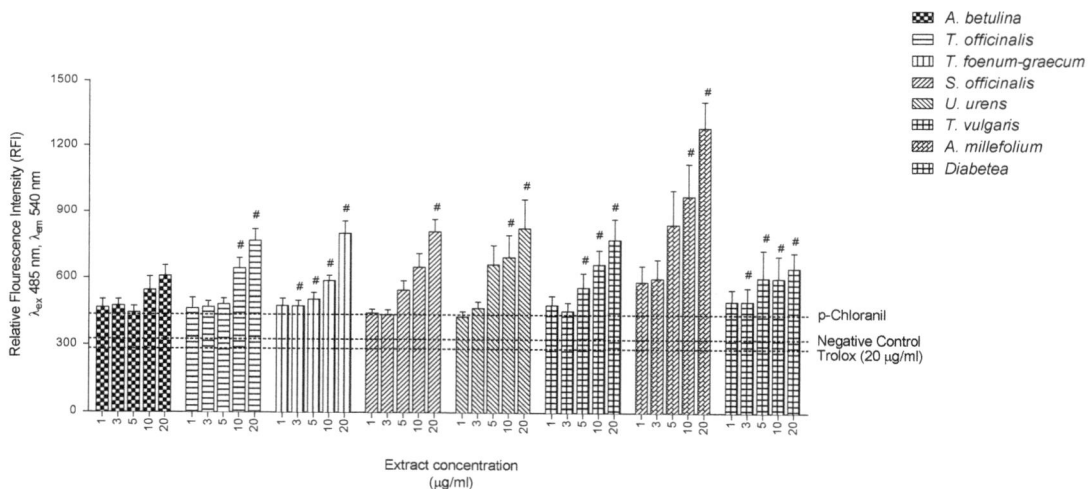

Fig. 2. Cell-based antioxidant activity of dichloromethane extracts tested at 1 to 20 µg/ml. Reactive oxygen species (ROS) were generated in Ea.hy926 endothelium cells using *p*-chloranil (20 µM in reaction). Each bar represents the mean fluorescence intensity ± SEM of triplicate (n = 9) tests. Significant (*p*<0.05) antioxidant activity of the plant extracts tested against *p*-chloranil (*), and overproduction of ROS compared to *p*-chloranil (#) was determined using the student's *t*-test. *p*-Chloranil, negative control and trolox are represented by dotted lines

antioxidant activity of the HW extract of *T. vulgaris* (6.7 µg/ml against ABTS$^{\bullet+}$) in the present study was comparable to that of trolox (4.4 µg/ml). The health benefits of *T. vulgaris* has been recognized and listed in the European and Hungarian pharmacopoeias [26].

The HW extract of *S. officinalis* possessed the second highest polyphenolic (58.3±1.6 mg GAE/g and 491.7±12.5 mg RE/g) content and antioxidant activities (IC$_{50}$: 16.9 µg/ml against DPPH$^{\bullet}$ and 13.9 µg/ml against ABTS$^{\bullet+}$). *S. officinalis* contains bioactive antioxidant flavonoids that are also found in *T. vulgaris*, such as: salvigenin, nevadensin, apigenin, cirsileol and cirsimaritin [35]. The antioxidant activity of *S. officinalis* has also been credited to flavonoid compounds such as carnosic acid and carnosol, as well as rosmarinic acid [36]. Although the HW extracts of *S. officinalis* was not as active against cell-free radicals as *T. vulgaris*, it significantly (*p*<0.05) attenuated cell-based ROS at all concentrations tested (Fig. 1). This indicates that both *T. vulgaris* and *S. officinalis* contain bioactive compounds with possible potent antidiabetic therapeutic activity.

The HW extract of *U. urens* displayed a significant (*p*<0.05) cell-free (IC$_{50}$ 27.0 µg/ml ABTS$^{\bullet+}$) and cell-based free-radical-mitigating activity at all dilutions tested (Table 2, Fig. 1). This could be ascribed to patuletin, an abundant and potent aglycon flavonol previously extracted from *U. urens* [37]. Patuletin is active at low concentrations (7.5 mg/kg body weight) in male Sprague-Dawley rats [38]. This phytochemical is lipophilic and readily crosses the cell membrane, making it easily available in the cytosol to exert its protective antioxidant action [38,39]. It has also been found to sustain the activity of the innate antioxidant defense system involving enzymes such as catalase, glutathione peroxidase and glutathione reductase [40]. A water extract of *U. urens* (1 mg/ml) was reported to contain activity against ABTS$^{\bullet+}$ and DPPH$^{\bullet}$ with greater action against ABTS$^{\bullet+}$ [41], which is expected due to the difference in assay affinity to hydrophilic extracts [21]. The antioxidant activity of flavonoids is attributed to their polyhydroxylated structure and the specific hydroxyl positions on the flavonoid backbone [42]. The catechol flavonoid structure has been identified as the required structure for the presence of antioxidant activity of any flavonoid, containing two phenyl rings and one pyrene ring [42,43]. Patelutin has been identified as a compound that possesses the structural requirements of such a bioactive antioxidant phytochemical [40].

The extracts of *T. foenum-graecum* had a low polyphenolic content (Table 1) and antioxidant activity (Table 2), which is supported by Kaviarasan et al. [44]. However, in an *in vivo* study, *T. foenum-graecum* seeds fed (5% w/w) to diabetic mice were shown to normalize the antioxidant defense response and decrease peroxidative damage [45]. This indicates that even though a low antioxidant activity is observed in *in vitro* studies (as is the current case), *in vivo* antioxidant activity may still be possible.

In contrast to the present findings, a hydro-alcoholic fraction of *A. millefolium* was found to be active against superoxide and hydroxyl radicals with IC$_{50}$ values of 0.82 and 0.26 µg/ml, respectively [46]. It has been reported that *A. millefolium* contains potent antioxidant compounds such as caffeic and *p*-coumaric acid [47]. The reason for the discrepancy found between the present study (Tables 1 and 2) and those carried out previously, may be attributed to the different assays used as well as the type of solvent used for extraction.

The extracts of *A. betulina* contained low polyphenolic content and antioxidant activity (Tables 1 and 2). Although the present study does not report a noteworthy antioxidant activity exerted by *A. betulina in vitro*, it may not be indicative of its *in vivo* and clinical activity. Diosmin and hesperidin are two main flavonoid compounds that have been isolated from the essential oil of *A. betulina*, which have been proven to act as antioxidant agents [48]. These flavonoids have been tested in the form of a micronised purified flavonoid fraction called Daflon 500 (90% diosmin and 10% hesperidin), and were found to have a long term antioxidant action on type 1 diabetic patients [49-51].

Most of the DCM extracts (except for *A. betulina*) as well as the HW extracts of *A. betulina*, *T. foenum-graecum*, *T. officinalis* and Diabetea had a significant (*p*<0.05) pro-oxidant activity in Ea.hy926 cells (Fig. 1). The overproduction of cellular-ROS was reported after cells were placed under certain biochemical or mechanical stress(es), either caused by unwanted environmental, chemical or pathological conditions [52]. The pro-oxidant activity of herb extracts have been linked to large doses / concentrations of antioxidant-type flavonoids and/or the presence of flavoniods containing specific structural modifications on its B-ring [53]. This could explain the pro-oxidant activity of *A. betulina*, *T. foenum-graecum*, *T. officinalis* and Diabetea, which are flavonoid-containing HW extracts. However, the flavonoid-rich HW extracts of *T. vulgaris* and *S. officinalis* had no pro-oxidant effect in Ea.hy926 cells, which may indicate that the pro-oxidant activity observed for the aforementioned plant extracts may not be due to a high concentration of flavonoids, but rather caused by flavonoids with specific structural modifications exerting pro-oxidant activity. Furthermore, all DCM extracts had a significant ($p<0.05$) pro-oxidant activity on Ea.hy926 cells, which could not be attributed to their flavonoid content since they were poor polyphenolic containing extracts.

A significant ($p<0.05$) correlation was observed between cell-free antioxidant activity and total polyphenolic content for the HW extracts (r = 0.98; results not shown). This confirms that the cell-free antioxidant activity exerted by polyphenols follows a linear dose-dependent (quantitative) model, which has previously been reported [48]. A significant ($p<0.05$) correlation between ABTS$^{\bullet+}$ and DPPH$^{\bullet}$ scavenging activity for HW extracts (r = 0.94) was found, suggesting that the mechanisms of ABTS$^{\bullet+}$ and DPPH$^{\bullet}$ scavenging activities of the individual extracts are similar. However, it should still be taken into account that the DPPH$^{\bullet}$ scavenging activity of the HW extracts were all lower than that of ABTS$^{\bullet+}$ attenuation due to the hydrophilic propensity of the ABTS$^{\bullet+}$ assay [24].

4. CONCLUSION

The traditional use of *T. vulgaris*, *S. officinalis* and *U. urens* as antidiabetic herbs is supported in the present study in terms of their significant *in vitro* cell-based antioxidant capacity. The most significant of these was the HW extract of *T. vulgaris*, which correlated with its polyphenolic content. The HW and DCM extracts of *T. foenum-graecum*, *T. officinalis* and *A. betulina* as well as Diabetea was associated with the overproduction of cellular ROS. The cell-free antioxidant activity of the HW extracts significantly correlated with their polyphenolic content, confirming a linear, dose-dependent antioxidant activity of polyphenols against cell-free radicals. However, it was shown that extracts with low polyphenol content, such as the DCM extracts of *T. foenum-graecum*, *S. officinalis*, *T. vulgaris*, *A. millefolium* and Diabetea also exerted significant antioxidant activity against ABTS$^{\bullet+}$. From this it can be concluded that such plant extracts contain non-polyphenolic compounds that are active against cell-free radicals or contain polyphenols with specific structural properties that are active at very low concentrations. This study showed that

the HW extracts of *T. vulgaris*, *S. officinalis* and *U. urens* contain bioactive compounds that may benefit patients with chronic hyperglycaemia. These individual herb extracts had more favourable activity than Diabetea, demonstrating that the polyherb mixture is not more active than its individual counterparts. However, before any recommendation can be made regarding the dosage concentration, regimen combination and administration of each, further testing is required. In addition to this, identification of the compounds responsible for this activity needs to be elucidated and subjected to further testing.

CONSENT

It is not applicable.

ETHICAL APPROVAL

It is not applicable.

COMPETING INTERESTS

Authors have declared that no competing interests exist.

REFERENCES

1. Cho NH, David Whiting D, Leonor Guariguata L, Montoya PA, Forouhi N, Hambleton I, Li R, Majeed A, Mbanya JC, Motala A, Narayan KMV, Ramachandran A, Rathmann A, Roglic G, Shaw J, Silink M, Williams DRR, Zhang P. IDF Diabetes Atlas. 6th edition. Edited by Guariguata L, Nolan T, Beagley J, Linnenkamp U, Jacqmain O. International diabetes federation; 2013.
Available:http://www.idf.org/diabetesatlas

2. Rolo AP, Palmeira CM:.Diabetes and mitochondrial function: Role of hyperglycemia and oxidative stress. Toxicol Appl Pharmacol. 2006;212:167-78.

3. Brownlee M. Biochemistry and molecular cell biology of diabetic complications. Nature. 2001;414:813-20.

4. Aruoma OI. Free radicals, oxidative stress, and antioxidants in human health and disease. J Am Oil Chem Soc. 1998;75:199-212.

5. Ali SS, Kasoju N, Luthra A, Singh A, Sharanabasava H, Sahu A, Bora U. Indian medicinal herbs as sources of antioxidants. Food Res Int. 2008;41:1-15.

6. Valko M, Rhodes CJ, Moncol J, Izakovic M, Mazur M. Free radical metals and

antioxidants in oxidative stress-induced cancer. Chemico Biologica Inter. 2006; 160:1–40.

7. Benzie IF, Strain J. The ferric reducing ability of plasma (FRAP) as a measure of "antioxidant power": The FRAP assay. Anal Biochem. 1996;239:70-6.

8. Pokorný J. Are natural antioxidants better– and safer–than synthetic antioxidants? Eur J Lipid Sci Tech. 2007;109:629-42.

9. McCune LM, Johns T. Antioxidant activity in medicinal plants associated with the symptoms of diabetes mellitus used by the indigenous peoples of the North American boreal forest. J Ethnopharmacol. 2002;82: 197-205.

10. Gryglewski RJ, Korbut R, Robak J, Swies J. On the mechanism of antithrombotic action of flavonoids. Biochem Pharmacol. 1987;36:317-22.

11. Yanishlieva NV, Marinova EM, Gordon MH, Raneva VG. Antioxidant activity and mechanism of action of thymol and carvacrol in two lipid systems. Food Chem 1999;64:59-66.

12. WHO. WHO Traditional Medicine Strategy 2002–2005. Geneva: World Health Organization;2002. WHO/EDM/TRM/2002.12.

13. Slinkard KS, Singleton VL. Total phenol analysis: automation and comparison with manual methods. Am J Enol Viticult. 1977; 28:49-55.

14. Quettier-Deleu C, Gressier B, Vasseur J, Dine T, Brunet C, Luyckx M, Cazin M, Cazin J-C, Bailleul F, Trotin F. Phenolic compounds and antioxidant activities of buckwheat (Fagopyrum esculentum Moench) hulls and flour. J Ethnopharmacol. 2000;72(1-2):35-42.

15. Re R, Pellegrini N, Proteggente A, Pannala A, Yang M, Rice-Evans C. Antioxidant activity applying an improved ABTS radical cation decolorization assay. Free Radic Biol Med. 1999;26(9-10):1231-7.

16. Gyamfi MA, Yonamine M, Aniya Y. Free-radical scavenging action of medicinal herbs from Ghana: Thonningia sanguinea on experimentally-induced liver injuries. Gen Pharmacol. 1999;32(6):661-7.

17. Szocs K. Endothelial dysfunction and reactive oxygen species production in ischemia/reperfusion and nitrate tolerance. Gen Physiol Biophys. 2004; 23:265-95.

18. Boissy RE, Trinkle LS, Nordlund JJ. Separation of pigmented and albino melanocytes and the concomitant evaluation of endogenous peroxide content using flow cytometry. Cytometry. 1989; 10(6):779-87.

19. Campbell MK, Farrell SO. Biochemistry. 6th ed. Canada: Brooks/Cole, Cengage Learning; 2008.

20. Spencer JP, Abd El Mohsen, Manal M, Rice-Evans C. Cellular uptake and metabolism of flavonoids and their metabolites: Implications for their bioactivity. Arch Biochem Biophys. 2004; 423(1):148-61.

21. Schlesier K, Harwat M, Böhm V, Bitsch R. Assessment of antioxidant activity by using different In vitro methods. Free Radic Res. 2002;36(2):177-87.

22. Galati G, Sabzevari O, Wilson JX, O'Brien PJ. Prooxidant activity and cellular effects of the phenoxyl radicals of dietary flavonoids and other polyphenolics. Toxicology. 2002;177:91–104.

23. Dorman H, Peltoketo A, Hiltunen R, Tikkanen M. Characterisation of the antioxidant properties of de-odourised aqueous extracts from selected Lamiaceae herbs. Food Chem. 2003;83(2):255-62.

24. Zaborowska Z, Przygonski K, Bilska A. Antioxidant effect of thyme (Thymus vulgaris) in sunflower oil. Acta Sci Pol Technol Aliment. 2012;11(3):283-91.

25. Rababah TM, Banat F, Rababah A, Ereifej K, Yang W. Optimization of extraction conditions of total phenolics, antioxidant activities, and anthocyanin of oregano, thyme, terebinth, and pomegranate. J Food Sci. 2010;75(7):626- 632.

26. Boros B, Jakabová S, Dörnyei Á, Horváth G, Pluhár Z, Kilár F, Felinger A. Determination of polyphenolic compounds by liquid chromatography–mass spectrometry in Thymus species. J Chromatogr. 2010;1217:7972–80.

27. Blum C, Kubeczka K-, Becker K. Supercritical fluid chromatography-mass spectrometry of thyme extracts (Thymus vulgaris L.). J Chromatogr. 1997;773(1-2):377-80.

28. Guillén MD, Manzanos MJ. Study of the composition of the different parts of a Spanish Thymus vulgaris L. plant. Food Chem. 1998;63(3):373-83.

29. Fecka I, Turek S. Determination of polyphenolic compounds in commercial herbal drugs and spices from Lamiaceae: Thyme, wild thyme and sweet marjoram by chromatographic techniques. Food Chem. 2008;108(3):1039-53.

30. Yanishlieva NV, Marinova EM, Gordon MH, Raneva VG. Antioxidant activity and mechanism of action of thymol and carvacrol in two lipid systems. Food Chem. 1999;64(1):59-66.

31. López-Mata MA, Ruiz-Cruz S, Silva-Beltrán NP, Ornelas-Paz JDJ, Zamudio-Flores PB, Burruel-Ibarra SE. Physicochemical, antimicrobial and antioxidant properties of chitosan films incorporated with carvacrol. Molecules. 2013;18(11):13735-53.

32. Cai Q, Rahn RO, Zhang R. Dietary flavonoids, quercetin, luteolin and genistein, reduce oxidative DNA damage and lipid peroxidation and quench free radicals. Cancer Lett. 1997;119(1):99-107.

33. Seelinger G, Merfort I, Schempp CM:.Antioxidant, anti-inflammatory and anti- allergic activities of luteolin. Planta Med. 2008; 74(14):1667-77.

34. Lee S, Umano K, Shibamoto T, Lee K. Identification of volatile components in basil (*Ocimum basilicum* L.) and thyme leaves (*Thymus vulgaris* L.) and their antioxidant properties. Food Chem. 2005; 91(1):131-7.

35. Cazzola R, Camerotto C, Cestaro B. Antioxidant, anti-glycant, and inhibitory activity against α-amylase and α-glucosidase of selected spices and culinary herbs. Int J Food Sci Nutr. 2011;62(2):175-84.

36. Chang SS, ostric-matijasevic B, Hsieh OA, Huang C. Natural antioxidants from rosemary and sage. J Food Sci. 1977; 42(4):1102-6.

37. Ataa S, Wafaa E, Youssry A. Flavonoids of *Urtica urens* L. and biological evaluation. Egypt J Pharm Sci. 1995;36:415–27.

38. Abdel-Wahhab MA, Said A, Huefner A. NMR and radical scavenging activities of patuletin from *Urtica urens* against aflatoxin B1. Pharm Biol. 2005;43(6):515-25.

39. Dearden JC. Partition and lipophilicity in quantitat ive structure activity relationships. Environ Health Perspect. 1985;61:203–28.

40. Kim SR, Park MJ, Lee MK, Sung SH, Park EJ, Kim J, Kim SY, Oh TH, Markelons GJ, Kim YC. Flavonoids of *Inula Britannica* protect cultured cotical cells from necrotic cell death induced by glutamate. Free Radic Biol Med. 2002;32:596–604.

41. Jimoh F, Adedapo A, Aliero A, Afolayan A. Polyphenolic and biological activities of leaves extracts of *Argemone subfusiformis* (Papaveraceae) and *Urtica urens* (Urticaceae). Int J. Trop Biol. 2010;58(4): 1517-31.

42. Das NP, Pereira TA. Effects of flavonoids on thermal autoxidation of palm oil: Structure-activity relationships. J Am Oil Chem Soc. 1990;67(4):255-8.

43. Amic D, Davidovic-Amic D, Bešlo D, Trinajstic N. Structure-radical scavenging activity relationships of flavonoids. Croat Chem Acta. 2003;76(1):55-61.

44. Kaviarasan S, Naik G, Gangabhagirathi R, Anuradha C, Priyadarsini K. *In vitro* studies on antiradical and antioxidant activities of fenugreek (*Trigonella foenum graecum*) seeds. Food Chem. 2007;103(1):31-7.

45. Genet S, Kale RK, Baquer NZ. Alterations in antioxidant enzymes and oxidative damage in experimental diabetic rat tissues: Effect of vanadate and fenugreek (*Trigonella foenum-graecum*). Mol Cell Biochem. 2002;236(1-2):7-12.

46. Trouillas P, Calliste C, Allais D, Simon A, Marfak A, Delage C, Duroux J-L. Antioxidant, anti-inflammatory and antiproliferative properties of sixteen water plant extracts used in the Limousin countryside as herbal teas. Food Chem. 2003;80(3):399-407.

47. Wojdyło A, Oszmiański J, Czemerys R. Antioxidant activity and phenolic compounds in 32 selected herbs. Food Chem. 2007;105(3):940-9.

48. Cornara L, La Rocca A, Marsili S, Mariotti MG. Traditional uses of plants in the Eastern Riviera (Liguria, Italy). J Ethnopharmacol. 2009;125(1):16-30.

49. Pari L, Srinivasan S. Antihyperglycemic effect of diosmin on hepatic key enzymes of carbohydrate metabolism in streptozotocin-nicotinamide-induced diabetic rats. Biomed Pharmacother. 2010; 64(7):477-81.

50. Campanero MA, Escolar M, Perez G, Garcia-Quetglas E, Sadaba B, Azanza JR. Simultaneous determination of diosmin and diosmetin in human plasma by ion trap liquid chromatography–atmospheric pressure chemical ionization tandem mass spectrometry: Application to a clinical pharmacokinetic study. J Pharm Biomed Anal. 2010;51(4):875-81.

51. Manuel y Keenoy B, Vertommen J, De Leeuw I. The effect of flavonoid treatment on the glycation and antioxidant status in Type 1 diabetic patients. Diabetes Nutr Metab. 1999;12(4):256-63.

52. Devasagayam T, Tilak J, Boloor K, Sane K, Ghaskadbi S, Lele R. Free radicals and antioxidants in human health: Current status and future prospects. JAPI. 2004;52:794-804.

53. Rietjens IM, Boersma MG, Haan Ld, Spenkelink B, Awad HM, Cnubben NH, van Zanden JJ, van der Woude H, Alink GM, Koeman JH. The pro-oxidant chemistry of the natural antioxidants vitamin C, vitamin E, carotenoids and flavonoids. Environ Toxicol Pharmacol. 2002;11(3):321-33.

22

In vitro Cytotoxicity and Antioxidation of a Whole Fruit Extract of *Liquidambar formosana* Exerted by Different Constituents

Jian Zhang[1,2*], Guixin Chou[1*], Zhijun Liu[3] and Gar Yee Koh[3]

[1]*Institute of Chinese Materia Medica, Shanghai University of Traditional Chinese Medicine, Shanghai, People's Republic of China.*
[2]*School of Perfume and Aroma Technology, Shanghai Institute of Technology, Shanghai, People's Republic of China.*
[3]*School of Renewable Natural Resources, Louisiana State University Agricultural Center, Baton Rouge, LA, United States of America.*

Authors' contributions

This work was carried out in collaboration between all authors. Authors JZ and GC designed the study. Author JZ performed fractionation, UPLC analysis, antioxidation study, literature search, and wrote the first draft of the manuscript. Authors ZL and GYK wrote the protocol and performed the cytotoxicity study. Authors ZL and GC revised the manuscript. All authors read and approved the final manuscript.

Editor(s):
(1) Marcello Iriti, Faculty of Plant Biology and Pathology, Department of Agricultural and Environmental Sciences, Milan State University, Italy.
Reviewers:
(1) Anonymous, UCSI University, Malaysia.
(2) Anonymous, National Research Center, Egypt.
(3) Anonymous, Yeni Yuzyil University, Turkey.

ABSTRACT

Aims: The fruit of *Liquidambar formosana Hance* under the name of Lu Lu Tong (LLT) has been used as a traditional Chinese medicine in China for thousands of years. This study was undertaken to attempt to illustrate some of the pharmacological effects by screening for its cytotoxic and antioxidant activities with *in vitro* assays.
Methodology: LLT extract was initially prepared with 95% aqueous ethanol, and then fractionated based on solvent polarity into three fractions of petroleum ether (LLT-P), dichloromethane (LLT-C), and methanol (LLT-M). human colon adenocarcinoma Cells HT-29 cultured in Dulbecco's Modified

Corresponding author: E-mail: jianzhang@sina.com, chouguixinzyb@126.com

Eagle's Medium were treated with LLT extracts in the concentration range of 0.39 µg/mL and 100 µg/mL and assayed by MTS. The antioxidant activities of each LLT fraction was reacted with a stable free radical of DPPH (1, 1-diphenyl-2-picrylhydrazyl) and ABTS•+ (2, 20-azino-bis (3-ethylbenzothiazoline-6-sulfonic acid) diamonium salt). Major constituents of three fractions were analyzed by UPLC-MS.

Results: Among the three fractions, LLT-M exhibited a strong antioxidant activity but the others had minimal or negligible effects. In contrast, the potent antioxidant fraction (LLT-M) showed essentially no cytotoxicity whereas the two fractions, LLT-P and LLT-C, were significantly cytotoxic.

Conclusion: Cytotoxicity and Antioxidant properties exhibited by LLT came from different constituents residing in different fractions of solvent affinity.

Keywords: Antioxidation; cytotoxicity; HT-29; fractionation; Liquidambar formosana.

1. INTRODUCTION

Four species are identified in the sweetgum genus of Liquidambar (Hamamelidaceae) with three residing in Asia and one in North America [1]. The mature fruit collected from the Chinese sweetgum tree Liquidambar formosana Hance is a Traditional Chinese Medicine (TCM) ingredient under the specific name of Lu Lu Tong (LLT). Despite the long history of use, its pharmacological mechanisms have not been fully and closely examined in modern scientific settings. In a multi-herb formulation of TCM, LLT has shown many pharmacological properties and was used to play the role of improving collateral circulation, amenorrhea [2], and arthralgia [3], promoting urinationtreating chronic renal diseases, removing numbness [4], reducing edema [5], relieving pain, activating collaterals, promoting blood circulation [6], and anti-inflammation and analgesics [7]. Oleanane triterpenoids in LLT exhibited a strong inhibition against the nuclear factor of activated T-cells and platelet aggregation induced by adenosine diphosphate [5,8]. LLT demonstrated the ability to reduce virus-induced cytopathic effects and virus yield in Madin-Darby canine kidney cells, and potently inhibited neuraminidase activity [9]. Among these triterpenes, lanostanes, cucurbitanes, and oleananes are probably the most interesting groups correlated to the immune responses and cancer or inflammation studies [10]. In addition to exerting cytotoxicity against cancer cells directly, antioxidation has become an approach for the prevention and therapy of diseases because oxidation was associated with the initiation and progression of cardiovascular, tumoral, and inflammatory conditions [11].

In recent natural product chemistry investigations, LLT was found to mainly contain triterpenoids such as betulinic acid, oleanolic acid, and lantanolic acid [6,12]. Other major constituents are tannins [13] and flavan glycosides [14]. In modern TCM, where each herbal ingredient is characterized by mostly one compound as qualitative index in China, betulinic acid is chosen to indicate LLT, [4] based primarily on chemical abundance, but not necessarily pharmacological activities responsible for reported bioactivities.

The North American species L. styraciflua, better known as sweetgum, was less used as an herbal medicine but more investigated in pharmacology. Sweetgum was found to possess anti-cancer properties, but little was known for the L. formosana species indigenous to China. TCM often uses the whole extract of all extractable constituents, while our objective is to narrow the whole extract to specific chemical constituents via fractionation. To assess the successful fractionation, fingerprinting analysis of each fraction is required. Subsequently, qualitative elucidation is needed to link chemical constituents to pharmacological activities. From this angle, this study was an expansion of traditional knowledge. In the meantime, antioxidation was screened for leaf extract [15], but not for the fruit. Based on the historical uses and exhibited pharmacological properties of limited scientific investigations, this study was undertaken to examine the dual pharmacological properties of antioxidation and cytotoxicity, and elucidate different constituents through phytochemical fractionation.

2. MATERIALS AND METHODS

2.1 Standards and Reagents

The human colon adenocarcinoma (HT-29) cell line was obtained from the American Type Culture Collection (Maryland, USA). Dulbecco's

Modified Eagle's Medium (DMEM), 10% fetal bovine serum (FBS), N-2-Hydroxyethylpiperazine-N′-2-ethanesulfonic Acid (HEPES), penicillin, streptomycin, sodium pyruvate, L-glutamine, and non-essential amino acids were purchased from Invitrogen Corporation (Carlsbad, CA, USA). Curcumin (used as positive control for the cytotoxicity assay) with purity of 96.4% was purchased from Chromadex Inc. (Irvine, CA, USA). The agents of 1, 1-diphenyl-2-picrylhydrazyl (DPPH), butylated hydroxytoluene (BHT) and 2, 2'-azino-bis (3-ethylbenzothiazoline-6-sulfonic acid) diamonium salt (ABTS) were purchased from Sigma-Aldrich China (Shanghai, China). Dichloromethane (CH_2Cl_2), petroleum ether, methanol, ethanol, formic acid were purchased from China National Medicine Group Shanghai Corporation (Shanghai, China). All chemicals and solvents were of analytical grade. Acetonitrile (Merck & Co. USA) and distilled water (Watson Group Shanghai Co., China) were of HPLC grade.

2.2 Preparation of *L. formosana* Extracts

Dried fruits of *L. formosana* (LLT) purchased from Kangqiao Herbal Material Company (Shanghai, China) were ground to particle sizes of approximately 5 mm, 500g of which was then extracted twice (1:10 w/v) with 5 L of 95% aqueous ethanol for 4 hours at 70°C. The solvent in the combined liquid extract (approximately 10 L) was then evaporated using a rotary evaporator (EYELA, Shanghai Ailang Co., Shanghai, China) under reduced pressure at 55°C to derive the ethanolic extract (30 g). This extract was then fractionated by silica gel (900 g, Particle size 100mesh, Qingdao Marine Chemical Factory, China) column chromatography. After loading the sample, the extract was sequentially eluted with petroleum ether, dichloromethane, and methanol. Solvent in each fractioned liquid extract was then evaporated to derive the fraction samples named as LLT-P, LLT-C, and LLT-M.

2.3 UPLC-MS Analysis

An ultra-performance liquid chromatography coupled with electrospray ionization mass spectrometry (UPLC-ESI-MS; Acquity-Quattro Premier, Waters Co.) was used to analyze LLTextracts. To perform the analyses, 10 mg each of LLT-P, LLT-C, and LLT-M samples was accurately weighed in 10 mL acetonitrile. The sample was extracted under sonication for 10 min and the solution was filtered through a 0.2 µm syringe filter prior to UPLC analysis. After a pretreatment procedure, the sample was separated on an Acquity UPLC BEH C18 column (20 ×100 mm, 1.7 µm) with a mobile phase consisting of A (acetonitrile with 0.1% formic acid, v/v) and B (distilled water with 0.1% formic acid, v/v). The gradient elution was designed as follows: from 0 to 15 min, a linear change for A from 5% to 25% (v/v); from 15 to 50 min, a linear change for A from 25% to 85% (v/v); and then hold A at 85% until 55 min, when the run was complete. Injection volume was kept at 5 µL and a flow rate was set at 0.20 mL/min. The column temperature was maintained at 30ºC. MS detection was performed by mass scan. The electrospray ionization source was applied and operated in both positive and negative ion modes (ESI±). The cone voltage was set at 40V and a full scan was obtained over the m/z range from 50 to 1000 Daltons to obtain total ion chromatography (TIC) for each sample.

2.4 Antioxidant Scavenging Activity

The antioxidant activities of each LLT sample was reacted with a stable free radical of DPPH (1, 1-diphenyl-2-picrylhydrazyl) and the DPPH radical scavenging activity was assayed using the modified method of Yosra [16]. Each extract sample was dissolved in ethanol to form its stock solution ranging from 1 to 10 mg/mL, 10 µL of which was transferred into 3 mL ethanol solution containing 0.1 mM of DPPH to allow reaction in an incubator at 30ºC. The scavenging activity of the DPPH radical was determined by UV spectrophotometer (757CR, Shanghai Precision Instrument Co., China) for the absorbance at 520 nm every 30 sec. for 15 min. Each LLT extract sample was reacted with the stable ABTS•$^+$ (2, 20-azino-bis (3- ethylbenzothiazoline-6-sulfonic acid) diamonium salt) radical cation and then assayed according to the modified method of Wang [15]. ABTS•$^+$ was produced by reacting ABTS with potassium persulfate ($K_2S_2O_8$). A stock solution of ABTS (7 mM) was prepared in phosphate-buffered saline (PBS, 50 mL). ABTS•$^+$ was produced by reacting stock (50 mL) with $K_2S_2O_8$ water solution (50 mL). The mixture was left to stand in the dark at room temperature for about 15 h before use. For the evaluation of antioxidant activity, the ABTS•$^+$ solution was diluted in PBS and equilibrated to 30°C to obtain an absorbance using UV spectrophotometer (757CRT, Shanghai Precision Instrument Co., China) at 730 nm. The mixture LLT sample solution (10 µL) with the ABTS•$^+$ solution (3 mL) were then assayed for absorbance at ambient temperature after 6 min. The antioxidant activity was expressed as percentage of scavenging activity on DPPH or ABTS•$^+$ radical of the samples:

Scavenging activity (%) =$[(Ac_{(0)}-A_{A(t)}) /Ac_{(0)}]\times 100$

Where $A_{C(0)}$ is the absorbance of the control (blank) at t=0 and $A_{A(t)}$ is the absorbance in the presence of the sample at t=15 min(DPPH) or t=6min(ABTS•$^+$). Ethanol was used as a blank control. All tests were in duplicate. The DPPH or ABTS radical scavenging activity of BHT was measured for comparison.

2.5 Cytotoxicity Screening Assay

The human colon adenocarcinoma (HT-29) cell line was maintained at 37°C in a humidified atmosphere with 5% CO_2. Cells were cultured in Dulbecco's Modified Eagle's Medium (DMEM) supplemented with 10% fetal bovine serum (FBS), N-2-Hydroxyethylpiperazine-N´-2-ethanesulfonic Acid (HEPES), penicillin-streptomycin, sodium pyruvate, L-glutamine, and non-essential amino acids. In vitro cell viability assays were conducted using the MTS (3-(4, 5-Dimethylthiazol-2-yl)   -5-   (3-carboxymethoxyphenyl) -2- (4-sulfophenyl) - 2H-tetrazolium) assay. HT-29 cells were added to 96-well plates at 1×10^4 cells/well, respectively, and allowed to adhere for 16 hours. For the activity screening assay, a single dose method was used. In this case, the stock solutions of LLT extracts were made in DMSO at 10 mg/mL then diluted to a final solution of 100 µg/mL that contained 1% DMSO with culture medium supplemented with 10% FBS. The stock solution of curcumin (positive control) was prepared at 1.5 mg/mL in DMSO then diluted to 15.0 µg/mL with culture medium and DMSO in the final solution was kept at 1% v/v. For the determination of IC_{50} (half maximal inhibitory concentration), a range of multiple doses were used. In this case, the cells were treated with LLT extracts in the range of 0.39 µg/mL to 100 µg/mL or with curcumin (positive control) in the range of 0.12 to 30.0 µg/mL in triplicate wells and incubated at 37°C for 72 hrs. DMSO in the final solutions was all kept at 1% v/v. On day three, a 20 µL aliquot of MTS solution premixed with phenazine methosulfate was added directly to each well and the plate was incubated at 37°C for another 2 hrs. Absorbance was measured at 490 nm using a Bio-Rad Microplate Absorbance Reader (iMark, Bio-Rad Co., Hercules, CA, USA). Percent viability was calculated as cell viability

relative to vehicle-treated control. The IC_{50} values were the average of at least two independent experiments.

2.6 Statistical Analysis

All data were analyzed using the paired Student's T-test (SAS, Cary, NC) and the means were compared. Significance of tests was set at $P < 0.05$ and data were expressed as mean ± SE (standard error) unless otherwise specified.

3. RESULTS AND DISCUSSION

3.1 Chromatographic Fingerprints Generated By UPLC-MS

Three samples were obtained from the fractionation and named LLT-P (8.2 g), LLT-C (10.7 g), and LLT-M (6.8 g), respectively. Eluting solvents of petroleum ether, dichloromethane, and methanol were used in a gradually increased polarity fashion. This sequential fractionation procedure resulted in the UPLC chromatographic fingerprints that showed variations in their peak occurrences and distribution.

Preliminary identification of major constituents in each of the three fractions was made based on UV and MS characteristics. Chromatographic fingerprints were developed for each fraction at wavelengths of 200-500 nm (Fig. 1). The number of identifiable peaks exhibited among the three fractions was more than thirty. Although same peaks appeared among the three fractions, differences in composition were obvious. Nine peaks were shown and numbered in the LLT-M fraction. The characteristic peaks were primarily detected in the first 10 min of the chromatogram. In a C18 reversed-phase column, the most polar constituents are predicted to elute first. This means LLT-M fraction contained more polar components. Peaks 2 and 3 showed absorptions at 203 to 205 nm and 254 to 262 nm, both of which highest peaks are characteristic of phenols. Mass fragments of m/z 181, m/z 137, and m/z 83 exhibited from these peaks are characteristic of phenols according to reference [17]. Those compounds with oxhydryl, carboxyl, carbonyl or methoxyl are subject to a logical loss by $[M-18]^+$, $[M-43]^+$, $[M-28]^+$, or $[M-30]^+$during ionization. Based on the predicted polarity as well as UV and MS spectra, these peaks are identified to be phenolic compounds (Fig. 2). There were no other obvious peaks after ten min of retention time, thus the LLT-M is characterized as the phenols-rich fraction.

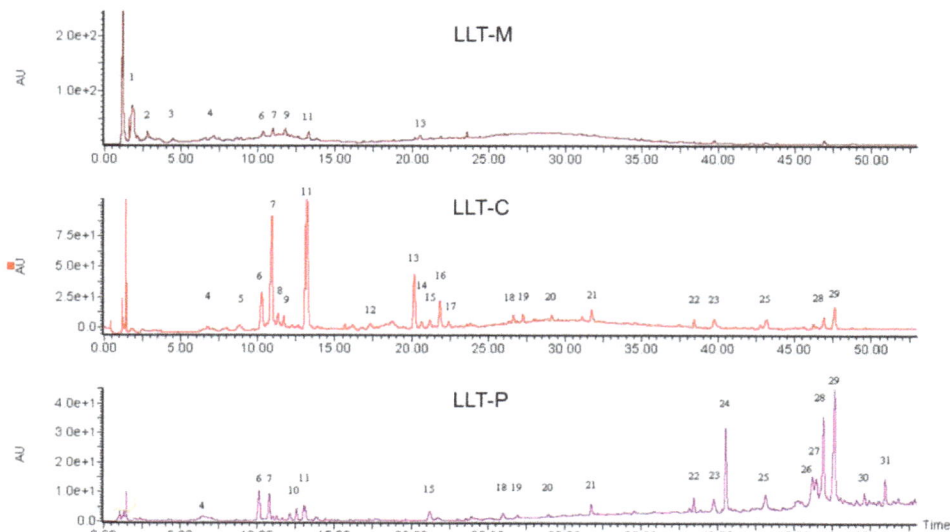

Fig. 1. Chromatographic fingerprints of three fraction extracts prepared from LLT at wavelengths of maximal absorption in the range of 200-500 nm. Upper: LLT-M; middle: LLT-C; and lower: LLT-P

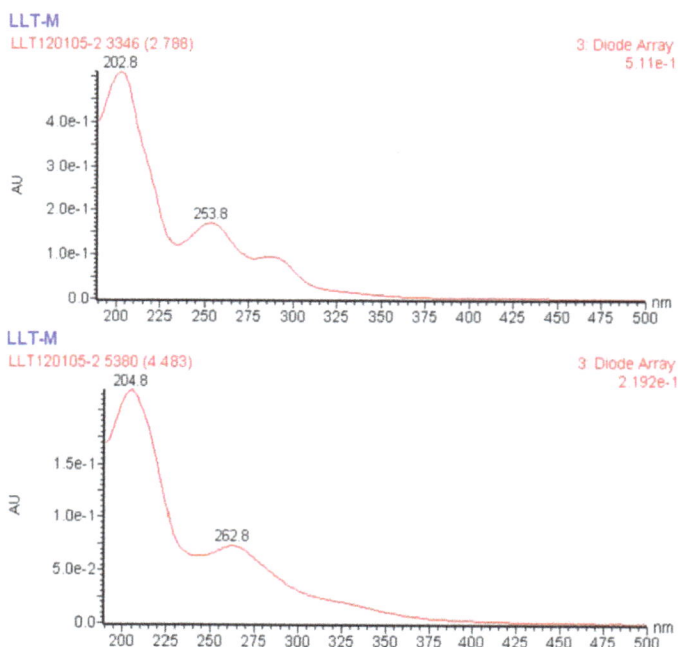

Fig. 2. UV spectrum of peak 2(upper) and peak 3(down) selected from the LLT-M fraction. UV absorption spectrum over the range of 200 and 500 nm of two representative peaks from one of the three fraction extracts prepared from the LLT

Twenty-two peaks were identified and numbered in the LLT-C fraction. Peak 7 showed two major absorption peaks at 216 nm and 309 nm; and Peak 11 showed two major absorption peaks at 245 nm and 342 nm. Dual absorption peaks between 216 nm and 245 nm and between 309

nm and 342 nm are characteristic of flavonoids (Fig. 3). UV spectra and MS fragments showed that the characteristics of those compounds matched flavone or isoflavone, flavonol, and chalcone [18]. Usually flavonoids produce mass fragments of $[A_1+H]^+$ m/z 121 (peak 6, peak 21),

B_1^+ m/z 102 (peak 13, peak 16, peak 21), and $[A_1\text{-}CO]^+$ m/z 92 (peak 6). Flavonols with one hydroxyl on the B ring produce a mass fragment of B_2^+ m/z 135 (peak 6) or B_2^+ m/z 165 (peak 7) when two hydroxyl groups are on the B ring. Those isoflavones with methoxyl group on the ring produce two mass fragments of m/z 181 (peak 7) and m/z 191 (peak 7, peak 11). Most of the peaks eluted between retention time of 10 and 35 min are flavonoids according totheir UV and MS spectra Similar as peak 7and peak 11. The LLT-C fraction displayed most abundant and numerous peaks during this period, thus is considered a flavonoids-rich fraction.

Twenty peaks were detected in the LLT-P fraction. Although some peaks eluted before 35 min, major peaks appeared after 35 min. Most non-polar compounds including triterpenoids typically elute during this period. Unless α, β-unsaturated ketones were linked in the side chain, UV absorption only occurs at 205 nm or shorter wavelengths for triterpenoids. The highest absorption for peaks 28 and 29 was at 193 nm (Fig. 4). Six oleanane or ursane types of triterpenoids were reportedly isolated and identified from *L. styraciflua* chloroform ($CHCl_3$) extract and *L. formosana* $CHCl_3$ extract [19,20]. Oleanolic acid and ursolic acid with [M-1]- m/z 454, betulinic acid with [M-1]- m/z 453, Betulonic acid have characteristic mass fragments of [M-1]- m/z 454, m/z 439, m/z 234,m/z 189, and other oleanane triterpenoids have characteristic mass fragments of [M-1]- m/z 471, m/z 469,m/z 453, m/z 409, m/z 301, m/z 234, m/z 189, and m/z 149 matching the data reported in the reference [21]. Oleanolic acid and ursolic acid generate of fracture fragment m/z 189 according to the inverse Dells - Alder rule. Those compounds (peak 22- peak 31) peaked similarly as peak 28 or peak 29 in this retention time period have shown spectral data characteristic of those found for triterpenoids [13]. Triterpenoids appeared to be most abundant in this fraction, thus the LLT-P is characterized as a triterpenoids-rich fraction.

Column chromatography was successful in separating phenols, flavonoids, and triterpenoids into the LLT-M, LLT-C, and LLT-P fractions, which were tested for bioactivities.

3.2 Effects on Antioxidant Activity

The scavenging abilities of various fractions against DPPH radical were concentration-dependent. Compared with the positive control BHT, the phenols-rich LLT-M fraction was found to be a more active DPPH radical scavenger than the other two fractions. The flavonoids-rich LLT-C fraction showed a similar scavenging capacity to that of BHT. In contrast, the triterpenoids-rich LLT-P fraction showed minimal scavenging activity to less than 20%, whereas the phenols-rich and flavonoids-rich fractions generated 35% and 58% scavenging activity, respectively (Fig. 5). This result is in agreement with the findings that the extracts richer in total phenolic compounds and total flavonoids are more potent DPPH radical scavengers [16,22]. The low radical scavenging activity displayed by the LLT-P fraction may have been the result of lacking abundant phenolic compounds and/or flavonoids.

Similar to the DPPH assay, the phenols-rich LLT-M fraction exhibited a stronger antioxidant activity than the positive control BHT and the flavonoids-rich LLT-C fraction. Once again, there was no difference in ABTS radical scavenging activity between the flavonoids-rich LLT-C fraction and the positive control BHT. The triterpenoids-rich LLT-P fraction showed weaker ABTS radical scavenging capacity than BHT or LLT-C (Fig. 6).

The antioxidant properties normalized and expressed by the inhibitory rate on 50 percentage concentration are summarized in Table 1. According to the two methods used for measuring antioxidant potency by the DPPH and ABTS radical assays, antioxidation capability was in the order of LLT-M > LLT-C > LL-T-P. Good linear correlations were reported between various antioxidant activities and contents of total phenols [23] or flavonoids [24]. These findings coincide with the results of this study.

Table 1. Antioxidant properties of IC_{50} by DPPH and ABTS radicals of the LLT fraction extracts

Sample	DPPH IC_{50} Value [a] (μg/mL)	ABTS IC_{50} Value [b] (μg/mL)
BHT [c]	54.34±0.86	32.08±0.48
LLT-P	89.08±0.83	35.81±0.17
LLT-C	70.34±0.03	31.28±0.27
LLT-M	25.00±0.03	10.71±0.02

[a] The inhibitory concentration at which DPPH radicals were scavenged by 50%. Results are expressed as the mean ±SD (n = 2) in each group.

[b] The inhibitory concentration at which ABTS radicals were scavenged by 50%. Results are expressed as the mean ±SD (n = 2) in each group.

[c] Used as Positive control. Tests were in two replications

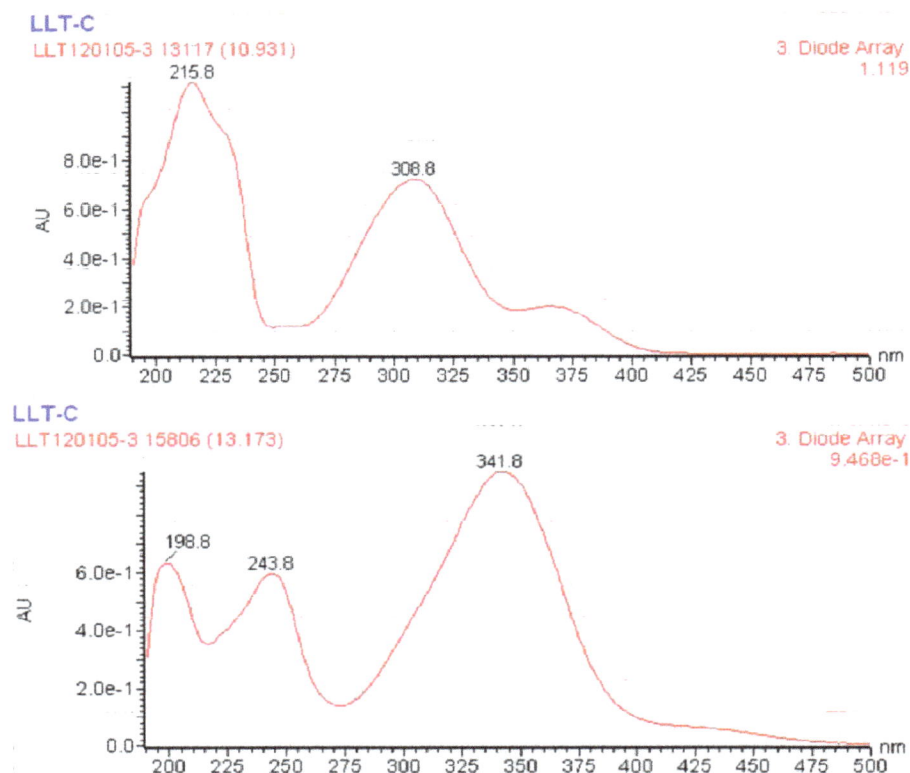

Fig. 3. UV spectrum of peak 7(upper) and peak 11(down) selected from the LLT-C fraction. UV absorption spectrum over the range of 200 and 500 nm of two representative peaks from one of the three fraction extracts prepared from the LLT

3.3 Effects on Cell Viability

At 100 µg/mL, the triterpenoids-rich LLT-P and flavonoids-rich LLT-C fractions inhibited the growth of HT-29 cells by 92.9% and 78.0%, respectively, whereas the phenols-rich LLT-M fraction had negligible cytotoxicity (Table 2). Curcumin (positive control) at 15.0 µg/mL inhibited 50.2%, similar to the report by Zhang [25]. The triterpenoids-rich fraction and flavonoids-rich fraction decreased the viability of HT-29 in a concentration-dependent manner between 12.5 µg/mL and 100 µg/mL with IC_{50} values of 50.9 µg/mL and 73.0 µg/mL, respectively (Fig. 7). The curcumin control displayed an IC_{50} of 11.90µg/mL between 0.12 and 30.0 µg/mL, in agreement with a previous finding of IC_{50} at 36.89 µM (13.58µg/mL) [25]. Further isolation of major triterpenoids and structural elucidation will enable the identification of responsible compounds. The IC_{50} value of 50.9 µg/mL was promising because this fraction is still a mixture of triterpenoids. As it becomes purer, it is generally predicted bioactivity would improve. Some triterpenoids isolated from the sweetgum tree were potently cytotoxic against 39 human cancer cell lines [21]. Triterpenoids of uvaol and oleanolic acid from multiple botanical sources were found to affect cell viability, proliferation, and cycle; entice apoptosis; and increase reactive oxygen species level and oxidative DNA damage to human MCF-7 breast cancer cell line [16]. The multiple bioactivities displayed by the triterpenoids oleanolic acid and its derivatives prompted wide-spread interests in pre-clinical and clinical studies for their anti-tumor, antioxidant, anti-inflammatory, and anti-angiogenic properties [26]. It will be interesting to know if triterpenes in the current study are some of these reported or new. Meanwhile, non-cancerous cells are needed to show that a cytotoxic compound targets cancer cells. For example, Hong [27] found that isolates from Genkwa Flos were almost 400 times more potent against cancer cells than non-cancerous cells. There were no reports on LLT's cytotoxicity against non-cancerous cells. When isolates from our LLT extracts are completed in future studies, it will be necessary to compare them with non-cancerous cells.

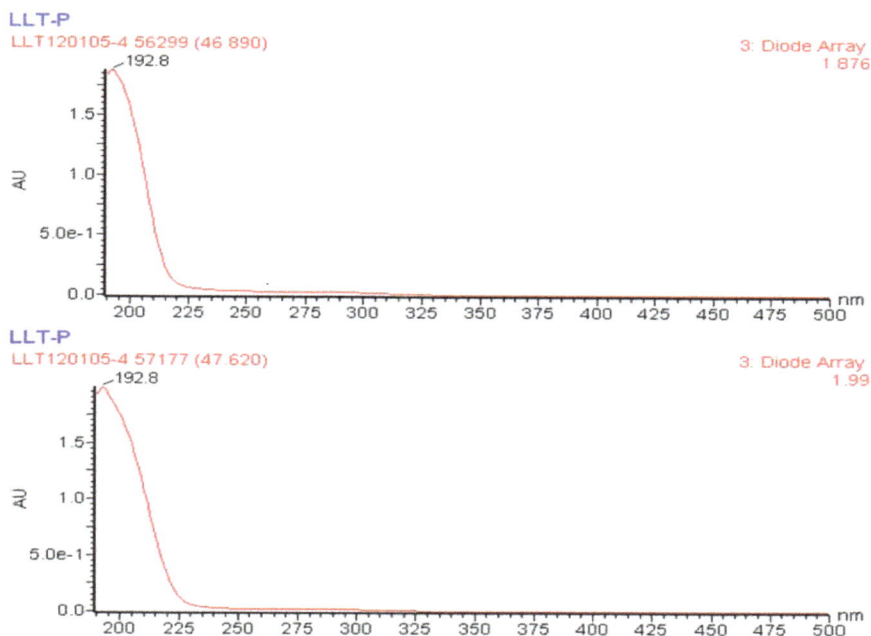

Fig. 4. UV spectrum of peak 28(upper) and peak 29(down) selected from the LLT-P fraction. UV absorption spectrum over the range of 200 and 500 nm of two representative peaks from one of the three fraction extracts prepared from the LLT

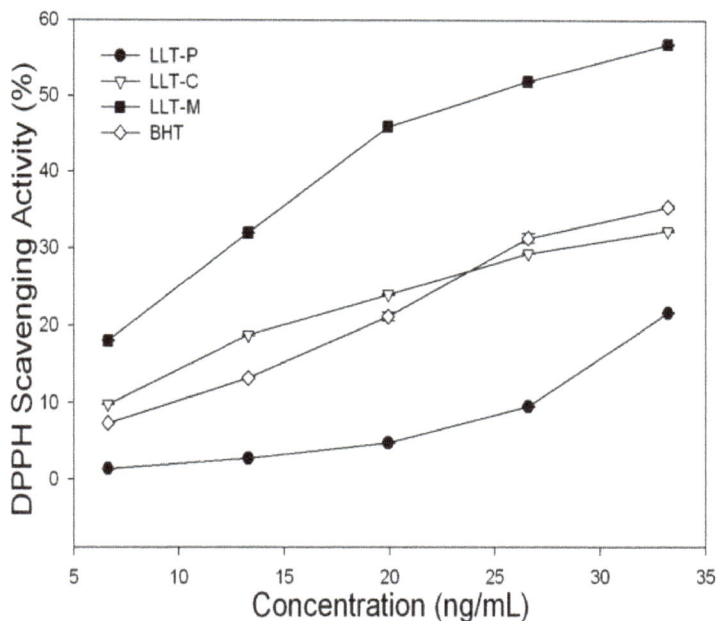

Fig. 5. Different DPPH free radical scavenging activity exerted by the fraction extracts of obtained from the fruit of *Liquidambar formosana*

LLT-M is the methanol fraction; LLT-C is the dichloromethane fraction; LLT-P is the petroleum ether fraction; and BHT is the positive control. Each data point is the mean ± SD of two replications. P < 0.05. The vertical bars across each data point represent one standard deviation.

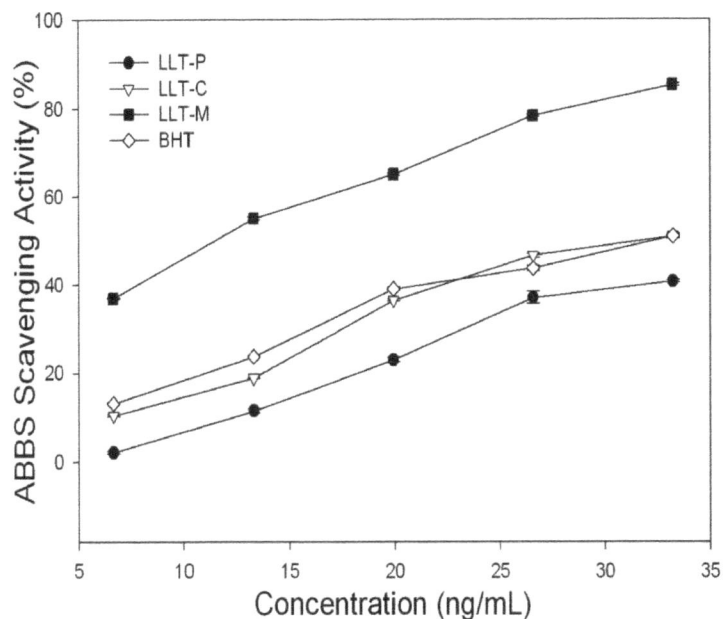

Fig. 6. Different ABTS free radical scavenging activity exerted by the fraction extracts of obtained from the fruit of *Liquidambar formosana*
LLT-M is the methanol fraction; LLT-C is the dichloromethane fraction; LLT-P is the petroleum ether fraction; and BHT is the positive control. Each data point is the mean ± SD of two replications. P < 0.05. The vertical bars across each data point represent one standard deviation

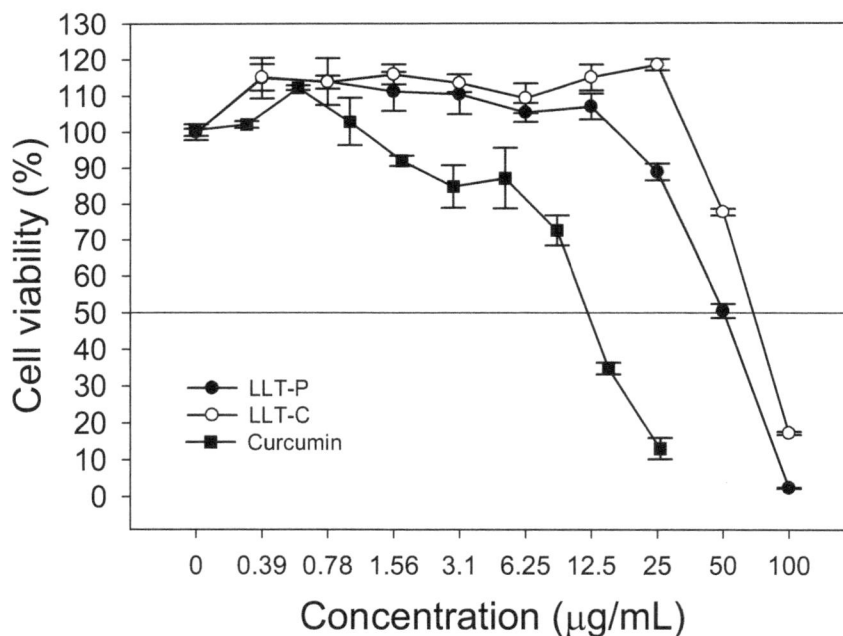

Fig. 7. Cell viability assay showing cytotoxicity of the two LLT fraction extracts against human colon adenocarcinoma cell line (HT-29) by MTS Assay
Absorbance was measured at 490 nm by a Bio-Rad Microplate Reader. Curcumin was used as a positive control. Each data point is the mean± SE of two independent experiments and vertical bars represent one standard error

In vitro Cytotoxicity and Antioxidation of a Whole Fruit Extract of Liquidambar formosana...

209

Table 2. Inhibition of human colon adenocarcinoma (HT-29) cell growth by LLT fraction extracts[a]

Sample	% Inhibition
LLT-P	92.86±0.57
LLT-C	78.01±0.32
LLT-M	0.00
Curcumin	50.20±2.84

[a] *HT-29 human colon cells were added to 96-well plates at 1×10^4 cells/well, respectively. The cells were treated with LLT extracts at the dose of 100 µg/mL (LLT-P, LLT-C and LLT-M) and curcumin (positive control) at the dose of 15 µg/mL in triplicate wells.*

4. CONCLUSION

Fractionation of a whole fruit extract using column chromatography techniques was successful in obtaining phenols-rich, flavonoids-rich, and triterpenoids-rich fractions, as indicated from the UV and MS analyses. Corresponding to compositional variations among the three fractions, bioactivities separated. In this study, the antioxidant activity of the *Liquidambar formosana* fruit extract came primarily from the methanol fraction (LLT-M). In contrast, cytotoxicity against a human colon cancer cell line came from the petroleum ether fraction (LLT-P) rich in triterpenoids and the dichloromethane fraction (LLT-C) rich in flavonoids, but not from the methanol fraction (LLT-M) rich in phenols. These interesting findings illustrate the versatility of a single herbal extract in exerting multiple activities of antioxidation and cytotoxicity. If both properties contribute to a concerted effect, chemo-preventive efficacy could be augmented significantly compared to the use of any single component such as the antioxidant fraction or the cytotoxic fractions. Further studies could be designed to elucidate responsible cytotoxic compounds in both fractions and consider the possibility of merging the two into one.

CONSENT

Not applicable.

ETHICAL APPROVAL

Not applicable.

COMPETING INTERESTS

Authors have declared that no competing interests exist.

REFERENCES

1. Ickert-Bond SM, Pigg KB, Wen J. Comparative infructescence morphology in *Liquidambar* (Altingiaceae) and its evolutionary significance. AM J Bot. 2005;92(8):1234-1255.

2. National pharmacopoeia commission of China, editors. Botanical drug pharmacopoeia of people's republic of China. 8th ed. Beijing: Chinese Medicine and Technology Press; 2010.

3. Huang Z, Fang J, Zen X, Zhang M, Liu D, Hung YY. Windproof passed winds the pill to match closed circuit lu tongsan to treat class the rheumatism arthritis 106 example clinical observations. CHIN Manipulation Rehabilitation Med. 2010;12(4):96-97.

4. Zhang QW, Zhang YX, Sun YR, Zhang D. Qualitative and quantitative methods of betulonic acid in fruits of *Liquidambar formosana*. China J CHIN Materia Medica. 2005;30(15):1168-1170.

5. Yang NY, Chen JH, Zhou GS. Pentacyclic triterpenes from the resin of *Liquidambar formosana*. Fitoterapia. 2011;82(6):927-931.

6. Liu ZL, Ni S, Liu H. Compositions and biological activities of *Liquidambar formosana*. NW Acta Pharmacol. 2009;24(6):513-515.

7. Liu T, Sun Y, Qin C, Wu ZL, Zhang Y, Li LF, et al. Anti-inflammatory and analgesic effects of liquidambaric acid. CHIN J Exp Tradit Med Formulae. 2006;12(12):45-47.

8. Nguyen TD, Lee IS, Cai SF, Shen GH, Kim YH. Oleanane triterpenoids with inhibitory activity against NFAT transcription factor from *Liquidambar formosana*. Biol Pharm Bull. 2004;27:426-428.

9. Tian L, Wang ZY, Wu H, Wang S, Wang Y, Wang YY, et al. Evaluation of the anti-neuraminidase activity of the traditional Chinese medicines and determination of

the anti-influenza a virus effects of the neuraminidase inhibitory TCMs *In vitro* and *In vivo*. J Ethnopharmacol. 2011;137(1):534-542.

10. Rios JL. Effects of triterpenes on the immune system. J Ethnopharmacol. 2010;128(1):1-14.

11. Rios JL, Recio MC, Escandell JM, Andujar I. Inhibition of transcription factors by plant-derived compounds and their implications in inflammation and cancer. Curr Pharn Design. 2009;15(26):1212-1237.

12. Cai Y, Ruan J. Studies on the chemical constituents from the leaf of *Liquidambar formosana* hance. Zhong Yao Cai. 2005;28(4):294-295.

13. Tsutomu H, Reiko K, Masao Y, Takuo O. Seasonal changes in the tannins of *Liquidambar formosana* reflecting their biogenesis. Phytochemistry. 1986;25(12):2787-2789.

14. Zhong RJ, Yuan H, Fu HZ, Zhou GP, Wu X, Zhang CH, et al. Three new compounds from the leaves of *Liquidambar formosana*. J Asian Nat Prod Res. 2013;15(12):1249-1255.

15. Wang K, Pan Y, Wang H, Zhang Y, Lei Q, Zhu Z, et al. Antioxidant activities of *Liquidambar formosana* hance. Med Chem Res. 2010;19:166-176.

16. Yosra A, Fernando W, Mari´a C. Antioxidant, anti-proliferative, and pro-apoptotic capacities of pentacyclic triterpenes found in the skin of olives on mcf-7 human breast cancer cells and their effects on DNA damage. J Agric Food Chem. 2011;59:121-130.

17. Xu RS. Editors Natural Product Chemistry. 2th ed. Beijing: Science Press; 2004.

18. Xiao CH. Editors. Traditional Chinese medicine chemistry. 1st ed. Shanghai: Shanghai Scientific and Technical Press; 2002.

19. Sakai K, Fukuda Y, Matsunaga S, Tanaka R, Yamori T. New cytotoxic oleanane -type triterpenoids from the cones of *Liquidamber styraciflua*. J Nat Prod. 2004;67:1088-1093.

20. Li C, Sun Y, Su Y. Chemical composition of fructus *Liquidambaris*. Acta Pharm sin. 2002;37(4):263-266.

21. Lai ZQ, Dong Y. Studies on the chemical constituents of the Lu Lu Tong. Acta Sci Natur Univ Sun YS. 1996;35(4):64-69.

22. Larrosa M, García-Conesa MT, Espín JC, Tomás-Barberán FA. Ellagic acid and vascular health. Mol Aspects Med. 2010;31(6):513-539.

23. Thind ST, Singh R, Kaur R, Rampal G, Arora S. *In vitro* antiradical properties and total phenolic contents in methanol extract fractions from bark of *Schleichera oleosa* (Lour.). Oken. Med Chem Res. 2011;20:254-260.

24. Hong Y, Lin S, Jiang Y. Variation in contents of total phenolics and flavonoids and antioxidant activities in the leaves of 11 eriobotrya species. Plant Foods Hum Nutr. 2008;63:200-204.

25. Zhang F, Koh GY, Jeansonne D, Hollingsworth J, Russo P, Liu Z, et al. A novel solubility-enhanced curcumin formulation showing stability and maintenance of anti-cancer activity. J Pharm Sci. 2011;100:2778–2789.

26. Nighat S, Athar A. Oleanolic acid and related derivatives as medicinally important compounds. J Enzyminhib Med CH. 2008;23(6):739-756.

27. Hong JY, Nam JW, Seo EK, Lee SK. Daphnane diterpene esters with anti-proliferative activities against human lung cancer cells from *Daphne genkwa*. Chem. Pharm. Bull. 2010;58(2):234-237.

Permissions

List of Contributors

Solomon Akinremi Makanjuola
Department of Food Science and Technology, Federal University of Technology, Akure, Nigeria

Victor Ndigwe Enujiugha
Department of Food Science and Technology, Federal University of Technology, Akure, Nigeria

Olufunmilayo Sade Omoba
Department of Food Science and Technology, Federal University of Technology, Akure, Nigeria

David Morakinyo Sanni
Department of Food Science and Technology, Federal University of Technology, Akure, Nigeria
Department of Biochemistry, Federal University of Technology, Akure, Nigeria

Iroha Ifeanyichukwu
Department of Pharmaceutical Microbiology and Biotechnology, Nnamdi Azikiwe University, P.M.B 5025, Awka, Nigeria

Ejikeugwu Chika
Department of Applied Microbiology, Ebonyi State University, P.M.B 053, Abakaliki, Nigeria

Nwakaeze Emmanuel
Department of Pharmaceutical Microbiology and Biotechnology, Nnamdi Azikiwe University, P.M.B 5025, Awka, Nigeria

Oji Anthonia
Department of Pharmaceutical Microbiology and Biotechnology, Nnamdi Azikiwe University, P.M.B 5025, Awka, Nigeria

Afiukwa Ngozi
Department of Pharmaceutical Microbiology and Biotechnology, Nnamdi Azikiwe University, P.M.B 5025, Awka, Nigeria

Nwuzo Agabus
Department of Pharmaceutical Microbiology and Biotechnology, Nnamdi Azikiwe University, P.M.B 5025, Awka, Nigeria

M. A. Al-Mamun
Protein Science Lab, Department of Genetic Engineering and Biotechnology, University of Rajshahi, Rajshahi-6205, Bangladesh

Rafica Akhter
Ali. Mohammad Eunus Laboratory, Department of Genetic Engineering and Biotechnology, University of Rajshahi, Rajshahi 6205, Bangladesh

A. Rahman
Ali. Mohammad Eunus Laboratory, Department of Genetic Engineering and Biotechnology, University of Rajshahi, Rajshahi 6205, Bangladesh

Z. Ferdousi
Department of Genetic Engineering and Biotechnology, University of Rajshahi, Rajshahi-6205, Bangladesh

Yousif Y. Bilto
Department of Biological Sciences, The University of Jordan, Amman, Jordan

Nessrin G. Alabdallat
College of Applied Medical Sciences, Majmaah University, Majmaah, Saudi Arabia

Okwute Simon Koma
Department of Chemistry, University of Abuja, P.M.B. 117, Gwagwalada, Federal Capital Territory, Abuja, Nigeria

Yakubu Rufa'i
Department of Chemistry, University of Abuja, P.M.B. 117, Gwagwalada, Federal Capital Territory, Abuja, Nigeria

Firdaus Mukhtar Quraishi
Department of Life Sciences, University of Mumbai, Vidyanagari Campus, Santacruz (E), 400 098, Mumbai, India

B. L. Jadhav
Department of Life Sciences, University of Mumbai, Vidyanagari Campus, Santacruz (E), 400 098, Mumbai, India

Neeti Kumar
Department of Life Sciences, University of Mumbai, Vidyanagari Campus, Santacruz (E), 400 098, Mumbai, India

Hemayet Hossain
BCSIR Laboratories, Bangladesh Council of Scientific and Industrial Research, Dhaka, Dr. Qudrat-EKhuda Road, Dhaka-1205, Bangladesh

Proity Nayeeb Akbar
BCSIR Laboratories, Bangladesh Council of Scientific and Industrial Research, Dhaka, Dr. Qudrat-EKhuda Road, Dhaka-1205, Bangladesh

Shaikh Emdadur Rahman
Pharmacy Discipline, Life Science School, Khulna University, Khulna-9208, Bangladesh

Sabina Yeasmin
Pharmacy Discipline, Life Science School, Khulna University, Khulna-9208, Bangladesh

Tanzir Ahmed Khan
Institute of Food Science and Technology, Bangladesh Council of Scientific and Industrial Research, Dhaka, Dr. Qudrat-E-Khuda Road, Dhaka-1205, Bangladesh

Md. Mahfuzur Rahman
Institute of Food Science and Technology, Bangladesh Council of Scientific and Industrial Research, Dhaka, Dr. Qudrat-E-Khuda Road, Dhaka-1205, Bangladesh

Ismet Ara Jahan
BCSIR Laboratories, Bangladesh Council of Scientific and Industrial Research, Dhaka, Dr. Qudrat-EKhuda Road, Dhaka-1205, Bangladesh

Antoine H. L. Nkuété
Department of Chemistry, Faculty of Science, University of Dschang, Dschang, Cameroon
Center of Proteomical and Biochemical Analyses, Genomic Sciences and Biotechnology, Catholic University of Brasilia, DF, Brazil

Ludovico Migliolo
Center of Proteomical and Biochemical Analyses, Genomic Sciences and Biotechnology, Catholic University of Brasilia, DF, Brazil
S-Inova, Biotechnology, Catholic University Dom Bosco, Campo Grande, Mato Grosso doSul, Brazil

Hippolyte K. Wabo
Department of Chemistry, Faculty of Science, University of Dschang, Dschang, Cameroon

Pierre Tane
Department of Chemistry, Faculty of Science, University of Dschang, Dschang, Cameroon

Octávio L. Franco
Center of Proteomical and Biochemical Analyses, Genomic Sciences and Biotechnology, Catholic University of Brasilia, DF, Brazil
S-Inova, Biotechnology, Catholic University Dom Bosco, Campo Grande, Mato Grosso doSul, Brazil

Malika Ait Sidi Brahim
Laboratory of Biotechnology, Protection and Valorization of Plant Resources; Phytochemistry and Pharmacology of Medicinal Plants Unit, Department of Biology, Faculty of Sciences Semlalia, Cadi Ayyad University, Marrakech, Association CNRST URAC35, Morocco

Mariam Fadli
Laboratory of Biology and Biotechnology of Microorganisms, Department of Biology,
Faculty of Science Semlalia, Cadi Ayyad University, Marrakech, Morocco

Mohamed Markouk
Laboratory of Biotechnology, Protection and Valorization of Plant Resources; Phytochemistry and Pharmacology of Medicinal Plants Unit, Department of Biology, Faculty of Sciences Semlalia, Cadi Ayyad University, Marrakech, Association CNRST URAC35, Morocco

Lahcen Hassani
Laboratory of Biology and Biotechnology of Microorganisms, Department of Biology,
Faculty of Science Semlalia, Cadi Ayyad University, Marrakech, Morocco

Mustapha Larhsini
Laboratory of Biotechnology, Protection and Valorization of Plant Resources; Phytochemistry and Pharmacology of Medicinal Plants Unit, Department of Biology, Faculty of Sciences Semlalia, Cadi Ayyad University, Marrakech, Association CNRST URAC35, Morocco

Kazadi Minzangi
Department of Biology, Research Centre in Natural Substances CRSN/Lwiro, Official University of Bukavu, RD Congo

Pius T. Mpiana
Faculty of Sciences, University of Kinshasa, P.O.BOX 190, Kinshasa XI, RD Congo

Bashwira Samvura
Department of Chemistry, Institute of Pedagogy Bukavu, RD Congo

Archileo N. Kaaya
Department of Food Technology and Nutrition, Makerere University, Kampala, Uganda

Matthäus Bertrand
MRI - Max Rubner-Institut, Bundesforschungsinstitut für Ernährung und Lebensmittel, Food
Department Working Group for Lipid Research, Schützenberg 12, 32756 Detmold, Germany

Justin N. Kadima
Department of Pharmacy, School of Medicine and Pharmacy, University of Rwanda, Rwanda

Emmanuel E. Essien
Department of Chemistry, University of Uyo, Akwa Ibom State, Nigeria

Nimmong-uwem S. Peter
Department of Chemistry, University of Uyo, Akwa Ibom State, Nigeria

Stella M. Akpan
Department of Chemistry, University of Uyo, Akwa Ibom State, Nigeria

Akintayo L. Ogundajo
Department of Chemistry, Natural Products Research Unit, Faculty of Science, Lagos State University, Badagry Expressway, P.M.B. 0001 LASU Post Office, Ojo, Lagos, Nigeria

Mutiu I. Kazeem
Department of Biochemistry, Antidiabetic Drug Discovery Group, Faculty of Science, Lagos State University, Badagry Expressway, P.M.B. 0001 LASU Post Office, Ojo, Lagos, Nigeria

Jude E. Evroh
Department of Chemistry, Natural Products Research Unit, Faculty of Science, Lagos State University, Badagry Expressway, P.M.B. 0001 LASU Post Office, Ojo, Lagos, Nigeria

Mayowa M. Avoseh
Department of Chemistry, Natural Products Research Unit, Faculty of Science, Lagos State University, Badagry Expressway, P.M.B. 0001 LASU Post Office, Ojo, Lagos, Nigeria

Isiaka A. Ogunwande
Department of Chemistry, Natural Products Research Unit, Faculty of Science, Lagos State University, Badagry Expressway, P.M.B. 0001 LASU Post Office, Ojo, Lagos, Nigeria

Sanjita Chanu Konsam
Department of Life Sciences, Manipur University, Canchipur, Imphal, India

Sanjoy Singh Ningthoujam
Department of Botany, Ghanapriya Women's College, Imphal, India

Kumar Singh Potsangbam
Department of Life Sciences, Manipur University, Canchipur, Imphal, India

Oladipupo A. Lawal
Department of Chemistry, Natural Products Research Unit, Faculty of Science, Lagos State University, Badagry Expressway, PMB 0001 LASU Post office, Ojo, Lagos, Nigeria

Isiaka A. Ogunwande
Department of Chemistry, Natural Products Research Unit, Faculty of Science, Lagos State University, Badagry Expressway, PMB 0001 LASU Post office, Ojo, Lagos, Nigeria

Andy R. Opoku
Department of Biochemistry and Microbiology, University of Zululand, KwaDlangezwa 3886, South Africa

Le T. Huong
Faculty of Biology, Vinh University, 182-Le Duan, Vinh City, Ngh An Province, Vietnam

Tran D. Thang
Faculty of Chemistry, Vinh University, 182-Le Duan, Vinh City, Ngh An Province, Vietnam

Isiaka A. Ogunwade
Natural Products Research Unit, Department of Chemistry, Faculty of Science, Lagos State University, Badagry Expressway Ojo, P.M.B. 0001, LASU Post Office, Ojo, Lagos, Nigeria

E. U. Asogwa
Kola Research Programme, Cocoa Research Institute of Nigeria, Ibadan, Oyo State, Nigeria

T. C. N. Ndubuaku
Kola Research Programme, Cocoa Research Institute of Nigeria, Ibadan, Oyo State, Nigeria

O. O. Awe
Biology Department, Adeyemi College of Education, Ondo, Ondo State, Nigeria

I. U. Mokwunye
Kola Research Programme, Cocoa Research Institute of Nigeria, Ibadan, Oyo State, Nigeria

Elijah I. Ohimain
Department of Biological Sciences, Ecotoxicology and Environmental Safety Research Unit, Niger Delta University, Bayelsa State, Nigeria

Tariwari C. N. Angaye
Department of Biological Sciences, Ecotoxicology and Environmental Safety Research Unit, Niger Delta University, Bayelsa State, Nigeria

Sunday E. Bassey
Department of Biological Sciences, Ecotoxicology and Environmental Safety Research Unit, Niger Delta University, Bayelsa State, Nigeria

Sylvester C. Izah
Department of Biological Sciences, Ecotoxicology and Environmental Safety Research Unit, Niger Delta University, Bayelsa State, Nigeria

F. O. Omoya
Department of Microbiology, Federal University of Technology, P.M.B. 704, Akure, Ondo State, Nigeria

A. O. Momoh
Department of Microbiology, Federal University of Technology, P.M.B. 704, Akure, Ondo State, Nigeria

O. A. Olaifa
Department of Microbiology, Federal University of Technology, P.M.B. 704, Akure, Ondo State, Nigeria

Sameera N. Siddiqui
Department of Biochemistry, Rashtrasant Tukdoji Maharaj Nagpur University, Nagpur-440033, Maharashtra, India

Mandakini B. Patil
Department of Biochemistry, Rashtrasant Tukdoji Maharaj Nagpur University, Nagpur-440033, Maharashtra, India

Winifred N. Okechi
Department of Pharmacology, University of Calabar, P.M.B. 1115, Calabar, Cross River State, Nigeria

Babatunde A. S. Lawal
Department of Pharmacology, University of Calabar, P.M.B. 1115, Calabar, Cross River State, Nigeria

Nnabugwu P. Wokota
Department of Pharmacology, University of Calabar, P.M.B. 1115, Calabar, Cross River State, Nigeria

Jibril Hassan
Department of Pharmacology, University of Calabar, P.M.B. 1115, Calabar, Cross River State, Nigeria

V. Paddy
Department of Pharmacology, Faculty of Health Sciences, University of Pretoria, Private Bag X323, Arcadia 0007, South Africa

J. J. van Tonder
Department of Pharmacology, Faculty of Health Sciences, University of Pretoria, Private Bag X323, Arcadia 0007, South Africa

V. Steenkamp
Department of Pharmacology, Faculty of Health Sciences, University of Pretoria, Private Bag X323, Arcadia 0007, South Africa

Jian Zhang
Institute of Chinese Materia Medica Shanghai University of Traditional Chinese Medicine, Shanghai, People's Republic of China
School of Perfume and Aroma Technology, Shanghai Institute of Technology, Shanghai People's Republic of China

Guixin Chou
Institute of Chinese Materia Medica Shanghai University of Traditional Chinese Medicine, Shanghai, People's Republic of China

Zhijun Liu
School of Renewable Natural Resources Louisiana State University Agricultural Center Baton Rouge, LA, United States of America

Gar Yee Koh
School of Renewable Natural Resources Louisiana State University Agricultural Center Baton Rouge, LA, United States of America